Presurgical Psychological Screening

Presurgical Psychological Screening

UNDERSTANDING PATIENTS, IMPROVING OUTCOMES

EDITED BY

Andrew R. Block and David B. Sarwer

AMERICAN PSYCHOLOGICAL ASSOCIATION

WASHINGTON, DC

Published by
American Psychological Association
750 First Street, NE
Washington, DC 20002
www.apa.org

To order
APA Order Department
P.O. Box 92984
Washington, DC 20090-2984
Tel: (800) 374-2721; Direct: (202) 336-5510
Fax: (202) 336-5502; TDD/TTY: (202) 336-6123
Online: www.apa.org/pubs/books
E-mail: order@apa.org

In the U.K., Europe, Africa, and the Middle East, copies may be ordered from
American Psychological Association
3 Henrietta Street
Covent Garden, London
WC2E 8LU England

Typeset in Goudy by Circle Graphics, Inc., Columbia, MD

Printer: Edwards Brothers, Ann Arbor, MI
Cover Designer: Berg Design, Albany, NY

The opinions and statements published are the responsibility of the authors, and such opinions and statements do not necessarily represent the policies of the American Psychological Association.

Library of Congress Cataloging-in-Publication Data

Presurgical psychological screening : understanding patients, improving outcomes / edited by Andrew R. Block and David B. Sarwer. — 1st ed.
    p. cm.
  ISBN 978-1-4338-1242-2 — ISBN 1-4338-1242-8 1. Surgery—Psychological aspects.
2. Patients—Psychology. 3. Medical ethics. I. Block, Andrew. II. Sarwer, David B.
  RD31.7.P74 2013
  617.08—dc23
                                    2012019879

British Library Cataloguing-in-Publication Data
A CIP record is available from the British Library.

Printed in the United States of America
First Edition

DOI: 10.1037/14035-000

For Adam
—*Andrew R. Block*

For Miranda and Ethan
—*David B. Sarwer*

CONTENTS

CONTRIBUTORS

Kelly C. Allison, PhD, Center for Weight and Eating Disorders, Perelman School of Medicine, University of Pennsylvania, Philadelphia

Jane E. Austin, PhD, Department of Psychology, William Paterson University, Wayne, NJ

Brooke Bailer, PhD, Center for Weight and Eating Disorders, Perelman School of Medicine, University of Pennsylvania, Philadelphia

Andrew R. Block, PhD, ABPP, Texas Back Institute, Plano

Diane B. V. Bonfiglio, PhD, Department of Psychology, Ashland University, Ashland, OH

Andrea Bradford, PhD, University of Texas, MD Anderson Cancer Center, Houston

Canice E. Crerand, PhD, Department of Surgery, Perelman School of Medicine, University of Pennsylvania; Division of Plastic and Reconstructive Surgery, Children's Hospital of Philadelphia, Philadelphia

M. Scott DeBerard, PhD, Department of Psychology, Utah State University, Logan

Robert R. Edwards, PhD, Departments of Anesthesiology and Psychiatry, Brigham and Women's Hospital, Boston, MA

Lucy F. Faulconbridge, PhD, Center for Weight and Eating Disorders, Perelman School of Medicine, University of Pennsylvania, Philadelphia

Sarah E. Fraley, MRC, Department of Rehabilitation Counseling, University of Texas Southwestern Medical Center, Dallas

Robert J. Gatchel, PhD, ABPP, Department of Psychology, University of Texas—Arlington

Jason T. Goodson, PhD, Department of Psychology, Utah State University, Logan

Kathryn Holloway, MD, Medical College of Virginia Hospital of Virginia Commonwealth University; Southeast Parkinson's Disease and Movement Disorders Research, Education, and Clinical Center, Hunter Holmes McGuire Veterans Affairs Medical Center, Richmond

Robert N. Jamison, PhD, Departments of Anesthesiology and Psychiatry, Brigham and Women's Hospital, Boston, MA

Kristin K. Kuntz, PhD, Department of Psychiatry, Ohio State University Wexner Medical Center, Columbus

Sarah K. Lageman, PhD, ABPP-CN, Parkinson's and Movement Disorders Center and Department of Neurology, Virginia Commonwealth University, Richmond

Leanne Magee, PhD, Division of Plastic and Reconstructive Surgery, Children's Hospital of Philadelphia, Philadelphia, PA

Melody Mickens, MS, Parkinson's and Movement Disorders Center and Department of Psychology, Virginia Commonwealth University, Richmond

Sarah J. Miller, PsyD, Department of Oncological Sciences, Mount Sinai School of Medicine, New York, NY

Guy H. Montgomery, PhD, Department of Oncological Sciences, Mount Sinai School of Medicine, New York, NY

Christine Rini, PhD, Department of Health Behavior, Gillings School of Global Public Health, University of North Carolina at Chapel Hill

David B. Sarwer, PhD, Center for Weight and Eating Disorders, Perelman School of Medicine, University of Pennsylvania, Philadelphia

Julie B. Schnur, PhD, Department of Oncological Sciences, Mount Sinai School of Medicine, New York, NY

Anna W. Stowell, PhD, Department of Psychology, University of Texas—Arlington

Eric Swanholm, PhD, Department of Anesthesiology and Pain Management, University of Texas Southwestern Medical Center, Dallas

Therese Verkerke, BA, Parkinson's and Movement Disorders Center and Department of Psychology, Virginia Commonwealth University, Richmond

Thomas A. Wadden, PhD, Center for Weight and Eating Disorders, Perelman School of Medicine, University of Pennsylvania, Philadelphia

ACKNOWLEDGMENTS

The concept for this book arose about 5 years ago as we began to see the field of presurgical psychological screening (PPS) gaining greater acceptance and utility for an ever-widening range of medical conditions. The final spark to develop this text occurred in 2009, when one of us (Block) took the oral examination to become board certified in clinical health psychology by the American Board of Professional Psychology (ABPP) and was asked a question about how to handle differing hypothetical situations for a patient who had undergone PPS for a cardiac transplant. At that moment, it was clear that the time had arrived for a comprehensive book on PPS. Thus, we would like to recognize ABPP, and particularly American Board of Clinical Health Psychology President John Robinson, for providing the inspiration for this book.

Andrew R. Block thanks the following surgeons at the Texas Back Institute, with whom he has worked for more than 20 years: Stephen Hochschuler, Ralph Rashbaum, Richard Guyer, Jack Zigler, Scott Blumenthal, Rey Bosita, Michael Hisey, Dan Bradley, Shawn Henry, Michael Duffy, Raj Arakal, Jessica Shellock, Izzy Lieberman, and Theodore Belanger. He also thanks the Texas Back Institute's chief executive officer, Trish Bowling, and chief development officer, Cheryl Zapata, for their constant support. Additionally, he thanks the following surgeons from other affiliations, who have been a source of much support and who have provided many referrals over the years: Jerry Lewis, Lew Frazier, John Peloza, Craig Callewart, Ken Reed, Steve Courtney, Andrew Park, Chun Lin, Renaud Rodrigue, Bob Bulger, and Rob Dickerman.

David B. Sarwer acknowledges several of his colleagues at the Perelman School of Medicine at the University of Pennsylvania, although space does not allow all to be named individually. First, he thanks Linton Whitaker, professor of surgery and founder and director of the Edwin and Fannie Gray Hall Center for Human Appearance, under whom he served as a postdoctoral fellow in 1995. Whitaker provided Sarwer both the initial opportunity to develop research and the guidance to promote it through the peer-reviewed literature as well as through regional, national, and international presentations. The psychological presence at the center has grown over the years. Canice E. Crerand and Leanne Magee currently serve as psychologists at the center and focus their work on reconstructive surgery, particularly with children and adolescents. Their excellent work is a source of great satisfaction and pride.

Noel Williams serves as director of the Bariatric Surgery Program. From the earliest days of the program, he and the other surgeons and members of the program have supported both the use of PPS and psychosocial and biomedical research with these patients. Sarwer also acknowledges his other colleagues at the Center for Weight and Eating Disorders in the Department of Psychiatry. First and foremost, Thomas A. Wadden, the Albert J. Stunkard Professor of Psychiatry, who is the director of the center and an internationally recognized scholar in the etiology and treatment of obesity, has served as Sarwer's primary professional mentor since 1995. Also, Kelly C. Allison, Robert Berkowitz, Lucy F. Faulconbridge, and Albert "Mickey" Stunkard, other current faculty members at the center, have contributed to his work and are both colleagues and friends. Sarwer thanks Rebecca Dilks, Scott Ritter, and Jacqueline Spitzer, also at the center, with whom he works closely on a daily basis and who play an instrumental role in the success of his research projects.

Finally, we express our great appreciation to Susan Reynolds, senior acquisitions editor, and Beth Hatch, development editor, at the American Psychological Association for all their many great suggestions and their care in producing the best possible book.

Presurgical Psychological Screening

INTRODUCTION

ANDREW R. BLOCK AND DAVID B. SARWER

A 46-year-old man cracks a lumbar vertebra after a fall from a ladder while working as a painter. Although his pain complaints seem excessive, and he has been taking more pain medication than prescribed, he undergoes a spinal fusion. The fusion heals correctly from the surgeon's perspective, but the patient continues to report high levels of pain, be disabled, and consume large quantities of narcotics.[1]

A 48-year-old woman with a body mass index of 43 kilograms per square meter, Type 2 diabetes and hypertension, and a history of psychiatric hospitalizations for depression, undergoes bariatric surgery. After an initial weight loss of 50 pounds in the first year after surgery, she regains 75 pounds in the next 18 months, and her depression returns.

We acknowledge the contributions of the following individuals to some of the concepts discussed in this chapter: Diana Jochai, Shawn T. Mason, and James A. Fauerbach.

[1]Details of the cases in this introduction have been altered to protect each patient's identity.

DOI: 10.1037/14035-001
Presurgical Psychological Screening: Understanding Patients, Improving Outcomes, Andrew R. Block and David B. Sarwer (Editors)

A 43-year-old executive with a family history of high blood pressure who has resisted the pleas of his physician that he stop working excessively and consuming cigarettes and alcohol, has kidney failure and undergoes renal transplant. Once he has recovered from the transplant, he returns to his preoperative lifestyle of working excessively, smoking, and drinking. He misses several medical appointments and, several months after the transplant, has a stroke.

These cases exemplify a not-infrequent outcome of surgery: Although the surgery is technically successful and achieves its physical aims of correcting the underlying medical condition, the patient does not experience improvement in symptoms. In extreme cases, the patient's condition may even worsen or new physical problems may arise. Moreover, cognitive difficulties or emotional distress may increase. Patients may even develop narcotic addiction as a result of efforts to control postoperative pain. In such cases, the surgery, on which all involved have pinned so much hope, turns out to be the impetus for a downward physical and emotional spiral.

When surgery is ineffective, not only are the consequences to the patient often dramatic and tragic, but the consequences for the surgeon, insurers, and even society can be significant. The surgeon may face the patient's anger or even litigation; insurers may face the costs of additional medical procedures; and society may face the costs of financially supporting the patient through Social Security Disability, Medicare, or Medicaid. Thus, maximizing the likelihood of successful surgical outcome is in everyone's interest.

These cases point to problems that arise when the surgical team focuses only on correcting physical pathology without regard to a complete understanding of the patient. In each of these cases, psychosocial factors—issues such as excessive pain sensitivity (Case 1), history of significant psychopathology (Case 2), or behavioral noncompliance (Case 3)—likely exerted negative influences on the surgery's results. A growing body of research has demonstrated that these and other patient characteristics can play a large role in determining the success or failure of many surgical procedures. Thus, although surgeons are always concerned with proper diagnosis of the underlying medical condition, treatment planning can be greatly enhanced by considering the patient's emotional state, behavioral tendencies, personality factors, and psychosocial environment.

Responding to the growing recognition of the complex amalgam of factors influencing surgical outcome, mental health clinicians (MHCs) are frequently included on the surgical treatment team. In some cases, MHCs simply help to support the patient's recovery through *psychoeducational services*—the provision of information and advice to the patient that can improve surgical results and avoid postoperative difficulties. Such services typically involve enhancing self-care skills and helping the patient to recognize and respond to problems (Rankin, Stallings, & London, 2005). Sometimes, they involve an assessment of the patient's ability to provide informed consent. However, in still other cases, the involvement of MHCs is much more primary because they now are being called on to conduct presurgical psychological screening (PPS) as part of the medical evaluation process.

PPS is, at its core, a risk assessment procedure—a projection of the extent to which psychological factors may influence surgery results, for better or worse. PPS is conducted with patients who have medical conditions that can potentially be ameliorated by surgery but for which research has demonstrated that objectively identifiable psychosocial factors can adversely influence surgery designed to treat the condition. PPS is conducted before the surgeon makes the decision to operate and often provides a key recommendation to the surgery team in making a final decision—whether to operate, delay the surgery, or avoid it altogether. As a result of the information obtained through PPS, the MHC can develop treatment plans, if necessary, to sufficiently overcome or mitigate psychosocial concerns and augment the likelihood of surgical success. Moreover, PPS results provide guidance to the treatment team in individualizing care. Additionally, if the treatment team decides to postpone or avoid surgery, PPS results can point to an alternative therapeutic course. Certainly, the MHC plays a psychoeducational role in the PPS process, providing the patient with helpful information and suggestions. However, when the MHC identifies psychosocial issues critical to the surgical decision and to patient management, the functions of PPS go far beyond psychoeducation.

In most cases, PPS results can provide input into the surgical decision. However, the specific issues examined vary widely across different types of surgery. In some cases, such as bariatric surgery (see Chapter 3, this volume) or organ transplantation (Chapter 1), one of the primary purposes is to identify potential challenges to patient compliance with treatment regimens and even to suggest means to test treatment adherence before surgery. In other cases, such as reconstructive plastic surgery (Chapter 8) and gynecologic surgery (Chapter 10), a primary focus of PPS is to determine the surgical procedure's impact on self-image and psychosocial status. Frequently, as in spine surgery (Chapter 2), temporomandibular disorder–related surgery (Chapter 7), and carpal tunnel surgery (Chapter 11), the patient's response to and interpretation of pain sensations are critically examined. Thus, although the overall goals of PPS are to provide the treatment team with information about potential psychosocial obstacles to surgical outcome and to provide interventions that can ameliorate such problems, the critical issues and means for achieving these goals are syndrome specific.

This text is intended to benefit treatment providers across disciplines who are concerned that surgical candidates have the best possible opportunity to obtain good results and to avoid negative surgical consequences. A mental health practitioner or student who reads this text will obtain basic knowledge of the major psychosocial concerns associated with each surgery type, learn general approaches to applying this knowledge in assessing risk for reduced or adverse surgical outcome, and appreciate behavioral treatment techniques that facilitate patient recovery and improvement. Surgeons and other medical providers will gain insight into the ways in which psychosocial issues can influence the outcome of surgery and, thus, understand how ignoring such issues can lead to failure of the surgery to produce desired results even when the surgery is performed correctly. Case managers and others involved in the third-party payment system will learn how inclusion of PPS in their treatment guidelines can help improve overall results and avoid failures.

In the remainder of this introduction, we first elaborate on the value PPS brings to the surgeon and treatment team. Next, we provide a broad overview of the PPS process, describing the means for identifying factors that may affect surgical outcome and the types of suggestions for surgery and patient management that are the primary functions of PPS. We then introduce the most frequently encountered psychosocial factors that influence surgical outcome across the spectrum of conditions covered in this text. We go on to discuss bioethical issues involved in PPS, as well as the value that conducting PPS brings to the MHC. We conclude with an explanation of the book's organization.

VALUE OF PRESURGICAL PSYCHOLOGICAL SCREENING FOR THE SURGEON

Why would a physician, highly trained in diagnosis and with superior surgical expertise and skills, consider the professional opinions of an MHC? Although surgeons often have a long history of success, they have not infrequently experienced unexpected failures—patients who did not improve, whose emotional states worsened, who became addicted to medications, or who developed significant complications. Thoughtful surgeons often go through a process of self-investigation when such failures occur, coming to the conclusion that such poor response might have been predicted. In such situations, the surgeon may be motivated to improve the process of patient selection—and when research has demonstrated that psychological factors play a strong role in influencing surgical outcome, taking such factors into account in determining when, and whether, to operate is natural. PPS, then, helps the surgeon to improve overall surgical results and to avoid problem patients—those whose lack of response creates protracted frustration and places extensive demands on the surgeon. Finally, when the physician has a gut feeling that the patient may not obtain good results, PPS can provide objective confirmation of such a feeling—or contradict it, with the recommendation that surgery proceed without undue influence from psychosocial factors.

At the same time, many medical institutions directly or indirectly support PPS. The general movement toward integrated, multidisciplinary treatment teams in many areas of medicine has brought more professionals to the decision-making process. Hospitals and health systems that champion quality assurance and minimization of medical errors typically support the inclusion of consultations that can minimize morbidity and mortality, with PPS falling into this category. In like fashion, use of PPS may reduce the likelihood of medical malpractice litigation because it demonstrates that the surgeon has been cautious in decision making, not simply operating unaware of psychosocial concerns that may affect surgical response. Moreover, insurance companies are increasingly requiring PPS as part of the diagnostic evaluation. Finally, in areas such as bariatric surgery, PPS is a formal requirement by third-party payers.

PROCESS OF PRESURGICAL PSYCHOLOGICAL SCREENING

The MHC must use a systematic process for PPS determinations, lest some information be missed or decisions be based on nonscientific factors, such as rapport, intuition, or pressure from the patient. In other words, the specific information to be obtained and the manner in which it is brought together to inform decisions about challenges to surgical success and other adjustments to the treatment plan must be as detailed, systematic, and concrete as possible. The MHC must recognize his or her responsibility to the patient—making decisions with great care for both short- and long-term impact on the patient, providing information about the bases for the decisions made, and, especially when the suggestion is to delay or avoid surgery, explaining how and why such decisions are in the patient's best interest. This explanation may be especially difficult when the patient (or family) sees no other option for recovery or improvement.

PPS, as emphasized throughout this text, is a multistep process, including

- information gathering from multiple sources, including patient (and perhaps family member) interviews, psychometric testing, and review of the course of the patient's medical condition and treatment;
- an empirically based assessment of the risks that psychosocial concerns may present to the outcome of the surgical procedure—that is, the extent to which the patient may have a diminished

likelihood of good response to the surgery and the factors that may exert such influences; and

- treatment suggestions, which should be given to both the medical team and the patient, including (a) procedures to be initiated before surgery that may improve the outcome of the procedure, (b) postoperative management, and (c) alternative treatments if the patient's psychosocial prognosis for surgery is poor or may result in the development of new problems.

In the following sections, we discuss these steps in detail.

Information Gathering

The first step in this process is to gather relevant information from multiple sources. The evaluator needs to keep in mind that one primary goal is to identify psychosocial *risk factors*—that is, elements of the patient's situation that have been empirically demonstrated to militate against good surgery results. Some of these data can be measured objectively, for example, medication use, vocational status, and cognitive function. Other factors are of a more subjective nature, for example, pain level, depressive symptoms, and stress. The most valid approach to gathering information, then, is one of *convergent validity*, wherein data from multiple sources are used to confirm or deny the presence of a particular issue. For example, pain level is best assessed through a combination of patient self-report, observation of behavioral limitations, changes in vocational ability, and narcotic medication use. The MHC, then, needs to take an unbiased, circumspect, and careful approach in accruing the data necessary to provide the most accurate and valid recommendation to the treatment team.

Medical Information

Most MHCs do not have specific medical training. Yet, for PPS to be of value, one must have knowledge of the proposed surgery: its appropriate indications; the physical, emotional, and cognitive demands it places on the patient; and actions patients must take for the surgery to be successful.

An invaluable primary source of information is available for each surgical candidate—the medical chart. For most of the conditions examined in this text, consideration of surgery comes as the terminus of an extended set of diagnostic procedures and other, less intensive medical interventions. Such protracted medical conditions carry with them significant stress and test the patient's strengths and ability to cope. The results of such efforts are often reflected in the medical chart. Here one finds a history of the patient's reaction to differing types of medical information, adherence to treatment suggestions, use of narcotic medications, even attitude toward the treatment team. Also, buried in the chart will often be discussion of alternative treatment strategies, explanations for delays in treatment (e.g., insurance authorization problems, patient procrastination), and even a running commentary on the physician's concerns, frustrations, and investigations into the patient's condition. Thus, the medical chart provides both objective and impressionistic information of critical importance in PPS.

Health Psychology Interview

The second component of information gathering for PPS, the health psychology interview, is at once both more comfortable for the MHC and more fraught with the possibilities of error and bias. Although psychologists' clinical training teaches techniques for building rapport, conveying empathy, and obtaining a comprehensive history, little can prepare one to elicit truthful information from a patient who is bent on avoiding disclosure for fear that expressing personal concerns or emotional distress may adversely influence the surgeon's decision to operate. Moreover, many patients coming to PPS are not well prepared by their surgeons for the referral and do not understand why the referral has occurred or how it can be of benefit to them. Thus, the evaluator is often initially met with the patient's resistance, anger, and confusion.

Conducting a successful PPS interview involves at least two key elements. First, the evaluator must normalize the screening situation—that is, help the patient to see that the evaluation is a routine part of the presurgical diagnostic workup and does not imply that the patient is crazy, making up symptoms, or a hypochondriac. Although the evaluator can acknowledge the basis for any reluctance to participate in the PPS interview, he or she can at the same time present the interview as a forum for discussing the medical condition, the psychological concerns it engenders, the patient's expectations for surgical outcome, and even other aspects of the patient's life and situation that may affect the success of surgery. Thus, normalizing the PPS interview demonstrates understanding of and empathy for the patient and invests the patient in the process of discussing emotional and psychosocial issues.

The second critical component of a PPS interview is to structure the interview format sufficiently that the MHC can obtain all information critical to reaching the final PPS recommendations, yet flexibly, so that the MHC can pursue issues of importance to the patient. Some relevant issues—for example, a history of sexual abuse or substance abuse—are quite sensitive, and the patient may not feel comfortable discussing them until a sense of trust and rapport has been established. Such feelings cannot be created by a mechanical or strict approach to the interview and may often not develop until near its end. The evaluator must at all times balance the need to probe deeply into emotionally laden issues with the requirement to obtain critical information. Having a preset, semistructured interview format may be key to striking this balance.

Psychometric Testing

Just as the medical diagnostic procedure involves both an examination by the physician and a battery of tests that examine the patient's condition in multiple ways, the process of PPS frequently demands the inclusion of standardized, scientifically validated psychometric testing. PPS involves a wide range of such tests. In some conditions, such as chronic pain, tests such as the Minnesota Multiphasic Personality Inventory—2 (Butcher, Dahlstrom, Graham, Tellegen, & Kaemmer, 1989) or a shorter alternative test, the Minnesota Multiphasic Personality Inventory—2—Restructured Form (Ben-Porath, 2012), that assess broad, general psychological characteristics are used. Often, more narrow measures of specific emotional conditions, such as the Beck Anxiety Inventory (Beck, Epstein, Brown, & Steer, 1988) or the Center for Epidemiological Studies Depression Scale (Radloff, 1977), are included, especially when brevity of testing is critical because of patients' weakened physical condition or limited cognitive capacity. For most conditions examined in this book, questionnaires aimed at assessing the patient's knowledge of and response to the specific medical conditions are available, such as the Transplant Evaluation Rating Scale (Twillman, Manetto, Wellisch, & Wolcott, 1993) in assessing bone marrow and stem cell transplant patients. Other frequently used questionnaires provide objective assessment of coping, expectancy, social support, substance abuse, and compliance.

Presurgical Psychological Screening Decision Making

The major decisions to be made in PPS concern whether the surgical outcome is expected to be affected by psychosocial factors, in what ways this might occur, and whether interventions exist that might improve surgical results. Thus, four possibilities flow out of PPS:

1. Surgery can proceed without significant concern that psychosocial factors will influence outcome.
2. If surgery proceeds, psychosocial factors may be expected to have an adverse impact on results. Therefore, preoperative psychological intervention is recommended.
3. Surgery should be delayed, if medically feasible, because untreated psychological factors are very likely to have a negative impact on surgical results. Elective surgery should only proceed in such a

case if psychological intervention is successful in reducing risk factors.

4. Surgery should be avoided altogether, if medically feasible, because of significant and often chronic psychosocial issues that cannot be improved.

PPS is a field in its early stages. Although a large and growing body of research exists on PPS in each of the medical conditions reviewed in this text, in most cases minimal standards exist for translating this research either into a specific determination of overall risk for problematic surgical results or into treatment plans to augment surgical outcome. The range of processes for considering the impact of psychosocial factors is quite broad. In screening for spine surgery, Block (see Chapter 2) has developed an algorithm that lists each potential risk factor, then quantifies and combines them, stratifying patients into one of five outcome prognosis levels ranging from good to poor. In most areas, however, the approach to determining the overall impact of psychological factors is less well defined and is still emerging. The chapters in this book provide the most current thinking on factors critical to recommending whether surgery will proceed, be delayed, or be avoided altogether.

Further complicating the determination of surgical prognosis is the fact that the outcome can and must be examined in many different ways. Although the most obvious concern is that the surgery achieve its physical objective—correcting, compensating for, or ameliorating the underlying medical condition—surgical success means much more. Patients' functional abilities should improve. They should be able to eliminate, if not dramatically reduce, narcotic use. They must be able to overcome emotional distress related to the medical condition and should certainly not experience a worsening of depression or anxiety. A cautionary example is found in data suggesting that the rate of suicide among women with breast implants is 2 to 3 times higher than that in the general population (see Chapter 12). Patients must comply with postoperative treatment regimens, lest any gains engendered by the surgery be lost. For each medical condition, the psychosocial risk factors that militate against positive outcomes in one area, such as improvement in emotional distress, may be quite different from those associated with improvement in another area, such as postoperative treatment adherence.

Regardless of the specific approach used, the MHC needs to be consistent in the choice of instruments and methods used to assess the patient and the manner in which the findings are translated, through the process of convergent validity, into specific concerns about the influence of psychosocial factors on surgical outcome and recommendations for individualizing the treatment plans. Such consistency is critical so that the MHC's projection of how the patient will fare in response to surgery rests on scientifically reliable data, not on bias or a desire to please either the patient or the physician. Patients' desire for the proposed surgery can range from ambivalent to desperate. Indeed, in some cases, such as organ transplantation, the difficult decision to advise against the surgery may be one of life versus death; however, in such cases, the very valuable and limited resources of transplantable organs cannot be wasted on a patient who is unlikely to comply with medical treatment regimens or obtain good results. Thus, the MHC's recommendations must always be objective, consistent, and research based.

Suggestions for Individualizing Treatment to Improve Surgical Outcome

PPS also points to targets for psychological intervention. Such treatments may be aimed directly at reducing the patient's emotional distress, often through a combination of psychotropic medications and cognitive–behavioral psychotherapy. Negative or maladaptive cognitions that become the focus of treatment often include *catastrophizing*—that is, the tendency to believe that things will inevitably worsen and to magnify symptoms and problems related to the medical condition. Brief interventions aimed at challenging such negative thoughts, replacing them with more realistic, behaviorally based ones, can significantly improve the patient's emotional state and motivation for the surgery.

In situations in which the MHC recommends delaying surgery, non-compliance with pre- and postoperative treatment regimens is often a major concern. When the PPS reveals the potential for such problems to occur, the MHC can devise or provide interventions designed to both test and improve patient compliance. For example, smoking cessation may be required before surgery can proceed. In the case of organ transplants, patients with a history of alcohol abuse may be required to be abstinent for 6 months before the transplant can proceed. Such compliance assessment measures are often accompanied by more common psychoeducational approaches, designed to inform the patient about the medical condition and ways in which surgical results may be improved.

Treatment Suggestions When Presurgical Psychological Screening Recommendation Is to Avoid Surgery

For most of the medical conditions covered in this book, one possible outcome of the PPS is a recommendation to avoid surgery, if medically feasible. This recommendation is only given in relatively unusual situations. Most often, such a recommendation is given if the patient has such a high level of psychosocial risk factors that preoperative intervention will not improve the likelihood of obtaining good surgical results. Examples of such situations include intractable substance abuse, documentable deceptive behavior, history of severe noncompliance with treatment recommendations, refusal to carry out necessary preoperative treatment requirements, expressed negative attitude toward the surgery, and psychosis. In all these cases, it is important that the MHC explain thoroughly to the patient the reasons for recommending against surgery. Recommendations should also be given for professional mental health treatment, self-help, or support groups.

PSYCHOSOCIAL FACTORS INFLUENCING SURGICAL OUTCOME

The various surgical procedures discussed in this text share many common goals—reduction of the emotional impact of the illness or disease, reduced reliance on medication, and improvement in quality of life, to name a few. However, the surgical interventions also have many, and somewhat disparate, targets. For some interventions, such as surgery for breast cancer, the primary goal is to stop the progression of a deadly disease. For others, such as organ transplantation, it is to prolong life. For still others, the goals are less physically critical but no less psychologically significant—reduction in pain (e.g., pain stimulators and implantable pumps) and even improvement in body image and self-esteem (e.g., cosmetic surgery), to name a few. Despite the wide range of conditions examined in this text, the reader will find that several psychological factors emerge as critical influences on surgical outcome.

Emotional Factors

Most of the medical conditions examined in this book are quite distressing, and they frequently engender strong emotions—depression, stress, and anger—in those who have them. For some patients, such reactive emotional issues are compounded with more long-standing affective problems such as anxiety disorders or recurrent depression. As the reader will see, presurgery emotional distress is often associated with reduced outcome of surgical intervention, especially when such distress is chronic and is not being adequately treated at the time of surgery. Patients with such recalcitrant emotional difficulties may, in fact, experience a worsening of their distress after surgery. However, even acute emotional distress may bode poorly for surgical outcome. For example, posttraumatic stress disorder, which is common among burn patients, is associated with increased length of hospitalization, heightened pain sensitivity, and cognitive deficits (see Chapter 8). In some cases, if the preoperative distress associated with many of the medical conditions discussed is sufficiently intense, a recommendation may be made that the surgical procedure be delayed until the patient is more stabilized.

Interpersonal Factors

All medical conditions occur in multiple interpersonal contexts. Family members and significant others are usually deeply affected and may respond to the patient with varying degrees of empathy, sympathy, or even anger. Such individuals may encourage the patient to seek treatment or, alternatively, may feel strongly that the surgery should be avoided. Some family members or friends may provide significant social support—help and assistance with tasks, as well as emotional support—and others may be cold and distant. Examining the responses of significant others to the patient, as well as the patient's support system, is often critical. For example, in organ transplantation, support from the family may strongly influence compliance with difficult postoperative medical regimens (see Chapter 1). Low levels of perceived social support among stem cell transplant patients are associated with increased risk for depression posttransplant (see Chapter 5). As the reader will see, to the extent that those involved with patients do not provide social support, are surrounded by chaotic events, or are inclined to provide reinforcement for the patient to remain sick or disabled, the surgery may be less likely to achieve its desired ends.

Coping

Medical conditions leading to surgery are, by their very nature, highly stressful events. They affect the patient's ability to function and lead a normal life, can lead to decreased self-worth, and can dramatically alter life plans. Uncertainty and worry about the outcome of the surgical procedure can weigh heavily on the patient. Yet, some meet the medical condition with a sense of challenge and optimism. As with so much else in life, the ways in which individuals cope with these medical conditions vary widely, and coping strategies have consistently been shown to influence the effectiveness of surgical procedures. For example, avoidant·coping is associated with poorer adjustment after surgery for breast cancer (see Chapter 9). For many of the conditions covered in this text, questionnaires and other condition-specific coping assessment strategies have been developed, the results of which are useful in predicting the patient's response to surgery and in individualizing treatment strategies.

Historical Factors

Each patient has a unique history—triumphs and failures, traumatic events, mistakes, and difficulties overcome. Many issues in the patient's past can give clues to his or her ability to respond well to surgery. Patients with a history of substance abuse may be at increased risk of narcotic dependence after some surgeries. Patients with a history of major mental health problems and psychiatric hospitalizations may be less well-equipped to deal with some postoperative stresses and issues of compliance. With many of the conditions examined in this text, one of the best ways to predict the patient's future response to surgery is to examine the past.

Compliance Influences

Surgery is most often only the most dramatic and obvious step in recovery from illness and injury. For the surgery to achieve its goals, patients must be active participants in their recovery. Appropriate use of medications, exercise, diet, follow-up visits with the medical treatment team, and many more activities are often critical for success. Patients must see themselves as part of a treatment team and adhere carefully to medical treatment recommendations, lest they fail to improve or their medical conditions relapse. Thus, to predict how patients will fare, it is important to understand how they have been involved with treatment providers—whether they have complied with recommendations, whether they have communicated symptoms and problems, and whether they have approached treatment providers in a cooperative or adversarial spirit.

Body Image

For a number of the conditions covered in this text, physical appearance and the patient's perception of his or her appearance play significant roles. The psychological construct of body image was initially, for the most part, reserved for discussion of eating disorders. In the 1990s, it blossomed to become of focal empirical and clinical interest for a variety of medical and surgical conditions. In some cases, such as amputation, patients may become socially avoidant or even experience stigmatization because of their appearance. In other cases, such as plastic surgery (both reconstructive and cosmetic) or bariatric surgery, patients' perceptions of their appearance are a strong motivating factor for surgery. In all these cases, understanding how patients consider their appearance, and the factors that can lead to acceptance of altered physiognomy and those that make adjustment to such conditions more problematic, becomes important. For example, the extreme body image dissatisfaction seen in people with body dysmorphic disorder is relatively common among candidates for cosmetic procedures, affecting approximately 15%, with most reporting no change or a worsening of their body image after surgery and a small minority becoming suicidal (see Chapter 3).

Pain Perception and Somatic Sensitivity

For many surgical procedures, the primary goal is the relief of pain. In some conditions, such as carpal tunnel syndrome, temporomandibular joint replacement, and spine injury, pain relief should occur if the surgical procedure corrects the underlying medical condition causing the pain. With stimulators and implantable pumps, the goal is to directly relieve pain without regard to fixing its cause. For all surgeries in which pain control is the primary goal, understanding the patient's pain sensitivity is critical—that is, whether the patient experiences pain and disability that far exceed the expected levels, given the nature of the underlying medical problem. In such surgeries, excessive pain sensitivity is associated with significantly reduced results (see Chapters 2, 4, 7, and 11).

Knowledge and Expectations

Surgery is a dramatic, life-altering event. To undergo the rigors of surgery—anesthesia, hours in the operating room with internal organs exposed, weeks or months of recovery—requires physical strength, psychological determination, and intellectual knowledge. Thus, gaining insight into the patient's understanding of the surgical procedure and his or her expectations for surgical outcome is important. For example, bone marrow and stem cell replacement patients who possess disease-related information, and the ability to apply it, are better able to adhere to self-care regimens (see Chapter 5). To the extent that the patient is overly optimistic about surgical results—expecting, for example, complete resolution of underlying medical problems—disappointment and dissatisfaction are likely to be experienced. Also important to consider is whether the patient's motivation for surgery is at least partly based on an expectation that changes brought about by surgery will be accompanied by changes in interaction with others. Bariatric surgery patients, for example, may expect surgery to lead to improved relationships or sexual function (see Chapter 3). Unfortunately, predicting how others will respond to patients' physical, functional, and emotional improvement is difficult. If the patient's motivation for surgery is primarily external—that is, expecting changes in the responses of others—rather than internal, surgical outcome may be diminished (see Chapter 12).

Financial Incentives

Many of the medical conditions examined in this text may have resulted from situations in which litigation can arise—industrial accidents, motor vehicle accidents, and exposure to environmental chemicals. Also, related issues may arise, such as workers' compensation cases or patients applying for Social Security Disability, in which financial benefits are greater for unsuccessful treatment than for an effective surgery. Certainly, it is the rare patient who would undergo surgery for the primary purpose of obtaining financial gain. Still, the evidence that financial incentives can influence surgical results is significant, as is the case in spine surgery, in which patients receiving workers' compensation or involved in litigation generally tend to obtain poorer results than those who are not involved in such situations (Chapter 2).

BIOETHICS

Despite all the benefits that PPS can provide to patients, surgeons, and third-party payers, the interests and desires of all these involved parties do not always coincide. For example, patients may feel that their own actions to control or improve health have failed and that the surgery will both provide a cure and obviate their role in health improvement. When the MHC recognizes that such expectations are unrealistic and may even undermine surgical effectiveness, then the stage for conflicting interests is set. The conflict between patients' goals and those of health care providers and insurers provide the greatest challenges to the MHC. They must be carefully considered and successfully navigated if the results are to be valid, meet the MHC's responsibilities, and provide the best possible results for the patient.

The potentially conflicting interests and needs that arise in PPS are perhaps best considered in relation to the ethical principles and standards set forth by the American Psychological Association (APA; 2010) in its "Ethical Principles of Psychologists and Code of Conduct," as well as in relation to medical ethics in general. In the remainder of this introduction, we consider several ethical challenges surrounding PPS, with an eye toward helping the MHC gain the ability to apply ethical principles to complex medical issues, in collaboration with other professionals who may not adhere to, or necessarily believe in, the ethical standards of the mental health professional. We frame our discussion around five major ethical constructs: self-determination, beneficence, nonmaleficence, justice, and informed consent. For more guidance, the reader is referred to the APA Ethics Code.

Self-Determination

Self-determination (see Principle E, Respect for People's Rights and Dignity; APA, 2010, p. 3) involves an individual's ability to determine how he or she is to be treated by others. It means that patients can freely act to define the treatment, outcomes, and processes used in their health care. Self-determination implies the ability to make reasonable informed decisions in one's self-interest. Issues of self-determination frequently arise in communicating surgical treatment plans. In cases that do not involve life-threatening issues, such as bariatric surgery and, to an even greater extent, cosmetic surgery, should the surgeon perform an operation on a patient just because the patient requests it? Or should the patient be asked to demonstrate some level of understanding about the potential medical and psychosocial risks and benefits of surgery? Moreover, if the ultimate outcome of the surgery depends on patient behaviors, such as compliance with medication or exercise regimens, should a patient with a documented history of noncompliance be allowed to undergo elective surgery? Ideally, PPS can enhance self-determination: It assists patients in deciding whether surgery is the best course of action, with the knowledge that their expectations, emotional state, and behavioral adherence to treatment regimens are likely to significantly influence results.

The issue of self-determination is particularly acute when one considers that some patients may engage in *impression management*, minimizing symptoms of psychopathology and, in some cases, producing invalid test results (Walfish, Vance, & Fabricatore, 2007). Impression management is most likely to occur if the patient is told that the MHC is a gatekeeper for the surgery and that only if the patient "passes" the PPS will surgery be allowed to proceed. When this occurs, the information obtained in the PPS may be of somewhat limited validity, allowing for a less accurate assessment of psychosocial risk.

Several actions can minimize this particular dilemma. First, the MHC can help the surgeon to properly frame the referral by informing the patient that PPS is not a pass–fail decision and that the results are like those of many other preoperative evaluations—they provide the surgeon with information that will allow him or her to weigh the benefits versus the risks and will lead to more appropriate treatment decisions. The timing of the referral is, therefore, also critical and ideally should occur after the physician has informed the patient about the surgery being considered but before the patient is scheduled for surgery. Second, the clinician conducting PPS must work hard to enlist patients as collaborators in the evaluation process, by helping them see the value that PPS can bring in improving surgical outcomes, improving overall health, and avoiding adverse surgical results. Finally, psychometric testing that assesses whether patients are minimizing, exaggerating, or correctly reporting symptoms can be included in the PPS battery. Such testing might include, for example, an examination of validity scales from the Minnesota Multiphasic Personality Inventory—2—Restructured Form.

Patient self-determination can also be defined in terms of negative and positive freedoms (Cohen, 2000). *Negative freedoms* include freedom from coercion by others, and *positive freedoms* are those that allow for self-determination, expression, and choice. In theory, patients who undergo most surgical procedures are able to exercise their self-determination by deciding whether to consent to treatment and arrive at the operating room on the day of surgery. However, this sense of self-determination may be influenced by the nature of the illness. In bariatric surgery, for example, the patient's sense of self-determination may be compromised by physicians who have informed the patient, "This is your last, best chance to control your weight" or have made statements such as "If you don't lose weight soon, you will die in the next 5 years" (Raper & Sarwer, 2008). Such subtle and more overt forms of coercion are challenges to self-determination and must be considered in giving the PPS recommendations.

Beneficence and Nonmaleficence

Beneficence (Principle A, Beneficence and Nonmaleficence; APA, 2010, p. 3) is a principle by which professionals provide what they believe is best for another person. Sometimes the professionals' idea of the best course of treatment may differ from that of the patient or family. Other times, it may vary across professional opinion, leading to significant ethical dilemmas for the clinician performing PPS. For example, in the case of a patient with a spine injury, the referring surgeon may be considering a multiple-level spinal fusion (a surgery with potential for significant benefits, but also one that requires substantial psychological stamina) when a different surgeon might also consider less invasive procedures for the same condition (either at the same institution or at a competing institution). Although it is clearly beyond the MHC's scope of training to determine which surgery may best help the patient, the PPS decision is often made within the context of conflicting medical opinions about the best treatment option. The clinician performing the PPS may be put in a position to say that a particular patient could handle a less invasive treatment, or one requiring less postoperative rehabilitation, but would be less able to handle a more demanding one, even if the referring surgeon does not perform such a more limited procedure.

Nonmaleficence (Principle A, Beneficence and Nonmaleficence; APA, 2010, p. 3) is the expectation that the professional will do everything possible to avoid harm, as embodied in APA Ethical Standard 3.04: "Psychologists take reasonable steps to avoid harming their clients/patients . . . and to minimize harm where it is foreseeable and unavoidable" (APA, 2010, p. 6). This issue is perhaps the most critical one in PPS because many of the surgeries discussed in this text, although they have the potential to reduce physical and psychological suffering, also have the potential to lead to no change or a worsening of symptoms. The issue of nonmaleficence is brought into sharpest focus when the patient has clear physical indications for the surgery but psychosocial factors decrease the likelihood of obtaining positive surgical results or increase the possibility of harm. Further complicating this issue may be pressure placed on the clinician by the surgeon, who may only be referring the patient for PPS because of insurance requirements and, therefore, may view an MHC's recommendation to delay or avoid surgery as an obstacle rather than an opportunity to help the patient. The MHC, then, is potentially faced with a conflict of interest (Standard 3.06): "Psychologists refrain from taking on a professional role when personal, scientific, professional, legal, financial or other interests could reasonably be expected to (1) impair their objectivity, competence or effectiveness" (APA, 2010, p. 6). The dilemma, then, becomes one of maintaining the surgeon as a referral source while helping the patient avoid the potential harm of surgery. Fortunately, the trust of the referring physician is bolstered by the recognition that short-term concerns about losing a surgery case because of psychological issues are balanced against more significant long-term benefits: It improves the surgeon's overall effectiveness, reduces the likelihood of dissatisfied patients, and brings value to the surgical field in general.

Justice

In bioethical decision making, *justice* (Principle D, Justice; APA, 2010, p. 3) involves treating patients fairly and providing them with the care they are entitled to receive. In many cases involving PPS the principle of justice raises significant dilemmas. For example, in the case of solid organ transplantation, in which organs are a limited commodity, determining entitlement for treatment can be difficult because the decision to use an organ may delay transplant for another patient. What is surprising to many people is that severity of illness, rather than the psychosocial and behavioral contributions to the disease, can determine where someone is positioned on a transplant list: The person with chronic alcoholism who has made no effort to maintain sobriety over the course of his lifetime may be placed higher on the list than the young patient in liver failure because of some rare disease if the person with chronic alcoholism is sicker.

For most clinicians, justice is considered in the context of a given doctor–patient relationship. At the same time, the professional may have a sense of the public health policy issues involved, wherein a professional may be called on to protect society and act to maximize fairness. When resources are scarce, does a patient's medical condition entitle him or her to a particular form of care, or should certain behavioral or other criteria be met in order to receive that care? When patient and societal goals are at odds, the MHC must carefully consider the issue of justice.

Informed Consent

Even a cursory review of bioethical issues is not complete without a discussion of informed consent (Standard 3.10; APA, 2010, p. 6). Informed consent has several components. First, the MHC must inform the patient, before conducting PPS, of (a) the reasons for the evaluation, (b) the types of information to be obtained, and (c) the possible uses of this information. The MHC should indicate that results will be used by the surgeon to develop the best possible treatment course for the patient while minimizing the risk of harming the patient. The patient must also be informed that honest answers to inquiries made in the PPS will ensure such results. Again, the patient needs to be informed that the surgeon makes the ultimate determination of the course of treatment but that PPS results may play a large role in making such a decision. Carefully informing the patient of all these issues will minimize the likelihood that the patient will take any legal action against the MHC, should he or she disagree with the MHC's recommendations.

However, the surgeon must impart, in a clear, understandable manner, the reasons for the surgery, the specific type of surgery, and the expected postoperative course. Also included in this aspect of the informed consent process should be information about the risks of the surgery and their likelihood of occurring, alternatives to the procedure that is planned, and the risks of the alternatives. Unfortunately, the MHC who performs PPS will often find that patients do not feel fully cognizant of the nature of the surgery and alternative treatments.

In most cases, research has shown that informed consent fails to be effective for two reasons: (a) surgeons' poor communication skills and (b) patients' preconceived notions and expectations (Gorney, 2006). Such problems are evident in the number of malpractice suits filed against surgeons stipulating failure to adequately obtain informed consent. Lawsuits focusing on informed consent often claim that the risks of procedures were not adequately communicated or that procedures were not adequately explained. An important distinction is made between ethically obtained informed consent and legally effective consent (Laneader & Wolpe, 2006). *Ethical consent* denotes a decision-making process based on mutual respect and full disclosure and usually describes a process of communication between practitioner and patient over time rather than an informed consent moment when a form is signed. The legal definition of informed consent focuses on the form and its discussion and mandates disclosure of what is "reasonably prudent."

Data have shown that informed surgery patients experience less anxiety, are more compliant with instructions, cope better with complications, and express greater satisfaction with results of the surgery (Redden, Baker, & Meisel, 1985). Primarily, the success of the informed consent process is based largely on effective communication (written and verbal) between the surgeon and the patient, as well as on the patient's ability to recall and understand the information provided. Plastic surgery patients have been shown to recall no more than 50% of potential complications delivered in writing (Goin, Burgoyne, & Goin, 1976); among bariatric surgery patients, only 36% could remember potential complications 1 year after surgery (Madan & Tichansky, 2005). Poor recall of information imparted during the informed consent process is best overcome by using multiple forms of communication and by allowing the patient and family multiple opportunities to learn about the procedure and raise relevant questions. Although providing informed consent about the surgery itself is outside the MHC's role, through careful questioning the MHC can certainly determine the extent to which patients have retained informed consent information and should alert the surgeon if the patient does not appear to understand or agree to the intended procedure.

PERSONAL AND PROFESSIONAL REWARDS OF CONDUCTING PPS

In this introduction, we have discussed at length the many benefits that PPS provides to patients, surgeons, insurers, and the public, as well as the ethical considerations that can arise when these different parties have conflicting objectives for PPS. Before explaining how the rest of this volume is organized, we must take a moment to explain how effectively conducting PPS benefits the MHC. The benefits are many, and the biggest rewards come from collaboration. PPS allows the MHC to be an integral member of a treatment team focused on the best overall care of the patient. It elevates the field of psychology, and the MHC, to a primary status in patient care. Perhaps even more important and satisfying is the knowledge that in conducting PPS, the MHC is collaborating with the patient to make the best possible choices about care and to maximize the patient's ability to obtain good treatment results. Unlike many areas of psychology, the benefits to the patient are concrete and observable—more rapid recovery, less use of medication, greater functional improvement, and avoidance of a worsening of condition. Thus, PPS brings a great sense of professional and personal satisfaction as physicians and surgery candidates seek out the MHC's opinion and expertise.

ORGANIZATION OF THIS BOOK

Each chapter in this book examines psychosocial influences on surgery for a specific medical condition. In general, the earlier chapters represent those areas in which PPS is already in common use: organ transplantation, spinal surgery, bariatric surgery, and pain control procedures. Conditions in which PPS is being used with increasing frequency represent the next group of chapters: stem cell and bone marrow implantation, deep-brain stimulation for Parkinson's disease, surgery for temporomandibular joint disorder, reconstructive surgery, breast surgery, and gynecologic surgery. The final chapters examine conditions for which PPS is beginning to be used but has not come into wide acceptance: carpal tunnel syndrome and cosmetic surgery. The Afterword suggests future directions for the field.

CONCLUSION

As surgical techniques and equipment evolve ever more rapidly, it is perhaps natural to think of surgery as a technological process: The surgeon carefully identifies the underlying medical condition and applies state-of-the-art procedures, and the condition is resolved. However, as the rapidly developing field of PPS demonstrates, it is critical that surgeons expand their vision beyond the physical causes of medical conditions. Emotional distress, substance abuse, personality disorders, and willingness to comply with medical regimens—all these and many other psychosocial issues can strongly influence the outcome of surgery. This text brings together the most current research and clinical practice in identifying such psychosocial influences on a wide range of surgical procedures. It is our hope that this book will increase the use and effectiveness of PPS so that patients can obtain the best possible treatment outcomes.

REFERENCES

American Psychological Association. (2010). *Ethical principles of psychologists and code of conduct* (2002, amended June 1, 2010). Retrieved from www.apa.org/ethics/code/index.aspx

Beck, A. T., Epstein, N., Brown, G., & Steer, R. A. (1988). An inventory for measuring clinical anxiety: Psychometric properties. *Journal of Consulting and Clinical Psychology, 56,* 893–897.

Ben-Porath, Y.S. (2012). *Interpreting the MMPI–2–F.* Minneapolis, MN: University of Minnesota Press.

Butcher, J. N., Dahlstrom, W. G., Graham, J. R., Tellegen, A, & Kaemmer, B. (1989). *The Minnesota Multiphasic Personality Inventory—2 (MMPI–2): Manual for administration and scoring*. Minneapolis, MN: University of Minnesota Press

Cohen, J. (2000). Patient autonomy and social fairness. *Cambridge Quarterly of Healthcare Ethics, 9*, 391–399.

Goin, M. K., Burgoyne, R. W., & Goin, J. M. (1976). Face lift operation: The patient's secret motivations and reactions to "informed consent." *Plastic and Reconstructive Surgery, 58*, 273–279. doi:10.1097/00006534-197609000-00002

Gorney, M. (2006). Professional and legal considerations in cosmetic surgery. In D. B. Sarwer, T. Pruzinsky, T. F. Cash, R. M. Goldwyn, J. A. Persing, & L. A. Whitaker (Eds.), *Psychological aspects of reconstructive and cosmetic plastic surgery: Clinical, empirical, and ethical perspectives* (pp. 315–327). Philadelphia, PA: Lippincott Williams & Wilkins.

Laneader, A., & Wolpe, P. R. (2005). Bioethical considerations in cosmetic surgery. In D. B. Sarwer, T. Pruzinsky, T. F. Cash, R. M. Goldwyn, J. A. Persing, & L. A. Whitaker (Eds.), *Psychological aspects of plastic surgery* (pp. 301–313). Philadelphia, PA: Lippincott Williams & Wilkins.

Madan, A. K., & Tichansky, D. A. (2005). Patients postoperatively forget aspects of preoperative patient education. *Obesity Surgery, 15*, 1066–1069. doi:10.1381/0960892054621198

Radloff, L. S. (1977). The CES-D Scale: A self-report depression scale for research in the general population. *Applied Psychological Measurement, 1*, 385–401. doi:10.1177/014662167700100306

Rankin, S. H., Stallings, K. D., & London, F. (2005). *Patient education in health and illness* (5th ed.). Philadelphia, PA: Lippincott Williams & Wilkins.

Raper, S. E., & Sarwer, D. B. (2008). Informed consent issues in the conduct of bariatric surgery. *Surgery for Obesity and Related Diseases, 4*, 60–68.

Redden, E. M., Baker, D. M., & Meisel, A. (1985). The patient, the plastic surgeon and informed consent: New insights into old problems. *Plastic and Reconstructive Surgery, 75*, 270–276. doi:10.1097/00006534-198502000-00023

Twillman, R. K., Manetto, C., Wellisch, D. K., & Wolcott, D. L. (1993). The Transplant Evaluation Rating Scale: A revision of the psychosocial levels system for evaluating organ transplant candidates. *Psychosomatics, 34*, 144–153.

Walfish, S., Vance, D., & Fabricatore, A. F. (2007). Psychological evaluation of bariatric surgery applicants: Procedures and reasons for delay or denial of surgery. *Obesity Surgery, 17*, 1578–1583. doi:10.1007/s11695-007-9274-0

1

TRANSPLANT RECIPIENTS AND ORGAN DONORS

KRISTIN K. KUNTZ AND DIANE B. V. BONFIGLIO

Organ transplantation has been a treatment for end-stage organ failure since the 1960s. Some transplant patients have been living with chronic illness for years, and others become acutely ill, resulting in the need for a lifesaving transplant. The long-term success of transplanted organs is largely dependent on patients' ability to effectively manage a complex medical regimen. Because of the shortage of available organs in relation to the need, it is vital that organs are allocated fairly and to those most likely to have an optimal outcome, both medically and psychologically.

In this chapter, we review the important components of the pre-transplant psychosocial evaluation. We discuss the psychosocial factors that have been linked to better and worse outcomes post–organ transplant and organ donation as well as ways to address these risk factors before transplant listing. The first part of the chapter focuses on the psychosocial evaluation of transplant recipients. Later, we discuss the psychosocial evaluation for individuals interested in donating an organ.

DOI: 10.1037/14035-002
Presurgical Psychological Screening: Understanding Patients, Improving Outcomes, Andrew R. Block and David B. Sarwer (Editors)

BACKGROUND

The scarcity of donated organs is evident from the discrepancy between the number of transplants performed and the number of individuals on the transplant waiting lists. Currently, more than 110,000 candidates are on the national waiting list for an organ in the United States (United Network for Organ Sharing, 2011). In the United States, 22,103 transplants were performed in 2010 using organs from deceased donors, and 6,559 transplants were performed using organs from living donors (Organ Procurement and Transplantation Network, 2011). The most recent report on deaths while waiting on the transplant list indicated that 7,182 patients died before receiving a transplant in 2008 (Organ Procurement and Transplantation Network, 2009b).

Patient survival after transplantation has increased yearly with the availability of more effective immunosuppressive medication and improved surgical technique. Survival rates vary depending on several factors, including which organ was transplanted, the recipient's ethnicity, and the recipient's age. General 1-year adjusted patient survival rates in the United States from 2007 are reported in Table 1.1 (Organ Procurement and Transplantation Network, 2009a).

WHY THE NEED FOR PSYCHOLOGICAL EVALUATION?

Because of the scarcity of organs and the great financial and medical resources used, individual cases are scrutinized to determine which patients would most benefit from transplantation. Also, there is an obligation to deceased donor families, to living donors, and to society to be good stewards

TABLE 1.1
National 1-Year Posttransplant Survival Rate

Organ type	Patient 1-year survival (%)	SE (%)
Kidney		
Deceased donor	96.5	0.2
Living donor	98.9	0.1
Pancreas	96.8	1.8
Liver		
Deceased donor	89.4	0.4
Living donor	91.7	1.7
Heart	89.2	0.7
Lung	82.7	1.0
Intestines	78.7	3.2

Note. Data from Organ Procurement and Transplantation Network (2009a).

of donated organs. Psychological and behavioral factors, including mental illness, substance abuse, and noncompliance, can contribute to morbidity and mortality posttransplant. Hence, a psychosocial assessment is usually performed as part of the comprehensive transplant evaluation. These assessments may be performed by social workers, psychologists, psychiatrists, or psychiatric nurses (Collins & Labott, 2007). The psychosocial evaluation is an opportunity to gather baseline information concerning psychological functioning, cognitive status, and quality of life that can be revisited over time. The overall purpose of the psychosocial evaluation in organ transplant is not necessarily to eliminate patients from becoming candidates but to identify any potential risk factors that would predict a difficult course during the transplant process or a less-than-optimal outcome (Huffman, Popkin, & Stern, 2003). The recognition of possible red flags allows for intervention before transplant, implementation of a care plan after transplant, or both.

ASPECTS OF THE ASSESSMENT

The pretransplant psychosocial assessment has several important components. A thorough psychosocial evaluation will assess coping resources; social support; history of or current mental illness; compliance; health behaviors, including tobacco, drug, and alcohol abuse or dependence; and decision-making capacity. Specific components of the evaluation often include a review of the patient's medical records, a semistructured interview with the patient, an interview with the patient's caregiver, and any testing of interest (i.e., cognitive, personality). Acquiring collateral information from the patient's other health care providers, such as the referring physicians or dialysis team, is important. In addition, transplant team members who have been working with the patient such as nurse coordinators, social workers, and physicians can also offer insight. The clinical interview must be very thorough and detailed. It would ideally be conducted after a patient has been provided with formal education about transplant.

Medical History

A common first step in the psychosocial evaluation for transplant is a review of the patient's medical records. This review informs the interviewer ahead of time and can help in determining the accuracy of the patient's self-report during the evaluation. The chart may have informative comments from the patient's physicians related to compliance and other psychosocial concerns (Collins & Labott, 2007). In addition, reviewing notes from other aspects of the transplant assessment, if available, can ensure that the patient is providing consistent information across providers.

During the interview, the patient should be able to demonstrate a basic level of knowledge about his or her condition and medications. More specifically, one should assess whether the patient can explain his or her diagnosis leading to transplant, including the date of first symptoms and date of diagnosis. The patient should be able to describe his or her symptom progression and the various treatments that have been used over the course of the illness. Prior surgeries and any complications should be discussed. This discussion can elicit how patients may have coped with prior setbacks related to their health. Any ongoing pain issues should be discussed, with an assessment for a history of opioid abuse. The interviewer should expect the patient to be able to name his or her current medications. The past or present use of home nursing or a home health aide can be an indicator of the patient's ability to care for him- or herself as well as a potential indicator that the patient lacks a support system. The interviewer must understand that medical symptomatology in end-stage organ failure can overlap with symptoms of psychiatric disorders (e.g., fatigue, appetite loss, sleep disturbance), so a thorough examination of the onset and frequency of symptoms must be conducted to distinguish between the two (Collins & Labott, 2007).

If a patient demonstrates difficulty with providing a thorough medical history, it can indicate problems with memory, organization, or health literacy. Compensatory strategies should be discussed with the patient. These strategies might include creating a binder to carry to appointments that is filled with important information such as dates of surgeries and a medication list. Often, a family member or friend can help to provide details of the patient's medical history and can be encouraged to attend future medical appointments with the patient. In some cases, this will be an indicator that a patient needs further education about his or her medical conditions, which can be communicated to the transplant team and to the patient's referring physician.

Compliance History

One of the primary reasons transplanted organs fail is because the patient does not follow the posttransplant regimen (Dew et al., 2001), and intractable noncompliance is considered to be a relative or absolute contraindication for most transplant programs (Levenson & Olbrisch, 1993). The posttransplant regimen includes taking multiple medications daily, including immunosuppressant drugs; having regular lab work; and attending clinic appointments. In addition, the patient must monitor his or her vital signs, check in with the transplant team regularly (i.e., before starting new medications prescribed by other practitioners, with any new medical symptoms or diagnoses), and follow infectious disease precautions because of his or her immunosuppressed state.

Noncompliance rates among transplant patients range from 20% to 50% across studies (Laederach-Hofmann & Bunzel, 2000). Some of the reasons patients report being noncompliant after transplant include difficulty affording medications, adverse side effects of medication, forgetting, psychological distress, and general perceived stress (Achille, Oulette, Fournier, Vachon, & Herbert, 2006; Jindal et al., 2009; Wainwright, Fallon, & Gould, 1999). Patients who felt indebted to their donors report better compliance (Achille et al., 2006).

In the pretransplant evaluation, compliance with the patient's current regimen is assessed. Questions relate to how often the patient takes medication daily and how often doses are missed (and reasons why they are missed). Also, assessing the patient's ability to manage medical appointments and any other components of the medical regimen, such as attending dialysis, is important. During the evaluation process and waiting time, the transplant center may require multiple tests and appointments. In addition, patients must be able to be easily contacted, must return calls promptly, and must keep the transplant team apprised of any changes in their medical and psychiatric health. Failure to do any of these can be a red flag for posttransplant care.

If a patient has demonstrated poor compliance with his or her medical regimen in the past or is currently demonstrating poor compliance, it is important to identify the barriers and help the patient problem solve. Medication noncompliance may mean implementing reminders such as an alarm and a pill box or increasing family support. In terms of noncompliance with appointments, the team can help the patient use calendars or daily planners, make reminder phone calls to family members (as well as the patient), or help the patient consider transportation options in the community. A compliance contract can set specific expectations the patient must meet for a specific amount of time before transplantation will be considered (Cupples & Steslowe, 2001). The benefits of setting specific goals in a contract include making the focus of the problem the behavior (not blaming the patient), making the patient take responsibility for his or her behavior, allowing the family to offer helpful support, and establishing a collaborative relationship versus a paternalistic one (Cupples & Steslowe, 2001).

Transplant Knowledge

Most transplant centers consider a lack of transplant knowledge to be a relative or absolute contraindication (Levenson & Olbrisch, 1993). To provide informed consent for transplantation, the patient must possess knowledge of the transplant procedure, including success rates, risks and benefits, and length of time of hospitalization and recovery (Collins & Labott, 2007). He or she should also be able to demonstrate knowledge of immunosuppression, rejection, and the lifetime need for medication. When applicable, the patient should be asked whether the possibility of using a living donor has been discussed and, if so, whether the patient has investigated this. In the evaluation of a patient's knowledge of transplant, any magical thinking, unrealistic expectations, fears, and concerns can be uncovered. It is important to note that some patients may have preexisting relationships with other transplant patients, which can affect their understanding of and attitude toward transplant in both positive and negative ways (Huffman et al., 2003).

If a patient seems to have cursory knowledge of transplant after being formally educated, his or her transplant coordinator must be informed. A patient may not be able to demonstrate transplant knowledge for various reasons, such as feeling overwhelmed with information, having poor attention and memory owing to organ failure, and having a learning disability (Collins & Labott, 2007). The transplant coordinator can arrange for a patient to receive further education, whether it is an individual session with the coordinator, physician, or both or whether it is having the patient return to a group education class. Support groups involving transplant professionals and posttransplant patients can also be a source of more education for a pretransplant patient.

Social Support

The availability of social support is a major determinant of a patient's psychosocial suitability for transplant. Research has shown that social support is positively associated with medication adherence and quality of life posttransplant (Cetingok, Hathaway, & Winsett, 2007; Chisholm-Burns, Spivey, & Wilks, 2010), whereas social instability has been found to be a predictor of poor outcomes in several studies of liver transplant patients (McCallum & Masterson, 2006). Both quality and quantity of social support should be assessed. The patient will need tangible support (e.g., transportation to appointments) as well as emotional support during the transplant process. During the evaluation, primary and secondary support providers should be named, and at least one support person should accompany the patient to transplant appointments. Caregivers' availability to be present before, during, and after the transplant should be assessed, which entails asking about whether they work and, if so, their ability to take sufficient time off to aid the patient immediately after surgery. Caregivers' health status should also be investigated to ensure that they are physically capable of providing care. If the caregivers have young children, a plan for child care should be determined. If possible, this information should be garnered from the caregiver directly and from the patient alone (see the Caregiver Interview section of this chapter). The dedication of the support system to the patient is vital to obtaining a successful outcome (Olbrisch, Benedict, Ashe, & Levenson, 2002).

When a patient reports a lack of support, it is important to investigate whether there is truly no one to provide care and support or whether the patient is simply uncomfortable asking for help or refuses to include others in the transplant process. Most transplant centers ask patients to bring support people to their transplant evaluation or to a formal family meeting before transplant listing, so that the caregivers can be educated about what the patient will experience; this way, the team can ensure that the patient has proper support. When a patient's support system appears to be truly lacking, the psychosocial team must work with him or her to find ways to increase it. Many forms of potential support for a patient are available, such as formal appointments with a mental health practitioner, transplant support groups (or support groups for the patient's underlying medical condition), religious organizations, neighbors, and extended family (Finn, 2000). In addition, some transplant programs have formal mentorship programs, and others match a patient for support on an as-needed basis. A one-on-one mentorship relationship between a pretransplant patient and a posttransplant patient can become a lasting source of support.

Behavioral Health

In this section of the interview, a patient's lifestyle habits are investigated. Appetite and dietary habits are discussed (which also adds to the compliance discussion because many pretransplant patients have dietary restrictions). Any large weight gains or losses are discussed as well as any needed changes in weight required for transplant (a patient may be asked to lose weight or gain weight to improve surgical outcome). If the patient needs to make a change in weight, his or her plan for doing so should be discussed. Quality and duration of sleep is assessed. Physical activity level is assessed by inquiring about daily activity and intentional exercise. Capturing a current picture of the patient's behavioral health can provide information on how his or her daily life has been affected by the illness.

During this portion of the interview, the interviewer can potentially intervene with strategies to improve a patient's quality of life. The patient may be encouraged to engage in light exercise, implement better sleep hygiene, or discuss dietary changes with a nutritionist.

Psychiatric History and Mental Health

In this section of the interview, a patient's psychiatric history is discussed, including any diagnoses, treatment (i.e., counseling, psychotropic medications), psychiatric hospitalizations, and suicide attempts. Current mood and coping are also assessed, as well as family history. This place in the assessment is when the results of any psychosocial measures can be discussed. With a patient who is currently under the care of a mental health professional, getting a letter from or having a conversation with that professional can provide the interviewer with additional insight into the patient's condition. Also, the transplant team and the outside mental health provider can come to an agreement on how the patient will be monitored throughout the transplant process, given that it can be a time of increased stress.

Contraindications for transplant based on psychiatric illness are not always agreed on between transplant centers (Levenson & Olbrisch, 1993). Some of the less controversial exclusionary conditions include active suicidal or homicidal ideation, active psychosis, dementia, and profound mental retardation (Huffman et al., 2003). The evaluation considers psychiatric factors to identify how a patient might cope with the ongoing stresses of managing a transplant, such as medical complications. A preexisting diagnosis of a mood or anxiety disorder is not necessarily grounds for excluding a patient from transplant but indicates a need for monitoring after transplant.

The time surrounding transplant can be emotionally turbulent for the patient and his or her family (Finn, 2000). In cases in which a patient is experiencing current psychological distress or has an extensive psychiatric history, he or she may be strongly encouraged to seek treatment if not already doing so. If at any time during the transplant experience a patient is identified as having trouble coping, most transplant teams have a mental health professional available for inpatient and outpatient consultation.

Substance History

Substance abuse or dependence can jeopardize the outcome of a transplant, so most centers have set guidelines in place for it (Olbrisch et al., 2002). Past and current substance use should be thoroughly assessed, with special attention paid to length of abstinence from illicit substances and factors protective against relapse. In a review examining psychosocial selection criteria for liver transplant, McCallum and Masterson (2006) found several variables to be associated with sustained abstinence, such as a stable social situation, no alcohol dependence in first-degree relatives, older than age 50, no failed rehabilitation programs, good medical compliance, and the absence of a severe mental disorder. Not surprisingly, pretransplant substance use is a predictor of posttransplant use despite patients' often having to demonstrate a period of abstinence before transplantation (Dew, DiMartini, et al., 2007).

When a patient presents with a history of substance abuse or dependence, it is up to the transplant team to decide what abstinence period, if any, the patient must demonstrate before transplant. Some transplant centers require the patient to attend formal rehabilitation, and others only require the patient to submit to random drug screening to demonstrate abstinence. Some transplant centers use the same policies across organs, and other centers have different abstinence requirements for different substances and different organs. For example, unlike with illicit drugs and alcohol, smoking cessation is not always required to receive organs other than hearts and lungs (Olbrisch et al., 2002).

Cognition and Mental Status

Cognitive functioning is assessed to identify any learning barriers that might interfere with a patient's ability to provide consent for transplant and to manage the transplanted organ. Various physiological reasons exist as to why a patient might present with cognitive impairment before transplant (e.g., hepatic encephalopathy, uremia, poor oxygen perfusion) and warrant examination (Olbrisch et al., 2002). In some cases a patient's cognitive function will improve after transplant, and in other cases the deficits will be more permanent. The Mini-Mental State Examination is an efficient way to detect any significant cognitive limitations (Huffman et al., 2003). More sensitive changes in cognition can be assessed by a full neuropsychological battery of tests. Some transplant centers have all patients complete neuropsychological testing to obtain a baseline measure of functioning that can be used to detect any postoperative changes (DiMartini, Dew, & Trzepacz, 2007).

A patient's problem-solving skills can be evaluated during the interview by presenting the patient with various scenarios that may occur after transplant. Questions such as "What would you do if you had unpleasant side effects from a medication?" and "What preparations would you make when going on vacation after your transplant?" can be an indicator of how well the patient can handle a complex medical regimen.

Cognitive impairment in the absence of an adequate support system can be a contraindication for transplant (Wise, 2008). When a patient does present with cognitive impairment, the social support system is closely examined to determine whether caregivers will be available to assist the patient. If a patient with mild cognitive impairment lives alone, home nursing is sometimes an option to help the patient with taking medication and organizing the regimen.

Psychosocial Measures

Often, psychosocial instruments are administered as part of the pre-transplant psychosocial assessment in conjunction with the assessment interview. Psychosocial measures may be used to screen patients before the interview to identify those who need further assessment in certain areas or to provide more information on those patients already identified as needing further examination (DiMartini et al., 2007). These tools may assess such areas as psychological distress, quality of life, social support, cognitive functioning, and adherence. Measures created specifically to assess suitability for transplant include the Psychosocial Assessment of Candidates for Transplant (Olbrisch, Levenson, & Hamer, 1989) and the Transplant Evaluation Rating Scale (Twillman, Manetto, Wellisch, & Wolcott, 1993).

Caregiver Interview

After the patient assessment is finished, it is helpful to have a separate interview with someone in the patient's support network, preferably the primary caregiver (Olbrisch et al., 2002), to assess the caregiver's opinions about the patient's transplant knowledge, how well the patient is coping with his or her illness, and whether the patient has needed much assistance in daily activities in recent times. Here, the interviewer can obtain another viewpoint about the patient's compliance history, illicit substance use, and cognitive functioning (Collins & Labott, 2007). The interview is also an opportunity to determine whether the caregiver can take the time to provide care after surgery and as needed throughout the patient's transplant course. The caregiver can discuss how he or she has been coping with the patient's illness and being a caregiver. It is important to remember that transplantation is a stressful process for the patient and for the support system, and the family may need as much support as the patient. In cases in which a patient presents urgently for transplantation and may even be unconscious, the caregiver provides the information that makes up the psychosocial evaluation (Olbrisch et al., 2002).

Impressions and Recommendations

After the medical chart has been reviewed, the patient and caregiver interviews are complete, and any testing has been reviewed, it is time to make a decision about a patient's suitability for transplant from a psychosocial perspective. For a patient with few to no psychosocial barriers to transplant, strengths can be described first, followed by any possible weaknesses. For a patient with multiple psychosocial barriers, the concerns can be described first, followed by the patient's strengths. The recommendations section of the evaluation lists what the patient can do to improve his or her candidacy and postoperative course. These recommendations are practical ones relating back to the points in the assessment section (e.g., psychotherapy, addiction counseling, improved compliance). Here is where the implementation of a compliance contract is noted. Finally, the assessment and the recommendations are shared with the transplant team, so that the entire unit is aware of the patient's psychosocial plan.

CASE STUDY

D. G. was a 29-year-old single Caucasian man referred for pre–kidney transplant psychological evaluation.[1] His medical history included end-stage renal disease secondary to hypertensive nephrosclerosis, and he had been on hemodialysis for 24 months. He also had anemia, hypertension, chronic neck pain of unknown origin, and a leg fracture in 1991. D. G.'s compliance with his medical regimen was poor. He reported that he "hardly ever" took his phosphorous binders unless he was feeling bloated (they were prescribed to be taken with each meal daily). He reported a history of adjusting his medications according to how he felt, and he admitted to not always following doctors' directions. He had a history of poor attendance at dialysis but had shown improvement in the past several months in hopes of being listed for transplant. He demonstrated a cursory level of knowledge about the transplant process and posttransplant responsibilities, despite having been through formal education.

D. G. had a high school education and had earned a license in welding. He worked as a structural welder for 7 years before being diagnosed with kidney disease. His worsening health led him to quit his job and start receiving disability. At the time of his evaluation, he was living in his deceased grandparents' home, which was in the process of being sold. He had not been looking for alternative housing and was unsure of where he would live after the house was sold. D. G. had a 7-year-old child whom he saw several weekends per month. He reported that his parents would be his caregivers after transplant, but he reported having a tumultuous relationship with his mother.

The behavioral health evaluation revealed more of D. G.'s difficulties. His body mass index was normal at 20.9. He reported that his appetite fluctuated, his sleep was erratic, and he did not get any regular exercise. He could not name any recreational activities other than spending time at a local bar where he met with his cousins and friends.

During the evaluation, D. G. minimized any psychiatric history, although his chart reflected a report of depression and anxiety 5 years earlier. In the past year, he admitted reporting depression to his nephrologist, who prescribed Lexapro. He said he only took it for 7 days but did engage in

---

[1]Details of this case have been altered to protect the patient's identity.

6 weeks of group therapy for depression, which he found to be helpful. D. G. had a legal history related to domestic violence and substance use, with the theme for all of his arrests being an inability to control his anger. When he was asked for alternative anger management strategies aside from violence, he was not able to generate adequate responses. D. G. reported currently experiencing moderately depressed mood and moderate levels of anxiety. His greatest stressors at the time of his evaluation were his unstable housing situation and his health. In terms of family psychiatric history, he was uncertain whether any psychiatric conditions ran in his family.

D. G. had a diagnosis of alcohol dependence, early partial remission; cannabis dependence, early full remission; and nicotine dependence, early full remission. He had a history of benzodiazepine abuse, taking more than was prescribed to him, which led to running out of his prescriptions early. He was getting narcotics from friends at times because no physician would give him narcotics for his neck pain. He never pursued any treatment for his substance use.

In summary, D. G. presented with psychosocial barriers to transplant, including poor compliance, a cursory understanding of transplant, an uncertain housing situation, a limited support system, substance dependence, and a lack of coping skills. During the caregiver interview, his parents were noticeably frustrated with D. G.'s personal choices and felt helpless as he engaged in self-destructive behaviors. Recommendations were communicated to the patient, his nephrologist, and the transplant team, including the need for the patient to demonstrate proper use of his medications as prescribed and no use of medications that had not been prescribed to him. He was asked to develop a plan for stable housing, to work on his relationship with his parents, and to identify secondary caregivers if possible. D. G. was instructed to seek substance rehabilitation that could also address his depression, anxiety, and anger. He was encouraged to return to the transplant center for more transplant education and reevaluation after having demonstrated compliance with these recommendations for 6 months.

D. G. returned to the transplant clinic 2 years after his initial evaluation. In that time, he had been seeing a licensed social worker for help with coping skills, was attending Alcoholics Anonymous meetings on a regular basis with a sponsor, and was working at a new part-time job through the Bureau of Vocational Rehabilitation. He had started a small woodworking business with his father and was living with his parents. He said his relationship with his mother had improved because he had started taking better care of himself. He had joined the YMCA and had started exercising regularly. D. G. said that working, concentrating on his woodworking hobby, and exercising had helped to improve his mood and anxiety. He had begun seeing a chiropractor to address his neck pain and no longer sought narcotics to manage it. He was able to demonstrate a clear understanding of his medications, and his dialysis center reported an improvement in his compliance. His parents were seen for a caregiver interview, and their attitude toward D. G. had markedly improved. They appeared to have become a stable support system for their son. The transplant team was updated on D. G.'s progress, and he was approved to be reevaluated medically for kidney transplant listing. The patient understood that if he received the transplant, he was expected to maintain the healthy behaviors he had been practicing throughout the rest of his life, and he was encouraged to contact a mental health professional for help if needed in the future.

WHEN A PATIENT IS NOT A TRANSPLANT CANDIDATE

When candidates are deemed unsuitable for transplant at the time of the evaluation, the consequences for the patient can be significant. In most cases, the transplant team recommends that the patient take steps to address the key concerns raised during the evaluation. For example, the team may ask the patient to complete a compliance contract (Cupples & Steslowe, 2001) or to demonstrate a period of abstinence from illicit substances with drug screens and possibly rehabilitation. After such time that the patient is able to address the team's concerns successfully, the transplant team may then reevaluate his or her suitability for transplant. The team must carefully consider the fact that the patient's medical hardship may be increased by any delays in listing. Some psychosocial issues may need to be addressed before listing (e.g., maintaining abstinence from substances or demonstrating compliance), whereas other barriers may be able to be addressed while a patient is on the waiting list (e.g., psychotherapy for an adjustment disorder related to the patient's illness).

Patients who are not able to or who choose not to take steps to address identified psychosocial barriers to transplant may need to continue with noncurative therapies. Options such as medication management, dialysis, or mechanical assist devices are often available to patients with end-stage organ failure. Such therapies may be associated, however, with greater mortality than transplant (Port, Wolfe, Mauger, Berling, & Jiang, 1993; Potapov et al., 2006).

LIVING DONOR EVALUATION

In addition to screening potential recipients of deceased donor organs, mental health professionals may also be called on to conduct presurgical evaluations of potential living kidney or liver donors. Living donors may be family members, nonrelated friends of the patient, or anonymous non-directed donors. Psychological evaluation of living organ donors presents the transplant team with a different set of challenges than evaluation of potential organ recipients. Here the purpose of the presurgical evaluation is to ensure the best possible outcome for the potential donor. Because the procurement of an organ from a healthy individual necessarily involves conducting major surgery on a healthy person, being particularly vigilant in identifying factors that might increase the risk of poor outcome is vital (Olbrisch, Benedict, Haller, & Levenson, 2001). Although the literature on living donor outcomes is not as fully developed as the literature on organ recipient outcomes, the literature available has suggested some areas that should be assessed. The evaluator is tasked with determining that the donor is free from significant psychopathology or substance abuse that might complicate the procedure and recovery, that the donor is capable of consenting to the procedure, and that the donor's decision is not inappropriately motivated.

It is important to assess for psychiatric conditions that may complicate the procedure or the donor's recovery. Carrying a psychiatric diagnosis usually does not automatically disqualify a donor, but it should prompt a close examination of the individual's current psychiatric stability and adherence to treatment regimen, if under psychiatric care (Rowley et al., 2009). The mental health professional should also assess the potential donor's drug and alcohol use, paying particular attention to the use of substances that might complicate healing and influence postsurgical pain. Many transplant centers require the donor to demonstrate a period of abstinence from substances before surgery to best prepare him or her for the procedure (Rodrigue et al., 2007).

The mental health professional must determine that the potential living donor is capable of providing informed consent to the transplant procedure. Informed consent implies that the potential donor has adequate knowledge of the procedure and its associated risks and that the potential donor is capable of voluntarily electing to engage in the procedure (Valapour, Kahn, Bailey, & Matas, 2011). Thus, the mental health professional is tasked first with determining to what degree the potential donor understands the procedure, including things such as potential complications of the surgery and the likely course of recovery (Rodrigue et al., 2007). It is important that the donor not only hold realistic expectations for how the process of donation may alter his or her own life but also understand likely outcomes and possible complications for the recipient (Dew, Jacobs, et al., 2007). If the potential donor is adequately knowledgeable, the mental health professional must then also determine that the donor can think rationally about the decision and its alternatives, effectively communicate his or her choices, and resist being unduly influenced by coercion (Dew, Jacobs, et al., 2007b).

Finally, the evaluator must carefully investigate the potential donor's motivations for considering donation. As already mentioned, the decision to donate must not be unduly influenced by coercion. However, the issue of coercion in living organ donation is complicated by direct life-and-death consideration, and thus various degrees of coercion and secondary gain must be considered (Papachristou et al., 2004). Donors may be influenced by the potential for moral or emotional reward, which may increase motivation and decrease psychological distress after donation (Papachristou et al., 2004). The decision to donate must not be financially motivated and should not be inappropriately motivated by desire for personal acclaim or to alter the dynamics of a personal relationship (Dew, Jacobs, et al., 2007).

Certainly, more research is needed to investigate whether other factors influence donor outcomes. As those factors are identified, it will be vital for the transplant team to include them along with previously identified factors in a thorough assessment to increase the likelihood of successful outcomes for donors.

CONCLUSION

The psychosocial evaluation is an important way of making certain an individual has the resources to manage the physical, emotional, and mental burden of the transplantation or donation (Wise, 2008). Several psychosocial factors have been shown to predict worse adjustment and outcomes in these patients. Identifying these psychosocial variables before transplant allows the transplant team to intervene before those outcomes occur (DiMartini et al., 2007). In some cases, it may even be determined that transplantation or donation is not the best procedure for certain individuals to undertake. Although these decisions can at times be difficult to make, the psychosocial evaluation is a valuable part of the multidisciplinary transplant and donor assessments.

REFERENCES

Achille, M. A., Oulette, A., Fournier, S., Vachon, M., & Herbert, M. J. (2006). Impact of stress, distress, and feelings of indebtedness on adherence to immunosuppressants following kidney transplantation. *Clinical Transplantation, 20,* 301–306. doi:10.1111/j.1399-0012.2005.00478.x

Cetingok, M., Hathaway, D., & Winsett, R. (2007). Contribution of post-transplant social support to the quality of life of transplant recipients. *Social Work in Health Care, 45,* 39–56. doi:10.1300/J010v45n03_03

Chisholm-Burns, M. A., Spivey, C. A., & Wilks, S. W. (2010). Social support and immunosuppressant therapy adherence among adult renal transplant recipients. *Clinical Transplantation, 24,* 312–320. doi:10.1111/j.1399-0012.2009.01060.x

Collins, C. A., & Labott, S. M. (2007). Psychological assessment of candidates for solid organ transplantation. *Professional Psychology: Research and Practice, 3,* 150–157. doi:10.1037/0735-7028.38.2.150

Cupples, S. A., & Steslowe, B. (2001). Use of behavioral contingency contracting with heart transplant candidates. *Progress in Transplantation, 11,* 137–144.

Dew, M. A., DiMartini, A. F., DeVito, D. A., Myaskovsky, L., Steel, J., Unruh, M., . . . Greenhouse, J. B. (2007). Rates and risk factors for non-adherence to the medical regimen after adult solid organ transplantation. *Transplantation, 83,* 858–873. doi:10.1097/01.tp.0000258599.65257.a6

Dew, M. A., Dunbar-Jacob, J., Switzer, G. E., DiMartini, A. F., Stilley, C., & Kormos, R. L. (2001). Adherence to the medical regimen in transplantation. In J. R. Rodrigue (Ed.), *Biopsychosocial perspectives on transplantation* (pp. 93–124). New York, NY: Kluwer. doi:10.1007/978-1-4615-1333-9_6

Dew, M. A., Jacobs, C. L., Jowsey, S. G., Hanto, R., Miller, C., & Delmonico, F. L. (2007). Guidelines for the psychosocial evaluation of living unrelated kidney donors in the United States. *American Journal of Transplantation, 7,* 1047–1054. doi:10.1111/j.1600-6143.2007.01751.x

DiMartini, A. F., Dew, M. A., & Trzepacz, P. T. (2007). Organ transplantation. In J. L. Levenson (Ed.), *Essentials of psychosomatic medicine* (pp. 285–312). Arlington, VA: American Psychiatric Publishing.

Finn, R. (2000). *Organ transplants: Making the most of your gift of life.* Sebastopol, CA: O'Reilly & Associates.

Huffman, J. C., Popkin, M. K., & Stern, T. A. (2003). Psychiatric considerations in the patient receiving organ transplantation: A clinical case conference. *General Hospital Psychiatry, 25,* 484–491. doi:10.1016/S0163-8343(03)00090-2

Jindal, R. M., Neff, R. T., Abbott, K. C., Hurst, F. P., Elster, E. A., Flata, E. M., . . . Cokor, D. (2009). Association between depression and nonadherence in recipients of kidney transplants: Analysis of the United States renal data system. *Transplantation Proceedings, 41,* 3662–3666. doi:10.1016/j.transproceed.2009.06.187

Laederach-Hofmann, K., & Bunzel, B. (2000). Noncompliance in organ transplant recipients: A literature review. *General Hospital Psychiatry, 22,* 412–424. doi:10.1016/S0163-8343(00)00098-0

Levenson, J. L., & Olbrisch, M. E. (1993). Psychosocial evaluation of organ transplant candidates: A comparative survey of process, criteria, and outcomes in heart, liver, and kidney transplantation. *Psychosomatics, 34,* 314–323. doi:10.1016/S0033-3182(93)71865-4

McCallum, S., & Masterson, G. (2006). Liver transplantation for alcoholic liver disease: A systematic review of psychosocial selection criteria. *Alcohol and Alcoholism, 41,* 358–363. doi:10.1093/alcalc/agl033

Olbrisch, M. E., Benedict, S. M., Ashe, K., & Levenson, J. L. (2002). Psychological assessment and care of organ transplant patients. *Journal of Consulting and Clinical Psychology, 70,* 771–783. doi:10.1037/0022-006X.70.3.771

Olbrisch, M. E., Benedict, S. M., Haller, D. L., & Levenson, J. L. (2001). Psychosocial assessment of living organ donors: Clinical and ethical considerations. *Progress in Transplantation, 11,* 40–49.

Olbrisch, M. E., Levenson, J. L., & Hamer, R. (1989). The PACT: A rating scale for the study of clinical decision making in psychosocial screening or organ transplant candidates. *Clinical Transplantation, 3,* 164–169.

Organ Procurement and Transplantation Network. (2009a). *OPTN/SRTR annual report: One year adjusted patient survival by organ and year of transplant, 1998 to 2007* [Data file]. Retrieved from http://optn.transplant.hrsa.gov/ar2009/111a_dh.htm

Organ Procurement and Transplantation Network. (2009b). *OPTN/SRTR annual report: Reported deaths and annual death rates per 1,000 patient-years at risk waiting list, 1999 to 2008* [Data file]. Retrieved from http://optn.transplant.hrsa.gov/ar2009/106_dh.htm

Organ Procurement and Transplantation Network. (2011). *Transplants by donor type* [Data file]. Retrieved from http://optn.transplant.hrsa.gov/latestData/rptData.asp

Papachristou, C., Walter, M., Dietrich, K., Danzer, G., Klupp, J., Klapp, B. F., & Frommer, J. (2004). Motivation for living-donor liver transplantation from the donor's perspective: An in-depth qualitative research study. *Transplantation, 78,* 1506–1514. doi:10.1097/01.TP.0000142620.08431.26

Port, F. K., Wolfe, R. A., Mauger, E. A., Berling, D. P., & Jiang, K. (1993). Comparison of survival probabilities for dialysis patients vs cadaveric renal transplant recipients. *JAMA, 270,* 1339–1343. doi:10.1001/jama.1993.03510110079036

Potapov, E. V., Jurmann, M. J., Drews, T., Pasic, M., Loebe, M., Weng, Y., & Hetzer, R. (2006). Patients supported for over 4 years with left ventricular assist devices. *European Journal of Heart Failure, 8,* 756–759. doi:10.1016/j.ejheart.2006.02.003

Rodrigue, J. R., Pavlakis, M., Danovitch, G. M., Johnson, S. R., Karp, S. J., Khwaja, K., . . . Mandelbrot, D. A. (2007). Evaluating living kidney donors: Relationship types, psychosocial criteria, and consent processes at US transplant programs. *American Journal of Transplantation, 7,* 2326–2332. doi:10.1111/j.1600-6143.2007.01921.x

Rowley, A. A., Hong, B. A., Martin, S., Jones, L., Vijayan, A., Shenoy, S., & Jendrisak, M. (2009). Psychiatric disorders: Are they an absolute contraindication to living donation? *Progress in Transplantation, 19,* 128–131.

Twillman, R. K., Manetto, C., Wellisch, D. K., & Wolcott, D. L. (1993). The transplant Evaluation Rating Scale: A revision of the psychosocial levels system for evaluating organ transplant candidates. *Psychosomatics, 34,* 144–153. doi:10.1016/S0033-3182(93)71905-2

United Network for Organ Sharing. (2011). *Transplant trends*. Retrieved from http://www.unos.org/

Valapour, M., Kahn, J. P., Bailey, R. F., & Matas, A. J. (2011). Assessing elements of informed consent among living donors. *Clinical Transplantation, 25*, 185–190. doi:10.1111/j.1399-0012.2010.01374.x

Wainwright, S. P., Fallon, M., & Gould, D. (1999). Psychosocial recovery from adult kidney transplantation: A literature review. *Journal of Clinical Nursing, 8*, 233–245. doi:10.1046/j.1365-2702.1999.00220.x

Wise, T. N. (2008). Update on consultation-liaison psychiatry (psychosomatic medicine). *Current Opinion in Psychiatry, 21*, 196–200. doi:10.1097/YCO.0b013e3282f393ae

2

SPINE SURGERY

ANDREW R. BLOCK

For the patient with intractable spine injury or disease, surgery may be the ultimate step toward returning to a happy and productive life. There have been many demonstrations of spine surgery effectiveness, such as that of Malter, Larson, Urban, and Deyo (1996), who found that patients receiving laminectomy or discectomy had significantly greater quality of life at 5 years postoperation than did patients provided nonoperative care alone. In a similar vein, Fritzell, Hagg, Wessberg, and Nordwall (2001) found that patients treated with spinal fusion had significantly greater pain reduction, improvement in function, and reduction in depression than did patients with similar diagnoses who were treated conservatively, primarily through physical therapy.

Spine surgery has three major goals: (a) Repair, replace, or minimize the impact of damaged or diseased physical structures; (b) improve the patient's ability to function; and (c) reduce the level of pain. Unfortunately, these goals are not always achieved. Large literature reviews have found that average

DOI: 10.1037/14035-003
Presurgical Psychological Screening: Understanding Patients, Improving Outcomes, Andrew R. Block and David B. Sarwer (Editors)

spine surgery success rates, measured in terms of reduced pain and improved function, range from 65% to 75% (Hoffman, Wheeler, & Deyo, 1993; Turner et al., 1992). Notwithstanding such less-than-overwhelming effectiveness, the number of patients undergoing spine surgery is quite large. According to the Agency for Healthcare Research and Quality (Lifton, 2008), U.S. hospitals discharged 575,000 spine surgery patients in 2005. The Dartmouth Atlas (Weinstein, Lurie, Olson, Bronner, & Fisher, 2006) indicated that the rate of patients undergoing spinal fusion—the most complex type of spine surgery and the one with the highest failure rate—quadrupled during the period from 1993 to 2003.

Failed spine surgery has profound effects on the patient, the surgeon, and third-party payers. The patient, of course, continues to remain disabled, with perhaps even greater pain, increased medication dependence, and more emotional difficulty than before the surgery. The surgeon is often left feeling the burden of heavy responsibility for the failure and may be in the position of having to provide long-term care for a patient who is less than pleased with the interventions. Finally, the economic impact of failed surgery can be significant, as demonstrated by a recent study showing that 28% of lumbar discectomy patients had unfavorable outcomes within 18 months of the procedure, with 80% of such patients undergoing repeat discectomy (average cost, $6,907) and 20% undergoing spinal fusion (average cost, $24,375; Sherman et al., 2010). Taken together, all these unfortunate consequences make spine surgery easy fodder for the popular media. For example, *Consumer Reports* ("Treatment Traps to Avoid," 2007) identified spine surgery as number one on their list of overused medical tests and treatments.

Many potential explanations exist for the failure of spine surgery. First, as Birkmeyer and Weinstein (1999) noted, spine surgeons lack a general consensus about indications for these procedures. This lack may perhaps explain why the rate of spine surgery in different areas of the country varies by as much as 8-fold (Weinstein et al., 2006). Second, spine surgeons' skill and experience vary widely, such that, in some hands, surgery may be a technical failure. Problems such as persistence of unrecognized lateral recess stenosis, a missed sequestered disc fragment, or spinal instability after fusion can lead to failure of the surgery to relieve pain (Oaklander & North, 2001). Most often, however, even when spine surgery is a clinical failure, it is, simultaneously, a technical success: The patient continues to experience disability and pain despite correction of the underlying pathophysiology. In such cases, the explanation for the limitations of spine surgery effectiveness most often rest on patient selection. A growing body of research, reviewed in the next section, has demonstrated that particular psychosocial factors can place patients at risk for poor surgery outcomes (Block, Gatchel, Deardorff, & Guyer, 2003; Celestin & Jamison, 2009; Gatchel & Mayer, 2008).

RISK FACTORS INFLUENCING SPINE SURGERY RESULTS

To best organize the range of potential challenges to spine surgery results, we divide risk factors into two categories: psychosocial and medical. These risk factors can combine to exert significant adverse effects on outcome.

Psychosocial Risk Factors

Many psychosocial factors challenge spine surgery results, and they have been assessed through multiple techniques—behavioral observation, psychometric testing, and detailed patient interview. As will be seen, in some studies, these psychosocial risk factors are stronger predictors of reduced spine surgery results than are the medical diagnostic tests that led to the surgery.

Emotions

The most widely explored set of psychosocial risk factors for poor surgery outcome are emotions—both acute reactions and chronic emotional states. Emotional risk factors have, in large part, been identified in research using the Minnesota Multiphasic Personality Inventory (MMPI) and its revision, the MMPI–2 (for reviews, see Block et al., 2003; Celestin, Edwards, & Jamison, 2009), although many studies have used different instruments for assessing similar emotion constructs.

Depression. Significant spine injury and disease almost inevitably lead to many adverse consequences: diminished functional abilities, loss of income, decreased sexual activity, and difficulties with sleep, to name just a few. Such effects can lead to a downward emotional spiral resulting in a major depressive episode, which occurs in as many as 85% of patients (Sørenson & Mors, 1988). Depressed individuals, in general, have long been known to be more likely to focus on negative than on positive events (Seligman, 1975), and depressed patients with chronic injuries are more likely both to interpret sensations as painful (Geisser & Colwell, 1999) and to be less able to recognize objective improvements in function (Kremer, Block, & Atkinson, 1983). It may come as no surprise, then, that several studies have found that spine surgery is less successful among depressed patients, including those with high scores on the MMPI–2 Depression scale (Block, Ohnmeiss, Guyer, Rashbaum, & Hochschuler, 2001), as well as other measures of depression (Chaichana, Mukherjee, Odogwa, Cheng, & McGirt, 2011; Schade, Semmer, Main, Hora, & Boos, 1999; Slover, Abdu, Hanscom, & Weinstein, 2006; Trief, Grant, & Fredrickson, 2000).

Pain Sensitivity. The major goal of spine surgery for most patients is reduction in the level of pain. Unfortunately, improvement in pain is impossible to assess directly because pain is a subjective experience. To the extent that a patient focuses on pain symptoms or experiences pain in excess of that expected for a particular physical condition, even a surgery that perfectly corrects underlying tissue damage may fail to achieve the goal of pain relief. This excessive pain focus, termed *pain sensitivity* and assessed by the MMPI–2's Hypochondriasis and Hysteria scales, has been shown in many studies to be associated with less positive spine surgery results. For example, Spengler, Ouelette, Battie, and Zeh (1990) gave the MMPI–2 to patients who were to undergo discectomy (i.e., removal of the herniated portion of a disc nucleus) and found that those who scored high on the Hypochondriasis and Hysteria scales had much poorer clinical outcomes than those who scored low on these dimensions. Across several studies, the MMPI–2's Hypochondriasis and Hysteria scales have shown the most consistent relationship with reduced spine surgery results (cf. Block et al., 2001; Herron, Turner, Ersek, & Weiner, 1992).

Anxiety. Anxiety and fear often accompany spine problems. Patients worry about their future ability to work, function, and return to normal lifestyle. They fear that certain activities will aggravate or worsen the physical damage to the spine. They worry about the surgery itself—whether it will improve their symptoms or create a whole new set of problems. Such reactive emotional distress can be particularly difficult for a patient who tends to be chronically anxious. Among the several MMPI–2 scales that assess anxiety, Psychasthenia has been found to have the stronger relationship to diminished spine surgery results (e.g., Block et al., 2001). Additional studies, using instruments other than the MMPI–2, have found that anxiety and fear, particularly fear of reinjury, are risk factors for less favorable spine surgery outcomes (den Boer, Oostendorp, Beems, Munneke, & Evers 2006; Trief, Ploutz-Snyder, & Fredrickson, 2006).

Anger. Patients with spine injuries have many reasons to feel angry. They may be angry at those they believe caused their injury or at themselves for getting injured and being unable to function well. They may be angry at insurance companies for problems with treatment authorization and with physicians for being unable to cure their problems. The injury-related pain itself can make an individual grumpy and irritable. Unfortunately, anger can have adverse consequences for recovery from a spine injury, from directly affecting the healing process through changes in immune system activity (Burns, 2006) to causing maladaptive lifestyle changes, such as poor health habits, lack of physical exercise, or excessive use of drugs or alcohol (Leiker & Haley, 1998). Several studies have found that the MMPI–2 clinical scale most directly associated with anger, the Psychopathic Deviancy scale, frequently accompanies a reduction in surgical effectiveness (e.g., Spengler et al., 1990).

Cognitive Coping

Patients vary in their ability to cope with spine injury. For some, the injury is just another of life's problems—one to be overcome with optimism and energy. Others may develop a strong sense of entitlement—feeling as though they should be coddled and not made to work. Some may come to believe that the injury represents the beginning of unending and worsening trauma—catastrophizing. Some patterns of coping, particularly catastrophizing, can be especially pernicious and lead to reduced outcome of spine surgery.

Gross (1986) administered the Coping Strategies Questionnaire preoperatively to 50 lumbar laminectomy candidates. She found that patients who obtained good results from surgery had indicated preoperatively that they felt better able to control the pain and were also more self-reliant. Other coping strategies assessed by the Coping Strategies Questionnaire, such as hoping and praying and catastrophizing, were associated with poor surgical outcomes. These results are consistent with those of several other studies demonstrating that more passive coping strategies and perceived lack of pain control tend to be associated with greater pain levels, higher opioid consumption, greater levels of depression, and poorer treatment outcome (e.g., den Boer et al., 2006; Turner & Clancy, 1986).

Historical Factors

The ways in which individuals respond to and cope with painful spine injuries are strongly influenced by their previous life experiences. Research has demonstrated a number of historic elements in the background of the spine surgery candidate that can negatively affect surgical recovery. One especially pernicious historical problem is a history of physical or sexual abuse or abandonment. Unfortunately, abuse is commonly found among patients with chronic back pain. Linton (1997), for example, in a general population survey, found that 46% of women with "pronounced" pain reported a history of sexual abuse. Schofferman, Anderson, Hinds, Smith, and White (1992) found an 85% failure rate of spine surgery among patients with a significant history of childhood abuse and abandonment, compared with a 5% failure rate among patients lacking such a traumatic history.

Additional historical factors may place a patient at risk for reduced spine surgery results. First, a long-term history of psychiatric problems (Block et al., 2001; Manniche et al., 1994) may indicate a patient who will have difficulty tolerating the stresses imposed by the surgery or whose emotional condition may devolve during the postoperative period. Second, a history of substance abuse may place a patient at risk because postoperative care most often involves provision of narcotic medication (Uomoto, Turner, & Herron, 1988).

Behavioral Factors

Pain behavior almost always occurs in a social context, communicating to observers that the patient is in distress. Observers, in turn, may react to such behavior with attempts to relieve the patient's pain, help him or her to avoid further problems, or be supportive of limitations in activity. Employers, and even the insurance system, may also inadvertently support pain behaviors through provision of disability benefits or time off work. Unfortunately, such solicitous responses from others, although well intentioned, may serve to reinforce or reward pain behaviors, increasing the likelihood that patients will continue to show and experience pain (Fordyce, 1976). Failure to alter reinforcement of pain behavior may contribute to prolonged disability after spine surgery and noninvasive treatment of spine injury. In other words, behavioral factors—the rewards for remaining disabled and the disincentives for recovery—may undo even the most technically effective surgery. Those behavioral factors that have been established as increasing the risk for poor spine surgery results include litigation (LaCaille, DeBerard, LaCaille, Masters, & Colledge, 2007), workers' compensation and disability (Carreon, Glassman, Kantamneni, Mugavin, & Djurasovic, 2010; Klekamp, McCarty, & Spengler, 1998), and solicitous responding by the patient's partner (Romano et al., 1995).

On consideration, however, such behavioral factors may be more complicated than they first appear. Consider, for example, the situation of a patient who is injured on the job and is unable to work. Such a patient receives not only medical benefits to cover treatment of the injury but at least partial wage replacement in the form of workers' compensation disability payments. Numerous studies have found that compared with patients without workers' compensation, those patients covered by workers' compensation often achieve poorer results from spine surgery, including lumbar discectomy (e.g., DeBerard, LaCaille, Speilmans, Colledge, & Parlin, 2009) and lumbar fusion (e.g., Carreon et al., 2010). Such outcome differences are particularly strong if the patient has an attorney involved in the case (cf. LaCaille et al., 2007). However, for workers' compensation disability payments to function as a reinforcer for pain and disability, the patient must, ipso facto, be unable to work, or else such payments would not be forthcoming. Several studies have shown that work status can significantly influence spine surgery outcome. For example, in one study patients who were working up to the time of surgery had a 10.5 times greater likelihood of working at 1-year follow-up than did those not working at the time of the surgery (Anderson, Schaegler, Cizek, & Leverson, 2006), an effect that was independent of workers' compensation status. Moreover, Dworkin, Handlin, Richlin, Brand, and Vannucci (1985) found that length of time out of work negatively influenced spine surgery outcome, even with workers' compensation status covaried out. Thus, although workers' compensation and other behavioral factors do negatively influence the outcome of various spine surgeries, such factors must be considered in the context of the patient's overall social and vocational situations.

Medical Risk Factors

The above-cited studies demonstrated that the outcome of spine surgery can be strongly influenced by psychosocial factors. However, physical features of each patient's case can also militate for or against good surgical results. Many such factors have been examined, and in conducting PPS, the mental health professional needs to consider the interaction of such medical and physical features with psychosocial concerns. I discuss the major medical risk factors encountered in the following sections.

Surgery Type

All surgery requires the destruction of tissue. To accomplish spine surgery, the spinal structure is exposed by cutting through overlying tissue. Bones, ligaments, intervertebral discs, and other structures become targets for removal or repair. The spine surgeon's charge is to determine the type of surgery that will most effectively overcome injury or insult to the spine while minimizing the amount of tissue that must be damaged. Block (1996) used the term *destructiveness* to categorize the extent to which spine surgery entails collateral tissue damage. Destructiveness is determined by (a) the amount of time tissues are exposed; (b) the amount of tissue destroyed or removed; and (c) the use of hardware or instrumentation, such as cages, screws, or disc replacements. Generally, more destructive surgeries are associated with poorer outcome and with higher reoperation rates (Franklin, Haug, Heyer, McKeefrey, & Picciano, 1994; Weinstein et al., 2006).

Pain Duration

Even though at least 70% of Americans experience at least one episode of moderate to severe back pain (Taylor & Curren, 1985), 80% to 90% of those having such an episode recover completely, whether they receive treatment or not (Spengler et al., 1986). For those whose pain becomes more protracted, the treatment options available are almost unlimited. Initially, the thought of spine surgery may appear as a forbidding yet distant option. Multiple treatments may be attempted, at great cost, and sometimes with increasing invasiveness. Although these treatments may result in resolution of symptoms, for some there is little to no relief—the pain may persist for months or even years. When, at last, a physician mentions the idea of surgery, a patient who has attempted and failed many less conservative treatments faces two contradictory facts. Knowing that previous treatments have proved unsuccessful often gives a patient greater confidence that surgery is the only viable option; however, there is strong evidence that the likelihood of achieving good results from spine surgery diminishes as pain becomes more protracted (Anderson et al., 2006; Junge, Dvorak, & Ahrens, 1995; Trief et al., 2000).

Number of Previous Spine Surgeries

Failure of spine surgery to adequately relieve pain or improve function opens up the possibility of additional surgical procedures. Sometimes such procedures are contemplated when the initial surgery has failed to achieve its physical goals (e.g., when a spinal fusion fails to solidify properly) or when the underlying condition repaired in the initial surgery returns (e.g., a recurrent intervertebral disc herniation after a laminectomy or discectomy). Sometimes the surgery, although effective, increases the chances of developing new causes of spine pain (e.g., an intervertebral disc at a level adjacent to the level of a spinal fusion can itself degenerate). Whatever the cause, the evidence of an inverse relationship between successful spine surgery outcome and the number of previous spine surgeries is clear (Ciol, Deyo, Kreuter, & Bigos, 1994; Mannion et al., 2007).

Previous Medical Problems

Spine surgery candidates have often had aggressive medical treatment for many other medical problems, and in cases in which this occurs, patients tend to fare more poorly with spine surgery. For example, Hoffman et al. (1993) found an inverse relationship between diminished laminectomy or discectomy outcome and number of previous hospitalizations, and Ciol et al. (1994) found that previous hospitalizations were associated with increased risk for lumbar spine reoperation. DeBerard et al. (2009) found that larger numbers of comorbid medical conditions predict poor outcome in discectomy patients (cf. Slover et al., 2006). Such multiple medical problems may reflect a general unhealthiness or may perhaps suggest that the patient is hypervigilant concerning medical symptoms, leading to more aggressive medical treatment.

Nonorganic Signs

As noted earlier, the surgeon's and patient's goals often differ. The surgeon is primarily interested in repairing or correcting physical damage. The patient's goals, however, are to reduce the pain and improve functional abilities that have been impaired by the underlying physical damage. However, patients vary widely in the extent to which they experience symptoms related to underlying conditions. Some are quite stoic, reporting low levels of pain in limited body areas and with minimal functional impact. Others are quite the opposite; their pain is exquisite and widespread and their ability to function almost nil. Such excessive symptoms, especially if inconsistent with underlying physical damage, are frequently called *nonorganic signs*. A standard procedure for eliciting such signs is often a component of the medical evaluation of spine surgery patients (Waddell, McCulloch, Kummel, & Venner, 1980), and the presence of such signs is associated with reduced spine surgery results (Dzioba & Doxey, 1984). Similarly, patients often complete a Pain Drawing as part of their evaluation, indicating the body locations where pain is experienced. When such drawings are inconsistent with the identified underlying physical pathology, patients are less likely to respond well to spine surgery (Voorhies, Jiang, & Thomas, 2007).

Smoking

Of all the many ways in which smoking can have adverse health consequences, one of the least expected is its impact on the spine. Smokers have increased likelihood of developing significant back pain (Hellsing & Bryngelsson, 2000). Smokers are also at increased risk for the development of lumbar and cervical disc disease (An et al., 1994). Most significant for the present context, several studies have shown that smoking appears to place the patient at increased risk for obtaining poor results from spine surgery (Andersen, Christensen, Laursen et al., 2001; Slover et al., 2006).

Obesity

Obesity has many implications for spine surgery. First, extra weight places additional mechanical stress on the support structures of the spine, which can increase pain. Second, severe obesity increases the amount of tissue that must be cut in surgery and, thus, increases the duration of the surgery. Moreover, in many cases obesity makes it more difficult to gain exposure to damaged spine structures. Finally, obesity often reflects a sedentary lifestyle, which may either preexist the spine problems or result from the physical limitations imposed by the pain. Either way, surgical success often depends on active lifestyle changes including weight loss. It is no wonder, then, that obesity has been found in several studies to be associated with diminished spine surgery results (Block et al., 2001; Gepstein et al., 2004; LaCaille et al., 2007).

Combining Risk Factors

Several laboratories, drawing on the body of research reviewed here, have developed "scorecards" cataloging psychosocial risk factors in an attempt to provide a prognosis concerning the outcome of spine surgery (e.g., Junge, Frohlich, & Ahrens, 1995; Manniche et al., 1994). Most of these studies have demonstrated that patients with high levels of psychosocial risk achieve success in about only 15% to 20% of cases. In a prospective study, Block et al. (2001) created such a scorecard listing both psychosocial and medical risk factors that have been identified to be associated with reduced spine surgery outcome. Medical and psychological risk factors were added separately, and a high-risk threshold was assigned for each category. Patients were predicted to have poor outcome if they scored above the high-risk threshold for both medical and psychological factors and were predicted to have good results if they fell below the threshold in both categories. Patients who scored above the threshold in one category and below the threshold on the other were predicted to have a fair outcome. Block et al. found that 44 of 53 patients in the poor prognosis category obtained poor clinical results from spine surgery (both laminectomy or discectomy and spinal fusion) compared with a clinical failure rate of 3 of 31 patients in the group with a good psychosocial prognosis and a rate of 23 of 120 patients in the fair prognosis group.

Block et al. (2003) revised the scorecard to create a presurgical psychological screening (PPS) algorithm. Figure 2.1 shows the algorithm and scorecard, which is completed for the case study in this chapter. The algorithm incorporates two major new processes:

1. The determination of surgical outcome prognosis involves three consecutive evaluative steps: psychosocial risk factors (listed in the Interview Risk Factors and Testing Risk Factors boxes), medical risk factors, and a new step termed adverse clinical features. The adverse features are nonquantifiable aspects of the patient's case that could be expected to have a negative impact on surgical outcome.
2. The algorithm now provides five levels of psychosocial prognosis for spine surgery.

Research is currently being conducted on the utility of an even newer version of this algorithm that incorporates the MMPI–2—Restructured Form (Ben-Porath & Tellegen, 2008) rather than the MMPI–2 in predicting the outcome of spine surgery (Block, Ben-Porath, Ohnmeiss, & Burchett, 2011). In this study, 155 patients who underwent spine surgery were assessed again at a mean of 141 days postoperation. Patients who were categorized as having a poor prognosis did not undergo surgery. Results demonstrated that those patients who fell into the fair and fair–poor prognosis categories reported significantly less pain relief and less functional improvement, were less satisfied with the surgical outcome, and reported higher levels of anger than did patients in the good and fair–good categories.

CATEGORY

5
4
3
2
1

PPS Algorithm

Total Psycho-social Risk — 8+ / 4-7 / 0-3

Total Medical Risk — 6+ / 0-5

Adverse Clinical Features — Present / Absent

Poor Discharge Recommended — 5

Poor Non-invasive Treatment — 4

Fair Compliance & Motivation Measures — 3

Good Post-Op Psych Treatment — 2

Good No psych Treatment — 1

© Andrew R. Block, Ph.D. 2001.

Interview Risk Factors

Factor	Pts
Job Dissatisfaction	2
Workers' Compensation	2 ✓
Litigation	2
Spousal Solicitousness	1
No Spouse Support	1
Abuse and Abandonment	1
Substance Abuse	
Current	2
Remote (older than 2 years)	1 ✓
Psych History	
Inpatient or long term	2
Outpatient or short term	1 ✓
Not working > 2 months	1 ✓

Testing Risk Factors (max 6 points)

Factor	Pts
Pain Sensitivity	
RC > 73, MLS > 79, NUC > 75, HPC > 71	2 ✓
Depression	
RCd > 6, RC2 > 65, EID > 62, SUI > 57	2 ✓
Chronic	
Reactive	1
Anger	
RC4 > 52, ANP > 54, AGG > 5	2
Anxiety	
RC7 > 54, STW > 60, AXY > 63	2
Depressed–Pathological	
4 RC scales > *SD* above mean	4
Low Self-Esteem	
K-r < 44, SFD > 60	1
Excessive Guardedness	
K-r > 64, L-r > 7	2
Catastrophizing	2
PAIRS > 75	1 ✓

Medical Risk Factors

Factor	Pts
Pain 6–12 months	
Pain > 12 months	2 ✓
Highly Destructive Surgery	2 ✓
Nonorganic Signs	2
Abnormal Pain Drawing	2
Prior Spine Surgeries	
2 or more	2 ✓
1	1
Prior Medical Problems	2
Smoking	2
Obesity	1 ✓

Adverse Clinical Features

Inconsistency
Medication Seeking
Staff Splitting
Compliance Issues
Threatening
Resignation
Deception
Personality Disorders

Figure 2.1. Presurgical psychological screening (PPS) algorithm for case study. Even if the total for the Testing Risk Factors box is greater than 6, the maximum score that can be used in the algorithm is 6 points. √ indicates the presence of the risk factor for M. C. RC1 = Restructured Clinical 1—Somatic Complaints; MLS = malaise; NUC = neurological; HPC = head pain complaints; RCd = Restructured Clinical—Demoralization; RC2 = Restructured Clinical 2—Low Positive Emotions; EID = emotional–internalizing dysfunction; SUI = suicide; RC4 = Restructured Clinical 4—Antisocial Behavior; RC7 = Restructured Clinical 7—Dysfunctional Negative Emotions; STW = stress–worry; AXY = anxiety; K-r = adjustment validity; SFD = self-doubt; L-r = Uncommon Virtues; PAIRS = Pain and Impairment Relationship Scale; post-op = postoperative; psych = psychiatric. Adapted from *The Psychology of Spine Surgery* (p. 108), by A. R. Block, R. J. Gatchel, W.W. Deardorff, and D. Guyer, 2003, Washington, DC: American Psychological Association. Copyright 2003 by the American Psychological Association.

CASE STUDY

M. C. was a 41-year-old woman with pain in the low back and both legs. She also had foot drop from nerve damage sustained in one of her previous surgeries.[1] She was injured in a slip and fall on the job as a restaurant manager, 2 years before the PPS. She had three previous laminectomy or discectomy procedures and was a candidate for lumbar spine fusion. She reported pain at a level of 7 to 9 on a 10-point scale. She had been disabled from her job since the time of the injury and, when evaluated, was mostly nonfunctional, spending her days reclining and getting little exercise. She had gained 50 pounds since the injury and slept an average of 4 hours per night. She was depressed and began taking 60 milligrams of duloxetine (Cymbalta) and 3 milligrams of alprazolam (Xanax) per day, which reduced her subjective symptoms of depression and anxiety. She was taking hydrocodone four times per day for pain, as well as muscle relaxers and anti-inflammatory medication. She was receiving Social Security disability benefits at the time of the surgery. She had been married twice, with her most recent marriage of 3 years' duration. She was raised in the foster care system and was not close to any of her foster parents. She did not report any history of mental health treatment.

Figure 2.1 displays the PPS algorithm for M. C. As can be seen, the patient scored 10 points in psychosocial risk factors and 7 points in medical risk factors, with no adverse clinical features. These scores placed her in Category 4, noninvasive treatment recommended. Psychological treatment was recommended for the purposes of helping her deal with maladaptive thoughts concerning her injury and for self-hypnosis training to improve self-esteem and pain management. These sessions were denied by her workers' compensation insurance carrier. Unfortunately, as sometimes happens, the surgeon decided to proceed with surgery, despite recommendations against it. At 2 years post-surgery, the patient was reporting Level 10 pain constantly and rated her satisfaction with the surgery as 0 on a 0–10 scale. She reported extreme depression and high levels of irritability and fear. Her hydrocodone use increased to eight times per day, and she continued on the Cymbalta and Xanax. She never returned to work and remains on Social Security disability.

CONCLUSION

Despite increasingly widespread use, the outcome of spine surgery is far from uniform. The studies reviewed in this chapter have indicated that psychosocial factors can strongly influence the outcome of spine surgery and

---

[1]Details of this case have been altered to protect the patient's identity.

may be at least partially responsible for such variable results. On the basis of such research, many insurance carriers, particularly within the workers' compensation system, are now requiring or strongly recommending PPS for spine surgery candidates.

Systematic approaches to examining adverse psychosocial factors, such as the algorithm described in this chapter, can be used to try to predict the outcome of spine surgery. For patients with high levels of psychosocial risk, alternative noninvasive treatments can be implemented, such as a multidisciplinary chronic pain management program, sparing them from invasive procedures likely to worsen their pain and functional disability. Chronic pain management programs have been demonstrated to be as effective as spine surgery in providing symptom improvement (Brox et al., 2003) and cost considerably less (Rivero-Arias et al., 2005). For patients whose profiles indicate medium levels of psychosocial risk, surgery can be delayed while they participate in behavioral treatments designed to test their motivation for engaging in the rehabilitation and improve their odds of obtaining satisfactory surgical results. Such cognitive–behavioral treatments could target medication reduction, smoking cessation, physical exercise programs, reframing of maladaptive thoughts, or psychological pain control techniques, such as hypnosis (see Block et al., 2003, for a complete discussion). Finally, patients with lower levels of psychosocial risk can proceed to surgery with greater confidence and reassurance that they should be able to achieve improvements in pain and function with relatively little influence from emotional and interpersonal concerns. Thus, PPS of spine surgery patients is a process that provides value to all: Surgeons improve their overall outcome; third-party payers experience reduced cost from avoiding both surgeries unlikely to be successful and the cost of reoperation; and most important, patients are given the treatments most likely to be effective while reducing the chances of worsening their conditions.

The mental health professional must recognize, however, that PPS is only one of many diagnostic procedures used in the evaluation of a spine surgery candidate. It is up to the surgeon to weigh the results of all these procedures and make the final determination about whether to proceed with the surgery. Sometimes spine surgeons will only come to fully appreciate PPS when poor outcome is seen in a patient whom the mental health professional found to have a high level of psychosocial risk.

PPS for spine surgery patients is a field that is continuing to gain acceptance by physicians, insurers, and patients. Continued research will further refine the critical variables that should be examined in PPS. Additionally, tools are being developed that will allow physicians to distinguish between those patients most likely to need a formal PPS and those who can proceed to surgery without the need for formal evaluation. For the present, PPS of spine surgery patients is an area, as with many others in this text, that provides significant value and makes intuitive sense but will require continued research and application before it will be used universally and systematically.

REFERENCES

An, H. S., Silveri, C. P., Simpson, M., File, P., Simmons, C., Simeone, A., & Balderston, R. A. (1994). Comparison of smoking habits between patients and surgically confirmed herniated lumbar and cervical disc disease and controls. *Journal of Spinal Disorders, 7,* 369–373. doi:10.1097/00002517-199410000-00001

Anderson, P. A., Schaegler, P. E., Cizek, D., & Leverson, G. (2006). Work status as a predictor of surgical outcome of discogenic low back pain. *Spine, 31,* 2510–2515. doi:10.1097/01.brs.0000239180.14933.b7

Anderson, T., Christensen, F. B., Laursen, M., Høy, K., Hansen, E. S., & Bünger, C (2001). Smoking as a predictor of negative outcome in lumbar spinal fusion. *Spine, 26,* 2623–2628. doi:10.1097/00007632-200112010-00018

Ben-Porath, Y., & Tellegen, A. (2008). *Minnesota Multiphasic Personality Inventory— 2 Restructured Form: Technical manual.* Minneapolis: University of Minnesota Press.

Birkmeyer, N. J., & Weinstein, J. N. (1999). Medical versus surgical treatment for low back pain: Evidence and clinical practice. *Effective Clinical Practice, 2,* 218–227.

Block, A. R. (1996). *Presurgical psychological screening in chronic pain syndromes: A guide for the behavioral health practitioner.* Mahwah, NJ: Erlbaum.

Block, A. R., Ben-Porath, Y. S., Ohnmeiss, D., & Burchett, D. (2011, November). *Presurgical psychological screening: A new algorithm, including the MMPI–2–RF, for predicting surgery results.* Presented at the 26th annual meeting of the North American Spine Society, Chicago, IL.

Block, A. R., Gatchel, R. J., Deardorff, W. W., & Guyer, D. (2003). *The psychology of spine surgery.* Washington, DC: American Psychological Association. doi:10.1037/10613-000

Block, A. R., Ohnmeiss, D. D., Guyer, R. D., Rashbaum, R., & Hochschuler, S. H. (2001). The use of presurgical psychological screening to predict the outcome of spine surgery. *The Spine Journal, 1,* 274–282. doi:10.1016/S1529-9430(01) 00054-7

Brox, J. I., Sørensen, R., Friis, A., Nygaard, Ø., Indahl, A., Keller, A., . . . Reikerås, O. (2003). Randomized clinical trial of lumbar instrumented fusion and cognitive intervention and exercises in patients with chronic low back pain and disc degeneration. *Spine, 28,* 1913–1921. doi:10.1097/01.BRS.0000083234.62751.7A

Burns, J. W. (2006). Arousal of negative emotions and symptom-specific reactivity in chronic low back pain patients. *Emotion, 6,* 309–319. doi:10.1037/1528-3542. 6.2.309

Carreon, L. Y., Glassman, S. D., Kantamneni, N. R., Mugavin, M. O., & Djurasovic, M. (2010). Clinical outcomes after posterolateral lumbar fusion in workers' compensation patients. *Spine, 35,* 1812–1817. doi:10.1097/BRS.0b013e3181c68b75

Celestin J., Edwards, R. R., & Jamison, R. (2009). Pretreatment psychosocial variables as predictors of outcomes following lumbar surgery and spinal cord stimulation: A systematic review. *Pain Medicine, 10,* 639–653. doi:10.1111/j.1526-4637.2009.00632.x

Celestin, J., & Jamison, R. (2009). Pretreatment psychosocial variables as predictors of outcomes following lumbar surgery and spinal cord stimulation: A systematic review. *Pain Medicine, 10,* 639–653. doi:10.1111/j.1526-4637.2009.00632.x

Chaichana, K. L., Mukherjee, D., Odogwa, O., Cheng, J. S., & McGirt, M. J. (2011). Correlation of preoperative depression and somatic perception with postoperative disability and quality of life after lumbar discectomy. *Journal of Neurosurgery Spine, 14,* 261–267. doi:10.3171/2010.10.SPINE10190

Ciol, M. A., Deyo, R. A., Kreuter, W., & Bigos, S. J. (1994). Characteristics in Medicare beneficiaries associated with reoperation after lumbar spine surgery. *Spine, 19,* 1329–1334. doi:10.1097/00007632-199406000-00005

DeBerard, M. S., LaCaille, R. A., Speilmans, G., Colledge, A., & Parlin, M. A. (2009). Outcomes and presurgery correlates of lumbar discectomy in Utah worker's compensation patients. *The Spine Journal, 9,* 193–203. doi:10.1016/j.spinee.2008.02.001

den Boer, J. J., Oostendorp, R. A. B., Beems, T., Munneke, M., & Evers, A. W. M. (2006). Continued disability and pain after lumbar disc surgery: The role of cognitive-behavioral factors. *Pain, 123,* 45–52. doi:10.1016/j.pain.2006.02.008

Dworkin, R. H., Handlin, D. S., Richlin, D. M., Brand, L., & Vannucci, C. (1985). Unraveling the effects of compensation, litigation and employment on treatment response in chronic pain. *Pain, 23,* 49–59. doi:10.1016/0304-3959(85)90229-5

Dzioba, R. B., & Doxey, N. C. (1984). A prospective investigation in the orthopedic and psychologic predictors of outcome of first lumbar surgery following industrial injury. *Spine, 9,* 614–623. doi:10.1097/00007632-198409000-00013

Fordyce, W. E. (1976). *Behavioral methods for chronic pain and illness.* St. Louis, MO: Mosby.

Franklin, G. M., Haug, J., Heyer, N. J., McKeefrey, S. P., & Picciano, J. F. (1994). Outcome of lumbar fusion in Washington State workers' compensation. *Spine, 19,* 1897–1904. doi:10.1097/00007632-199409000-00005

Fritzell, P., Hagg, O., Wessberg, P., & Nordwall, A. (2001). Volvo Award Winner in Clinical Studies: Lumbar fusion versus nonsurgical treatment for chronic low back pain: A multicenter randomized controlled trial from the Swedish Lumbar Spine Study Group. *Spine, 26,* 2521–2532. doi:10.1097/00007632-200112010-00002

Gatchel, R. J., & Mayer, T. G. (2008). Psychological evaluation of the spine patient. *Journal of the American Academy of Orthopaedic Surgeons, 16,* 107–112.

Geisser, M., & Colwell, M. (1999). Chronic back pain: Conservative approaches. In A. R. Block, E. F. Kremer, & E. Fernandez (Eds.), *Handbook of pain syndromes* (pp. 169–190). Mahwah, NJ: Erlbaum.

Gepstein, R., Shabat, S., Arinzon, Z. H., Berner, Y., Catz, A., & Folman, Y. (2004). Does obesity affect the results of lumbar decompressive spinal surgery in the elderly? *Clinical Orthopaedics and Related Research, 426,* 138–144. doi:10.1097/01.blo.0000141901.23322.98

Gross, A. R. (1986). The effect of coping strategies on the relief of pain following surgical intervention for lower back pain. *Psychosomatic Medicine, 48,* 229–241.

Hellsing, A. L., & Bryngelsson, I. (2000). Predictors of musculoskeletal pain in men: A twenty-year follow-up from examination at enlistment. *Spine, 25,* 3080–3086. doi:10.1097/00007632-200012010-00016

Herron, L., Turner, J. A., Ersek, M., & Weiner, P. (1992). Does the Millon Behavioral Health Inventory (MBHI) predict lumbar laminectomy outcome? A comparison with the Minnesota Multiphasic Personality Inventory (MMPI). *Journal of Spinal Disorders, 5,* 188–192. doi:10.1097/00002517-199206000-00007

Hoffman, R. M., Wheeler, K. J., & Deyo, R. A. (1993). Surgery for herniated lumbar discs: A literature synthesis. *Journal of General Internal Medicine, 8,* 487–496. doi:10.1007/BF02600110

Junge, A., Dvorak, J., & Ahrens, S. (1995). Predictors of bad and good outcomes of lumbar disc surgery: A prospective clinical study with recommendations for screening to avoid bad outcomes. *Spine, 20,* 460–468. doi:10.1097/00007632-199502001-00009

Klekamp, J., McCarty, E., & Spengler, D. (1998). Results of elective lumbar discectomy for patients involved in the workers' compensation system. *Journal of Spinal Disorders, 11,* 277–282. doi:10.1097/00002517-199808000-00001

Kremer, E. F., Block, A. R., & Atkinson, J. J. (1983). Assessment of pain behavior: Factors that distort self-report. In R. Melzack (Ed.), *Pain management and assessment* (pp. 165–171). New York, NY: Raven Press.

LaCaille, R. A., DeBerard, M. S., LaCaille, L. J., Masters, K. S., & Colledge, A. L. (2007). Obesity and litigation predict workers' compensation costs associated with interbody cage lumbar fusion. *The Spine Journal, 7,* 266–272. doi:10.1016/j.spinee.2006.05.014

Leiker, M., & Hailey, B. J. (1988). A link between hostility and disease: Poor health habits? *Behavioral Medicine, 14,* 129–133. doi:10.1080/08964289.1988.9935136

Lifton, J. (2008). The spine files: Demand for spine surgeons. *Spine, 8,* 1042–1044. doi:10.1016/j.spinee.2008.01.002

Linton, S. J. (1997). A population-based study of the relationship between sexual abuse and back pain: Establishing a link. *Pain, 73,* 47–53. doi:10.1016/S0304-3959(97)00071-7

Malter, A. D., Larson, E. B., Urban, N., & Deyo, R. (1996). Cost-effectiveness of lumbar discectomy for treatment of herniated intervertebral disc. *Spine, 21,* 1048–1054. doi:10.1097/00007632-199605010-00011

Manniche, C., Asmussen, K. H., Vinterberg, H., Rose-Hansen, E. B. R., Kramhoft, J., & Jordan, A. (1994). Analysis of preoperative prognostic factors in first-time surgery for lumbar disc herniation, including Finneson's and modified Spengler's score systems. *Danish Medical Bulletin, 41*, 110–115.

Mannion, A. F., Elfering, A., Staerkle, R., Junge, A., Gorb, D., Dvorak, J., . . . Boos, N. (2007). Predictors of multidimensional outcome after spinal surgery. *European Spine Journal, 16*, 777–786. doi:10.1007/s00586-006-0255-0

Oaklander, A. L., & North, R. B. (2001). Failed back surgery syndrome. In J. D. Loeser, S. H. Butler, C. R. Chapman, & D. C. Turk (Eds.), *Bonica's management of pain* (3rd ed., pp. 1540–1549). Philadelphia, PA: Lippincott Williams & Wilkins.

Rivero-Arias, O., Campbell, H., Gray, A., Fairbank, J., Frost, H., & Wilson-MacDonald, J. (2005). Surgical stabilisation of the spine compared with a programme of intensive rehabilitation for the management of patients with chronic low back pain: Cost utility analysis based on a randomised controlled trial. *British Medical Journal, 330*, 1239–1245. doi:10.1136/bmj.38441.429618.8F

Romano, J. M., Turner, J. A., Jensen, M. P., Friedman, L. S., Bulcroft, R. A., Hops, H., & Wright, S. F. (1995). Chronic pain patient-spouse interactions predict patient disability. *Pain, 63*, 353–360. doi:10.1016/0304-3959(95)00062-3

Schade, V., Semmer, N., Main, C. J., Hora, J., & Boos, N. (1999). The impact of clinical, morphological, psychosocial and work-related factors on the outcome of lumbar discectomy. *Pain, 80*, 239–249. doi:10.1016/S0304-3959(98)00210-3

Schofferman, J., Anderson, D., Hinds, R., Smith, G., & White, A. (1992). Childhood psychological trauma correlates with unsuccessful lumbar spine surgery. *Spine, 17*(6, Suppl.), S138–S144.

Seligman, M. E. P. (1975). *Helplessness: On depression, development, and death.* San Francisco, CA: W. H. Freeman.

Sherman, J., Cauthen, J., Schoenberg, D., Burns, M., Reaven, N. L., & Griffith, S. L. (2010). Economic impact of improving outcomes of lumbar discectomy. *The Spine Journal, 10*, 108–116. doi:10.1016/j.spinee.2009.08.453

Slover, J., Abdu, W. A., Hanscom, B., & Weinstein, J. N. (2006). The impact of comorbidities on the change in Short-Form 36 and oswestry scores following lumbar spine surgery. *Spine, 31*, 1974–1980. doi:10.1097/01.brs.0000229252.30903.b9

Sørenson, L. V., & Mors, O. (1988). Presentation of a new MMPI-2 scale to predict outcome after first lumbar discectomy. *Pain, 34*, 191–194. doi:10.1016/0304-3959(88)90165-0

Spengler, D. M., Bigos, S. J., Martin, N. A., Zeh, J., Fisher, L., & Nachemson, A. (1986). Back injuries in industry: A retrospective study. I. Overview and cost analysis. *Spine, 11*, 241–245. doi:10.1097/00007632-198604000-00010

Spengler, D. M., Ouelette, E. A., Battie, M., & Zeh, J. (1990). Elective discectomy for herniation of a lumbar disc: Additional experience with an objective method. *Journal of Bone & Joint Surgery, 72*, 230–237.

Taylor, H., & Curren, H. M. (1985). *The Nuprin pain report*. New York: Louis Harris and Assoc.

Treatment traps to avoid. (2007). *Consumer Reports, 72*(11), 12.

Trief, P. M., Grant, W., & Fredrickson, B. (2000). A prospective study of psychological predictors of lumbar surgery outcome. *Spine, 25*, 2616–2621. doi:10.1097/00007632-200010150-00012

Trief, P. M., Ploutz-Snyder, R., & Fredrickson, B. E. (2006). Emotional health predicts pain and function after fusion: A prospective multicenter study. *Spine, 31*, 823–830. doi:10.1097/01.brs.0000206362.03950.5b

Turner, J. A., & Clancy, S. (1986). Strategies for coping with chronic low back pain: Relationship to pain and disability. *Pain, 24*, 355–364. doi:10.1016/0304-3959(86)90121-1

Turner, J. A., Ersek, M., Herron, L., Haselkorn, J., Kent, D., Ciol, M. A., & Deyo, R. (1992). Patient outcomes after lumbar spinal fusions. *JAMA, 268*, 907–911. doi:10.1001/jama.1992.03490070089049

Uomoto, J. M., Turner, J. A., & Herron, L. D. (1988). Use of the MMPI and MCMI in predicting outcome of lumbar laminectomy. *Journal of Clinical Psychology, 44*, 191–197. doi:10.1002/1097-4679(198803)44:2<191::AID-JCLP2270440216>3.0.CO;2-B

Voorhies, R. M., Jiang, X., & Thomas, N. (2007). Predicting outcome in the surgical treatment of lumbar radiculopathy using the Pain Drawing Score, McGill Short Form Pain Questionnaire, and risk factors including psychosocial issues and axial joint pain. *Spine, 7*, 516–524. doi:10.1016/j.spinee.2006.10.013

Waddell, G., McCulloch, J. A., Kummel, E., & Venner, R. M. (1980). Nonorganic physical signs in low-back pain. *Spine, 5*, 117–125. doi:10.1097/00007632-198003000-00005

Weinstein, J. N., Lurie, J. D., Olson, P. R., Bronner, K. K., & Fisher, E. S. (2006). United States' trends and regional variations in lumbar spine surgery: 1992–2003. *Spine, 31*, 2707–2714.

3

BARIATRIC SURGERY

DAVID B. SARWER, KELLY C. ALLISON, BROOKE BAILER,
LUCY F. FAULCONBRIDGE, AND THOMAS A. WADDEN

Obesity is currently one of the biggest public health issues in the United States and many Westernized countries. Approximately one third of the U.S. population is obese, and another one third is overweight and at risk for developing obesity in the future (Flegal, Carroll, Kit, & Ogden, 2012). Although many treatments for excess body weight are available, many are limited in the amount of resultant weight loss, the occurrence of weight regain over time, or both.

Bariatric surgery holds great promise for the successful treatment of obesity. The weight losses seen with surgery are much greater and far more durable than those obtained with more conservative weight loss treatments, such as self-directed diets or commercial weight loss programs (Sjöström et al., 2004). The improvements in morbidity and mortality are similarly impressive, with a substantial majority of patients with diabetes, hyperlipidemia, hypertension, and obstructive sleep apnea experiencing partial or

DOI: 10.1037/14035-004
Presurgical Psychological Screening: Understanding Patients, Improving Outcomes, Andrew R. Block and
David B. Sarwer (Editors)

complete resolution (Buchwald et al., 2004). However, many individuals who present for bariatric surgery do so with a range of psychosocial and behavioral issues. As a result, almost all bariatric surgery programs in the United States (and most insurance companies) require patients to undergo a psychological evaluation before surgery. These evaluations are designed to identify psychiatric conditions that may contraindicate bariatric surgery as well as provide patients with psychoeducation regarding the postoperative dietary, behavioral, and lifestyle changes that they will need to make.

We begin this chapter with an overview of the research on the psychosocial characteristics of individuals who present for bariatric surgery. This literature has been used to inform recommendations for the presurgical psychological screening (PPS) of these patients. The recommended features of these evaluations are detailed, and a case example is presented to illustrate the use of PPS with bariatric surgery patients.

THE OBESITY PROBLEM

Obesity is defined by an individual's body mass index (BMI), which evaluates a person's weight relative to his or her height. BMI is calculated as weight in kilograms divided by height in meters squared. For example, a person with a weight of 100 kilograms and a height of 2 meters squared would have a BMI of 25.0 kg/m^2. Individuals with a BMI between 18.5 and 24.9 kg/m^2 are considered to be of normal weight. People with a BMI between 25.0 and 29.9 kg/m^2 are overweight. People with a BMI $\geq$ 30 kg/m^2 are clinically obese, with Obesity Classes 1 and 2 defined as BMIs of 30.0 to 34.9 kg/m^2 and 35.0 to 39.9 kg/m^2, respectively. Those who have a BMI $\geq$ 40.0 kg/m^2 are extremely (or morbidly) obese (Obesity Class 3). Although obesity is often perceived as an aesthetic issue, it is a significant medical condition. The presence of obesity increases the risk for many medical conditions, including cardiovascular disease, Type 2 diabetes, hypertension, sleep apnea, musculoskeletal problems, and several forms of cancer (Khaodhiar, McCowen, & Blackburn, 1999).

COMMON TREATMENTS FOR OBESITY

A wide range of recommended treatments for weight loss are available. They include self-directed diets, commercial weight loss programs, dietary counseling, physical activity, hospital-based programs, low-calorie diets, over-the-counter and FDA-approved weight loss medications, and residential weight loss facilities. Many of these approaches include behavioral modification strategies. Most approaches encourage patients to self-monitor their food intake with the goal of reducing caloric intake by 500 to 1,000 calories per day, often by reducing portion sizes and decreasing their intake of foods high in fat and sugar. In addition, patients are instructed to increase physical activity by as much as 150 minutes a week. This approach has been shown to produce a weight loss of approximately 8% to 10% within the first 4 to 6 months of treatment (National Heart Lung and Blood Institute, 1998). Unfortunately, weight regain after all of these treatments is common. Patients often begin to regain weight within the first year or 2 of the onset of treatment; most have regained all of their weight within 5 years (Karlsson, Taft, Ryden, Sjöström, & Sullivan, 2007). For these and other reasons, people have had a greater interest in weight loss treatments that produce larger and more durable weight losses, such as those seen with bariatric surgery.

BARIATRIC SURGERY

Bariatric surgery is presently reserved for individuals with a BMI $\geq$ 40 kg/m^2 or those with a BMI $\geq$ 35 kg/m^2 in the presence of major weight-related health conditions such as diabetes, high blood pressure, or heart disease (Mechanick et al., 2008; National Heart, Lung, and Blood Institute, 1998). Recent statistics have suggested that approximately 6% of Americans have a BMI $\geq$ 40 kg/m^2, including approximately one in every six African American women (Flegal et al., 2012). Although the rate of individuals with a BMI $\geq$ 30 kg/m^2 doubled between 1986 and 2000, the number of people with a BMI $\geq$ 40 kg/m^2 increased by a factor of seven (Sturm, 2007). More than 25 million adults currently meet the National Institutes of Health criteria for bariatric surgery.

The most common surgical procedures include laparoscopic adjustable gastric banding (LAGB) and Roux-en-Y gastric bypass (RYGB). In both procedures, weight loss is induced by restricting food intake. The LAGB procedure restricts food intake through the surgical insertion of a silicone band around the top portion of the stomach. When constricted, this band reduces stomach capacity, slows digestion, and increases satiety. The RYGB reduces food intake by creating a small pouch from the top portion of the stomach by surgically separating it from the bottom portion. The small intestine is then attached to this pouch to enable drainage. RYGB is also thought to induce weight loss through changes in gut peptides and food malabsorption (Guijarro et al., 2007). The RYGB, performed laparoscopically, is the current procedure of choice in the United States. Within the past several years, the sleeve gastrectomy, which reduces stomach capacity and food intake by removing the major curve of the stomach to make the stomach more sleeve or banana shaped, has become an increasingly popular alternative to the LAGB procedure.

Twelve to 18 months after surgery, individuals typically lose 25% to 35% of initial body weight with RYGB procedures and 20% to 25% with LAGB (Mechanick et al., 2008). Weight loss with both procedures is associated with significant improvements in obesity-related comorbidities; at least eight studies have documented decreased mortality among bariatric surgery patients compared with individuals who have not undergone surgery (Buchwald et al., 2004; Christou et al., 2004; Flum & Dellinger, 2004; MacDonald et al., 1997; Maggard et al., 2005; Pories et al., 1995; Sjöström et al., 2004, 2007).

Bariatric surgery is associated with significant improvements in psychosocial status. Most psychosocial characteristics—including symptoms of depression and anxiety, health-related quality of life, self-esteem, and body image—improve dramatically in the first year after surgery (Herpertz, Kielmann, Wolfe, Hebebrand, & Senf, 2004; Mitchell & de Zwaan, 2005; Sarwer, Wadden, & Fabricatore, 2005; van Hout, Boekestein, Fortuin, Pelle, & van Heck, 2006). Many of these benefits appear to endure through the first 4 postoperative years.

Although most studies have suggested that the psychosocial outcomes of bariatric surgery are largely positive, these experiences are not universal. Among the greatest causes for concern are recent findings that have suggested that postoperative bariatric surgery patients have a higher-than-expected rate of suicide, approximately twice that of similarly obese individuals who do not undergo surgery (e.g., Adams et al., 2007). Other concerns include suboptimal weight losses or weight regain, dietary nonadherence, and a range of psychosocial issues, as detailed later (Sarwer, Dilks, & West-Smith, 2011). For these reasons, and because of the psychological and social issues often experienced by people with extreme obesity who present for surgery, candidates for surgery are almost universally required to undergo PPS.

Before bariatric surgery, candidates are required to complete several medical evaluations (Mechanick et al., 2008). These evaluations typically include a medical history and physical examination, cardiac clearance, sleep study, and upper gastrointestinal examination. The PPS also takes place during this preparatory period. These evaluations are primarily designed to assess a patient's relative risks for surgery. At the same time, interactions with multiple members of the multidisciplinary team allow for a greater understanding of patients' motivations for surgery as well as their knowledge and understanding of the operation they plan to have, its potential risks and benefits, and the changes they must make in their eating and lifestyle habits.

PRESURGICAL PSYCHOLOGICAL SCREENING
BEFORE BARIATRIC SURGERY

Almost all bariatric surgery programs in the United States have candidates undergo PPS, which is typically performed by a psychologist or social worker. In general, the evaluation serves two purposes (Wadden & Sarwer, 2006). First, it can identify potential contraindications to surgery, such as substance abuse, poorly controlled depression, or other major mental illness. The evaluation can also help to identify potential postoperative challenges and facilitate behavioral changes that can enhance postoperative weight maintenance. Although published recommendations are available regarding the structure and content of these evaluations (e.g., Heinberg et al., 2010; Sogg, 2007; Wadden & Sarwer, 2006), consensus guidelines have yet to be established.

Almost all evaluations rely on clinical interviews with patients; approximately two thirds also include measures of psychiatric symptoms, objective tests of personality or psychopathology, or both (Fabricatore, Crerand, Wadden, Sarwer, & Krasucki, 2006). Some use questionnaires that are sent to the patient before the evaluation, which are then used to structure the interview. One example of such a questionnaire is the Weight and Lifestyle Inventory (Wadden & Foster, 2006), which assesses the patient's knowledge of bariatric surgery, weight and dieting history, and eating and activity habits and identifies potential obstacles and resources that may influence postoperative outcomes. Other mental health professionals use personality assessment tools or other paper-and-pencil measures of psychological symptoms or psychopathology, such as the Beck Depression Inventory—II (Beck & Steer, 1993) or more comprehensive measures, such as the Minnesota Multiphasic Personality Inventory—2 (Butcher, Dahlstrom, Graham, Tellegen, & Kaemmer, 1989) or the Millon Behavioral Medicine Diagnostic (Millon, Antoni, Millon, Meagher, & Grossman, 2001).

GENERAL PSYCHOSOCIAL CONSIDERATIONS

Several general psychosocial issues should be considered in candidates for bariatric surgery. These issues include the motivations for and expectations about surgery; quality of life, self-esteem, and body image; romantic and sexual relationships; and the possible experience of stigmatization or discrimination as a result of extreme obesity.

Motivations and Expectations

Most patients begin to consider bariatric surgery as a way to improve the health problems associated with their extreme obesity. At the same time, many are motivated to improve their physical appearance and body image. It is important that patients seek surgery for improvements in their health and well-being and not primarily for appearance-based reasons. Many individuals find it surprising that most patients who undergo bariatric surgery remain clinically obese even with a successful outcome; few patients return to a "normal" BMI (Mechanick et al., 2008).

As noted earlier, the weight losses associated with all of the bariatric surgical procedures dwarf those typically seen with more conservative weight loss treatments. In spite of this, individuals who present for bariatric surgery often have unrealistic expectations about the amount of weight they will lose. Although these unrealistic expectations were once thought to put individuals at risk for weight regain, it appears that they may be unrelated to weight losses after bariatric surgery (White, Masheb, Rothschild, Burke-Martindale, & Grilo, 2007). However, these unrealistic expectations may be associated with postoperative psychosocial complications, as we detail later.

Quality of Life, Self-Esteem, and Body Image

Individuals interested in bariatric surgery may have expectations about the impact of surgery on other areas of their lives. Numerous studies have shown a relationship between excess body weight and decreases in both health-related and weight-related quality of life (e.g., Fabricatore, Wadden, Sarwer, & Faith, 2005; Kolotkin et al., 2008; Sarwer et al., 2010).

For some individuals, the degree of obesity can have a dramatic impact on their self-esteem. Obesity may be more likely to affect women's self-esteem, in part because of society's overemphasis on thinness as a criterion for physical beauty. As a result, the positive relationship between BMI and body image dissatisfaction is not surprising (Sarwer, Dilks, & Spitzer, 2011). Although many individuals both anticipate and experience improvements in body image after bariatric surgery, for some the massive postoperative weight loss may result in the development of loose or sagging skin of the abdomen, thighs, legs, and arms that may increase body image dissatisfaction (Sarwer & Fabricatore, 2008). It may lead some patients to present to a plastic surgeon for body-contouring surgery, which is undertaken by approximately 55,000 individuals each year (American Society of Plastic Surgeons, 2011).

Marital and Sexual Relationships

Similarly, men and women interested in bariatric surgery should consider the potential impact of their weight loss on their marital and sexual relationships. Intuitively, most people presume that these relationships will improve with weight loss. However, body weight can play a much more complex role in close relationships. Some partners may feel threatened or jealous witnessing a partner's weight loss. Similarly, little is known about the relationship between excess body weight and sexual function. Studies have suggested that obesity is associated with impairments in sexual functioning (Sarwer, Lavery, & Spitzer, 2012). Although this relationship is not surprising, the potential mechanisms for these difficulties in functioning—physiological, psychological, or some combination of the two—are less well established.

Stigmatization and Discrimination

Finally, it is important to consider the potential impact of stigmatization and discrimination on people who present for bariatric surgery. Obesity, and extreme obesity in particular, can contribute to the experience of discrimination. Obese individuals are less likely to complete high school, are less likely to marry, and earn less money than average-weight people. Obese people are frequently subjected to discrimination in many settings, including educational, employment, and even medical settings (Puhl & Brownell, 2001). These experiences may be even more common among those with severe obesity.

CONDUCTING THE EVALUATION

At the start of the evaluation, patients are typically informed about the nature and purpose of the interview. They are told that the information will be used to generate a letter, sent to the patient's surgeon and forwarded to the patient's insurance company, that will summarize the evaluation and the mental health professional's recommendations. Sharing the summary with the patient at the end of the evaluation is also useful, although it is not always possible if the interviewer needs to contact the patient's mental health provider to confirm psychiatric status and appropriateness for surgery.

Much of the evaluation focuses on patients' psychiatric status and history, as with most mental health assessments. Between 20% and 60% of people with extreme obesity who pursue bariatric surgery have a psychiatric illness. In a study of 288 bariatric surgery candidates who were assessed by the Structured Clinical Interview for DSM Disorders, 38% received a current Axis I diagnosis and 66% were given a lifetime diagnosis (Kalarchian et al., 2007). The presence of psychopathology is believed to have a negative impact on postoperative outcome. In an observational study, patients with a lifetime diagnosis of any Axis I clinical disorder, particularly mood or anxiety disorders, experienced smaller weight losses 6 months after RYGB than those who had never had an Axis I disorder (Kalarchian et al., 2008). Bariatric surgery patients with two or more psychiatric diagnoses were found to be significantly more likely to experience weight loss cessation or weight regain after 1 year than those with no or one diagnosis.

Mood Disorders

Several studies have suggested a bidirectional relationship between obesity and depression (e.g., Anderson, Cohen, Naumova, & Must, 2006; Goodman & Whitaker, 2002; Herva et al., 2006; Pine, Goldstein, Wolk, & Weissman, 2001; Roberts, Deleger, Strawbridge, & Kaplan, 2003; Stice, Presnell, Shaw, & Rohde, 2005), and it is now well-established that obese individuals are at higher risk for current and lifetime depression than non-obese individuals. Roberts, Kaplan, Shema, and Strawbridge (2000) found the point prevalence rate of depression among obese adults older than age 50 to be 14%, compared with 7.5% among normal-weight adults.

People with extreme obesity are at even greater risk for depression. Extremely obese individuals were almost 5 times more likely to have experienced an episode of major depression in the past year than average-weight individuals (Onyike, Crum, Lee, Lyketsos, & Eaton, 2003). Men with Class 3 obesity were 38% more likely to experience current depression and 40% more likely to have a lifetime history of depression than were normal-weight men (Zhao et al., 2009). Women with Class 3 obesity were 31% more likely to experience current depression and 53% more likely to have a lifetime history of depression.

Individuals who present for bariatric surgery typically endorse an elevated number of symptoms of depression. Faulconbridge et al. (2012) found that approximately three quarters of surgery candidates reported minimal to mild symptoms of depression, with a mean score on the Beck Depression Inventory—II of 14.1 ($SD = 10.0$). These symptoms are generally not of clinical concern unless patients report suicidal ideation. Other candidates for bariatric surgery score in the moderate to severe range of symptoms of depression but report no history of depression or other emotional complications. They often deny that they feel depressed or believe that their dysphoria is attributable to their obesity-related complications. This weight-related depression is not uncommon in candidates for surgery, but the mental health professional should confirm that the patient does not have a true mood disorder.

For people with significant symptoms of depression, even after accounting for conditions associated with their weight, mental health treatment is recommended. Depending on the patient's functioning and life circumstances (e.g., relationship with primary care physician, access to mental health treatment), patients are encouraged to speak with their primary care physician about the use of pharmacotherapy or should be provided with a mental health referral. Patients are reminded that the goal of this treatment is to optimize their psychological functioning so that they are best prepared to take on the postoperative dietary and behavioral demands of bariatric surgery.

Suicidality is of particular concern with people interested in bariatric surgery. In the general population, obese women are more likely to experience suicidal ideation and to make suicide attempts than their normal-weight counterparts (Carpenter, Hasin, Allison, & Faith, 2000). People with extreme obesity have also been found to be more likely to attempt suicide than people in the general population (Dong, Li, Li, & Price, 2006; Mather, Cox, Enns, & Sareen, 2009; Tindle et al., 2010). Thus, obesity itself is a risk factor for suicidality, but bariatric surgery may have an independent relationship with suicide. Adams et al. (2007) examined mortality and causes of death among 7,925 postoperative bariatric surgery patients and 7,925 nonpatient controls who were matched for age, gender, and BMI (assessed before surgery in the surgery group and through self-report on driver's license applications in the control group). All-cause mortality was significantly reduced among surgery patients compared with controls. However, nearly twice as many surgery patients ($n = 43$) as controls ($n = 24$) died by suicide. In the absence of additional information on the relationship between bariatric surgery and suicide, these findings underscore the importance of ensuring that patients who have psychiatric disorders receive appropriate mental health care before and after bariatric surgery.

Anxiety Disorders

Anxiety disorders are also common among bariatric surgery candidates. In the study by Kalarchian et al. (2007), almost 24% of surgery candidates were found to have an anxiety disorder. The most common disorder was social anxiety disorder, found in 9% of patients. In a society that puts such a premium on physical appearance and thinness, it is not surprising that a significant minority of people with extreme obesity report increased anxiety in social situations. Despite these rates of anxiety disorders, no evidence has suggested that they contraindicate surgery. However, intuitive thought and clinical experience suggest that uncontrolled anxiety may have a negative impact on postoperative recovery as well as the patient's ability to adhere to the postoperative diet.

Eating Disorders

Disordered eating is common among candidates for bariatric surgery and is a likely contributor to the development of extreme obesity. Many patients have reported that they engage in eating for emotional reasons. Others have formally recognized eating disorders. The most commonly recognized eating disorder among bariatric surgery patients is binge-eating disorder. Although initial reports suggested that as many as half of all bariatric surgery patients had binge-eating disorder, more recent studies have indicated that the full disorder occurs in approximately 5% of patients (e.g., Allison et al., 2006; Colles, Dixon, & O'Brien, 2007). Fewer than 1% of patients have bulimia nervosa (Allison et al., 2006). Just fewer than 10% of candidates for bariatric surgery have night eating syndrome, which is characterized by a delayed circadian pattern of eating demonstrated by evening hyperphagia (i.e., consumption of at least 25% of intake after the evening meal), and/or two or more nocturnal ingestions per week (i.e., waking up from sleep to eat; Allison et al., 2010).

Disordered eating before bariatric surgery has been of particular concern because of its potential negative association with postoperative weight losses. Early studies of this issue suggested that the presence of binge eating was associated with either suboptimal weight losses or premature weight regain after bariatric surgery (Hsu, Betancourt, & Sullivan, 1996, 1997; Kalarchian et al., 2002; Mitchell et al., 2001). Other studies, however, have suggested that binge eating is unrelated to postoperative weight loss (Busetto et al., 2002; Gorin et al., 2008) at least in the 1st year after surgery (Wadden et al., 2011). Thus, the presence of binge eating is at present not considered an absolute contraindication to bariatric surgery. It is, however, considered a potential poor prognostic indicator of postoperative weight maintenance, because this behavior may be linked to postoperative grazing and loss of control over eating (Colles, Dixon, & O'Brien, 2008).

Patients who report binge eating or night eating on a regular basis are often recommended for mental health treatment with the goal of being able to demonstrate an ability to control or eliminate the behavior before surgery. In contrast, bulimia nervosa is a contraindication to bariatric surgery. Patients with this disorder would seem to be at high risk of excessive vomiting after surgery with its attendant effects on oral health, electrolyte balance, and cardiac function. These individuals are referred to psychotherapy and are reevaluated before being recommended for bariatric surgery.

Substance Abuse

A minority of bariatric surgery patients report a history of substance abuse. Approximately 10% of patients report a history of illicit drug use or alcoholism. Kalarchian et al. (2007) found that fewer than 2% of surgery candidates met criteria for a current substance abuse disorder. By contrast, the *Diagnostic and Statistical Manual of Mental Disorders* (4th ed., text rev.; American Psychiatric Association, 2000) estimated the point prevalence of just one such disorder, alcohol dependence, at approximately 5%. Regardless of the actual rate, active use or abuse of illegal drugs or alcohol is widely considered a contraindication to bariatric surgery.

Of particular concern is the risk associated with postoperative substance use and abuse. Two concerns regarding postoperative substance use are prominent in the media, if not in the scientific literature: changes in alcohol metabolism and addiction transfer. A limited number of studies have shown that patients experience alcohol intoxication more quickly, and with smaller amounts of alcohol, after RYGB (Hagedorn, Encarnacion, Brat, & Morton, 2007; Klockhoff, Näslund, & Jones, 2002). *Addiction transfer* is a popular term created by the mass media that refers to the idea that patients who undergo bariatric surgery may develop addictions to substances, gambling, sex, and so forth to replace their preoperative addiction to food. *Addiction transfer* is not an accepted clinical or scientific term. The term and construct have several shortcomings, as detailed by Sogg (2007). Chief among these is that the view of food as an addictive substance, or eating as an addictive behavior, is by no means supported by scientific consensus. Additionally, the notion that a treated symptom (e.g., compulsive eating) will resurface in a different form (e.g., compulsive drinking or shopping) has little support.

Thought Disorders

As with any surgical population, individuals with thought disorders present for bariatric surgery. Although little is known about the postoperative outcome of these patients, our bariatric surgery program at the University of Pennsylvania Health System has successfully operated on individuals with a history of schizophrenia and dissociative identity disorder when these patients have been through a long period of psychiatric stability that is confirmed by their mental health professional in the community.

Sexual Abuse

A modest association appears to exist between sexual abuse and obesity (Gustafson & Sarwer, 2004). Studies have suggested that between 16% and 32% of bariatric surgery candidates report a history of sexual abuse, which appears to be higher than estimates from the most rigorous studies of the general population (e.g., Grilo et al., 2005; Gustafson et al., 2006). Interestingly, several studies have suggested that a history of previous sexual abuse is unrelated to weight loss after bariatric surgery (Clark et al., 2007; Grilo et al., 2006; Larsen & Geenen, 2005). Nevertheless, patients with a history of sexual abuse often struggle with a range of psychological issues after bariatric surgery, including body image, sexual, and romantic relationship issues.

Although predicting which patients will struggle with these issues may be impossible, the preoperative psychological evaluation presents an opportunity to discuss these issues with patients and inform them that they may experience some postoperative psychological distress.

Psychiatric History

Studies have found that between 16% and 40% of patients report ongoing mental health treatment at the time of bariatric surgery (Clark et al., 2003; Friedman, Applegate, & Grant, 2007; Larsen et al., 2003; Sarwer et al., 2004). The most common treatment is the use of antidepressant medications, which are often prescribed and managed by primary care physicians. Unfortunately, little is known about how these medications interact with the different surgical procedures (Sarwer et al., 2010). Potentially dramatic changes in absorption of medications may occur because of a reduction in gastrointestinal surface area and other changes. Rapid changes in body weight and fat mass may also affect the efficacy and tolerability of antidepressant medications. To date, little guidance has been available on the peri- or postoperative management of these medications.

For patients who are under the care of a mental health provider, the professional who is conducting the evaluation for bariatric surgery should contact that provider. The current provider should confirm that the patient is stable from a psychosocial perspective and appropriate for surgery at the present time. For medical and legal reasons, these contacts with outside professionals should be documented in the letter sent to the bariatric surgeon.

At present, the relationship between preoperative psychological status and history and postoperative outcomes is unclear. As noted earlier, some studies have suggested that preoperative psychopathology and eating behavior are unrelated to postoperative weight loss (Delin, Watts, & Bassett, 1995; Larsen & Torgersen, 1989); others have suggested that preoperative psychopathology may be associated with untoward psychosocial outcomes, but not with poorer weight loss (Busetto et al., 2002; de Zwaan et al., 2002). Unfortunately, the complex relationship between obesity and psychiatric illness, as well as a number of methodological issues within this literature, make drawing definitive conclusions difficult. It may be that psychiatric symptoms that are largely attributable to weight, such as symptoms of depression and impaired quality of life, may be associated with more positive outcomes, whereas those symptoms representative of psychiatric illness that are independent of obesity are associated with less positive outcomes (Herpertz et al., 2004). Nevertheless, most mental health professionals who perform these assessments agree that significant psychiatric issues contraindicate bariatric surgery. Typically cited contraindications include active substance abuse, active psychosis, bulimia nervosa, and severe, uncontrolled depression. Nevertheless, even the presence of severe psychopathology must be balanced with the severity of the patient's health issues.

Weight Loss History

Many candidates for bariatric surgery are "dieting veterans" who have made multiple attempts with a range of more conservative weight loss treatments (Gibbons et al., 2006). Some have truly exhausted their more conservative treatment options and, coupled with the degree of obesity and related health problems, see bariatric surgery as their best (and perhaps last) chance to successfully control their weight. A small minority of patients, however, have not participated in any organized weight loss programs before surgery. As a result, they do not have the fund of dietary knowledge seen in other patients. With these patients, it is often useful to recommend some preoperative dietary counseling as well as attendance in the program's preoperative support group to help provide additional education on the dietary requirements of bariatric surgery.

Family Support

The decision to seek bariatric surgery is a significant one, not only for the patient but also for his or her family members. Thus, patients are asked about living arrangements, their satisfaction with their spouse (partner), and other intimate relationships and whether family members and friends support the decision to undertake surgery. In rare cases, family members may be opposed to surgery or may try to sabotage the candidate's weight loss efforts. Candidates who report they are dissatisfied with their marriage (or other intimate relationship) are informed that surgery and weight loss are unlikely to resolve these problems. It is also useful to ensure that patients have identified relatives or friends who will assist in their care in the initial days after surgery.

Timing of Surgery

The timing of surgery in relationship to other life events should be assessed to ensure that the candidate has chosen an appropriate time to undergo surgery, relatively free of stressors such as starting a new job, changing homes, or getting a divorce. Ideally, the patient should have 3 to 4 weeks to undergo the operation, recover from it physically, and begin to adopt new lifestyle habits, the most important of which is adhering to the postoperative diet.

Concluding the Evaluation

The evaluation should conclude with a brief summary of the interviewer's findings concerning the patient's weight and dieting histories, eating and activity habits, social and psychological status, and readiness for bariatric surgery. The ultimate recommendation regarding surgery should be communicated clearly to the patient, although it may be delayed pending contact with the patient's mental health professional.

In general, approximately 70% of patients are unconditionally recommended for surgery (Sarwer et al., 2004). Other patients are recommended to undergo additional treatment (mental health, dietary, or both) and are asked to return for further evaluation, typically in about 3 months. Most patients who follow these treatment recommendations ultimately have bariatric surgery. A patient's inability to follow these recommendations is likely a poor prognostic sign regarding the ability to make the dietary and behavioral changes required by bariatric surgery.

Case Example

This case report illustrates a woman who is appropriate for surgery from a physical perspective but may not be ready from a psychosocial perspective.[1]

M. V. is a 28-year-old European American woman. She is 61 inches tall, weighs 270 pounds, and has a BMI of 51 kg/m^2. She reported a high school education and is employed as a dispatcher for a police and fire department. She is single and lives with her grandparents and 3-year-old daughter. She indicated that she has plans to marry her boyfriend in a few months.

M. V. has a strong family history of obesity and remembered first being overweight at age 12. She reported that she is currently below her highest adult weight of 278 pounds, reached last year. She was able to lose 8 pounds in the past several weeks in preparation for surgery. M. V. reported a history of sleep apnea as well as spinal fusion surgery that still leaves her in a good deal of physical discomfort on a daily basis.

M. V. reported typically eating three meals and one to two snacks each day. She reported eating large amounts of high-calorie foods on a regular basis, such as fast food. She also reported drinking large amounts of sweetened beverages regularly. She displayed little awareness of the impact of these behaviors on her weight. She denied any history of binge eating or night eating, as well as any history of purging or other compensatory behaviors after overeating.

---

[1]Details of this case have been altered to protect the patient's identity.

M. V. has had depression, anxiety, and panic attacks for the past 5 years. She reported that she was involved in a car accident (which contributed to her current issues with her back) and broke off an engagement. She indicated that she subsequently went through a period of time in which she craved love and estimated that she had approximately 25 sexual partners in 2 years. She also reported ending three other engagements. She described how she has recommitted to her religion, found a new romantic partner, and put these issues behind her. She also reported that she has not had a panic attack in 3 years. She indicated that she is currently taking 75 milligrams per day of venlafaxine hydrochloride extended release (Effexor XR), as prescribed by her primary care physician. She otherwise denied a history of psychiatric treatment past or present. She denied a history of psychiatric hospitalizations.

Her Beck Depression Inventory—II score was 14, suggestive of mild symptoms of depression. She described her mood as "not happy" and attributed it to a fox that was making noise in her backyard the previous night. Her affect was flat, and she was quite guarded throughout the evaluation. She appeared to have an expressionless stare at several points in the evaluation and became quite defensive when asked about her social history. She displayed little awareness of the degree of turbulence in her life over the past few years or of how she presented herself to others. She denied any symptoms of depression, anxiety, or excessive stress on questioning. She denied any suicidal ideation.

In some respects, M. V. is a good candidate for bariatric surgery. Her BMI is > 40, and she has a history of weight-related comorbidities (sleep apnea). Her family history, coupled with her own childhood onset of overweight, provides evidence for a biological predisposition to obesity. She has tried a several more conservative weight loss efforts without success, and her chronic back injury is unlikely to improve without significant weight loss, thereby further limiting her ability to engage in physical activity and prevent additional weight gain as she gets older.

Her psychosocial history and current presentation, however, are of concern. Although she did not report severe symptoms of depression or anxiety, she has clearly dealt with some significant stressors in the past few years and engaged in a pattern of self-defeating behaviors. Although she believes that her symptoms are well controlled by medication and that she has put these issues behind her, her chronological age and lack of insight into her behavior suggest that these issues may be unresolved. There is concern that they may reappear postoperatively and interfere with her ability to make the dietary and behavioral changes required for surgery.

To obtain additional information about her history, M. V.'s primary care physician was contacted by phone. He indicated that he also finds her presentation to be guarded and defensive and said that he had no knowledge of the significant psychosocial stressors in her life over the past few years. Because of these issues, it was recommended that M. V. begin psychotherapy before surgery and return for further evaluation in 3 to 4 months.

CONCLUSION

The popularity of bariatric surgery has grown dramatically in the past decade. Given the current obesity problem in the Western world, coupled with the general efficacy of the procedures, it is likely to increase in popularity in the future. Almost all patients in the United States are currently required to undergo a preoperative mental health evaluation before surgery, and these evaluations are widely considered to be a critical part of the preoperative evaluation process. Although mental health professionals rarely recommend against or outright deny surgery, the evaluation plays a critical role in helping patients prepare for surgery as well as identifying some of the psychosocial issues that they may encounter postoperatively. Furthermore, from the surgeon's and hospital's perspective, the evaluation is also an important part of the risk management process. As the problem of extreme obesity continues to grow unchecked, an increasing number of mental health professionals will likely become involved in not only the preoperative evaluation of patients but their postoperative care as well.

REFERENCES

Adams, T. D., Gress, R. E., Smith, S. C., Halverson, R. C., Simper, S. C., Rosamond, W. D., . . . Hunt, S. C. (2007). Long-term mortality following gastric bypass surgery. *The New England Journal of Medicine, 357,* 753–761. doi:10.1056/NEJMoa066603

Allison, K. C., Lundgren, J. D., O'Reardon, J. P., Geliebter, A., Gluck, M. E., Vinai, P., . . . Stunkard, A. J. (2010). Proposed diagnostic criteria for night eating syndrome. *International Journal of Eating Disorders, 43,* 241–247.

Allison, K. C., Wadden, T. A., Sarwer, D. B., Fabricatore, A. N., Crerand, C., Gibbons, L., . . . Williams, N. (2006). Night eating syndrome and binge eating disorder among persons seeking bariatric surgery: Prevalence and related features. *Obesity, 14*(Suppl. 2), 77S–82S. doi:10.1038/oby.2006.286

American Psychiatric Association. (2000). *Diagnostic and Statistical Manual of Mental Disorders* (4th ed., text rev.). Washington, DC: Author.

American Society of Plastic Surgeons. (2011). *Report of the 2010 Plastic Surgery Statistics.* Retrieved from http://www.plasticsurgery.org/Documents/news-resources/

statistics/2010-statisticss/Top-Level/2010-US-cosmetic-reconstructive-plastic-surgery-minimally-invasive-statistics2.pdf

Anderson, S. E., Cohen, P., Naumova, E. N., & Must, A. (2006). Association of depression and anxiety disorders with weight change in a prospective community-based study of children followed up into adulthood. *Archives of Pediatrics & Adolescent Medicine, 160*, 285–291. doi:10.1001/archpedi.160.3.285

Beck, A. T., & Steer, R. A. (1993). *BDI–II: Beck Depression Inventory: Manual.* San Antonio, TX: Harcourt Brace.

Buchwald, H., Avidor, Y., Braunwald, E., Jensen, M. D., Pories, W., Fahrbach, K., & Schoelles, K. (2004). Bariatric surgery: A systematic review and meta-analysis. *JAMA, 292*, 1724–1737. doi:10.1001/jama.292.14.1724

Busetto, L., Segato, G., De Marchi, F., Foletto, M., De Luca, M., Caniato, D., & Enzi, G. (2002). Outcome predictors in morbidly obese recipients of an adjustable gastric banding. *Obesity Surgery, 12*, 83–92. doi:10.1381/096089202321144649

Butcher, J. N., Dahlstrom, W. G., Graham, J. R., Tellegen, A., & Kaemmer, B. (1989). *The Minnesota Multiphasic Personality Inventory—2 (MMPI–2): Manual for administration and scoring.* Minneapolis: University of Minnesota Press.

Carpenter, K. M., Hasin, D. S., Allison, D. B., & Faith, M. S. (2000). Relationships between obesity and DSM-IV major depressive disorder, suicide ideation, and suicide attempts: Results from a general population study. *American Journal of Public Health, 90*, 251–257. doi:10.2105/AJPH.90.2.251

Christou, N. V., Sampalis, J. S., Liberman, M., Look, D., Auger, S., MacLean, A. P., & MacLean, A. D. (2004). Surgery decreases long-term mortality, morbidity, and health care use in morbidly obese patients. *Annals of Surgery, 240*, 416–424. doi:10.1097/01.sla.0000137343.63376.19

Clark, M. M., Balsiger, B. M., Sletten, C. D., Dahlman, K. L., Ames, G., & Sarr, M. G. (2003). Psychosocial factors and 2-year outcome following bariatric surgery for weight loss. *Obesity Surgery, 13*, 739–745. doi:10.1381/096089203322509318

Clark, M. M., Hanna, B. K., Mai, J. L., Gaszer, K. M., Graner Krochta, J., McAlpine, D. E., . . . Sarr, M. G. (2007). Sexual abuse survivors and psychiatric hospitalization after bariatric surgery. *Obesity Surgery, 17*, 465–469. doi:10.1007/s11695-007-9084-4

Colles, S. L., Dixon, J. B., & O'Brien, P. E. (2007). Night eating syndrome and nocturnal snacking: Association with obesity, binge eating, and psychological distress. *International Journal of Obesity, 31*, 1722–1730. doi:10.1038/sj.ijo.0803664

Colles, S. L., Dixon, J. B., & O'Brien, P. E. (2008). Grazing and loss of control related to eating: Two high-risk factors following bariatric surgery. *Obesity, 16*, 615–622. doi:10.1038/oby.2007.101

Delin, C. R., Watts, J. M., & Bassett, D. L. (1995). An exploration of the outcomes of gastric bypass surgery for morbid obesity: Patient characteristics and indices of success. *Obesity Surgery, 5*, 159–170. doi:10.1381/096089295765557962 de Zwaan, M., Lancaster, K. L., Mitchell, J. E., Howell, L. M., Monson, N., Roerig, J. L., & Crosby, R. D. (2002). Health related quality of life in morbidly obese patients: Effect of gastric bypass surgery. *Obesity Surgery, 12*, 773–780. doi:10.1381/096089202320995547

Dong, C., Li, W. D., Li, D., & Price, R. A. (2006). Extreme obesity is associated with attempted suicides: Results from a family study. *International Journal of Obesity, 30*, 388–390. doi:10.1038/sj.ijo.0803119

Fabricatore, A. N., Crerand, C. E., Wadden, T. A., Sarwer, D. B., & Krasucki, J. L. (2006). How do mental health professionals evaluate candidates for bariatric surgery? Survey results. *Obesity Surgery, 16*, 567–573. doi:10.1381/096089206776944986

Fabricatore, A. N., Wadden, T. A., Sarwer, D. B., & Faith, M. S. (2005). Health-related quality of life and symptoms of depression in extremely obese persons seeking bariatric surgery. *Obesity Surgery, 15*, 304–309. doi:10.1381/0960892053576578

Faulconbridge, L. F., Wadden, T. A., Jones-Corneille, L. R., Sarwer, D. B., Fabricatore, A. N., Pulcini, M. E., & Williams, N. (2012). *Changes in symptoms of depression and quality of life in obese individuals with binge eating disorder treated with bariatric surgery or lifestyle modification.* Manuscript in preparation.

Flegal, K. M., Carroll, M. D., Kit, B. K., & Ogden, C. L. (2012). Prevalence of obesity and trends in the distribution of body mass index among US adults, 1999–2010. *JAMA, 307*, 491–497. doi:10.1001/jama.2012.39

Flum, D. R., & Dellinger, E. P. (2004). Impact of gastric bypass operation on survival: A population based analysis. *Journal of the American College of Surgeons, 199*, 543–551. doi:10.1016/j.jamcollsurg.2004.06.014

Friedman, K. E., Applegate, K. L., & Grant, J. (2007). Who is adherent with preoperative psychological treatment recommendations among weight loss surgery candidates? *Surgery for Obesity and Related Diseases, 3*, 376–382. doi:10.1016/j.soard.2007.01.008

Gibbons, L. M., Sarwer, D. B., Crerand, C. E., Fabricatore, A. N., Kuehnel, R. H., Lipschutz, P. E., . . . Wadden, T. A. (2006). Previous weight loss experiences of bariatric surgery candidates: How much have patients dieted prior to surgery? *Surgery for Obesity and Related Diseases, 2*, 159–164. doi:10.1016/j.soard.2006.03.013

Goodman, E., & Whitaker, R. C. (2002). A prospective study of the role of depression in the development and persistence of adolescent obesity. *Pediatrics, 110*, 497–504. doi:10.1542/peds.110.3.497

Gorin, A. A., Niemeier, H. M., Hogan, P., Coday, M., Davis, C., DiLillo, V. G., . . . Yanovski, S. Z. (2008). Binge eating and weight loss outcomes in overweight and obese individuals with type 2 diabetes: Results from the Look AHEAD trial. *Archives of General Psychiatry, 65*, 1447–1455. doi:10.1001/archpsyc.65.12.1447

Grilo, C. M., Masheb, R. M., Brody, M., Toth, C., Burke-Martindale, C. H., & Rothschild, B. S. (2005). Childhood maltreatment in extremely obese male and female bariatric surgery candidates. *Obesity Research, 13,* 123–130. doi:10.1038/oby.2005.16

Grilo, C. M., White, M. A., Masheb, R. M., Rothschild, B. S., & Burke-Martindale, C. H. (2006). Relation of childhood sexual abuse and other forms of maltreatment to 12-month postoperative outcomes in extremely obese gastric bypass patients. *Obesity Surgery, 16,* 454–460. doi:10.1381/096089206776327288

Guijarro, A., Suzuki, S., Chen, C., Kirchner, H., Middleton, F. A., Nadtochiy, S., . . . Meguid, M. M. (2007). Characterization of weight loss and weight regain mechanisms after Roux-en-Y gastric bypass in rats. *American Journal of Physiology: Regulatory, Integrative and Comparative Physiology, 293,* R1474–R1489. doi:10.1152/ajpregu.00171.2007

Gustafson, T. B., Gibbons, L. M., Sarwer, D. B., Crerand, C. E., Fabricatore, A. N., Wadden, T. A., . . . Williams, N. N. (2006). History of sexual abuse among bariatric surgery candidates. *Surgery for Obesity and Related Diseases, 2,* 369–374. doi:10.1016/j.soard.2006.03.002

Gustafson, T. B., & Sarwer, D. B. (2004). Childhood sexual abuse and obesity. *Obesity Reviews, 5,* 129–135. doi:10.1111/j.1467-789X.2004.00145.x

Hagedorn, J. C., Encarnacion, B., Brat, G. A., & Morton, J. M. (2007). Does gastric bypass alter alcohol metabolism? *Surgery for Obesity and Related Diseases, 3,* 543–548

Heinberg, L. J., Ashton, K., & Windover, A. (2010). Moving beyond dichotomous psychological evaluation: The Cleveland Clinic Behavioral Rating System for weight loss surgery. *Surgery for Obesity and Related Diseases, 6,* 185–190.

Herpertz, S., Kielmann, R., Wolfe, A. M., Hebebrand, J., & Senf, W. (2004). Do psychosocial variables predict weight loss or mental health after obesity surgery? A systematic review. *Obesity Research, 12,* 1554–1569. doi:10.1038/oby.2004.195

Herva, A., Laitinen, J., Miettunen, J., Veijola, J., Karvonen, J. T., Laksy, K., & Joukamaa, M. (2006). Obesity and depression: Results from the longitudinal Northern Finland 1966 Birth Cohort Study. *International Journal of Obesity, 30,* 520–527. doi:10.1038/sj.ijo.0803174

Hsu, L. K. G., Betancourt, S., & Sullivan, S. P. (1996). Eating disturbances before and after vertical banded gastroplasty: A pilot study. *International Journal of Eating Disorders, 19,* 23–34. doi:10.1002/(SICI)1098-108X(199601)19:1<23::AID-EAT4>3.0.CO;2-Y

Hsu, L. K. G., Betancourt, S., & Sullivan, S. P. (1997). Eating disturbances and outcome of gastric bypass surgery: A pilot study. *International Journal of Eating Disorders, 21,* 385–390. doi:10.1002/(SICI)1098-108X(1997)21:4<385::AID-EAT12>3.0.CO;2-Y

Kalarchian, M. A., Marcus, M. D., Levine, M. D., Courcoulas, A. P., Pilkonis, P. A., Ringham, R. M., . . . Rofey, D. L. (2007). Psychiatric disorders among bariatric surgery candidates: Relationship to obesity and functional health status. *The American Journal of Psychiatry, 164,* 328–334. doi:10.1176/appi.ajp.164.2.328

Kalarchian, M. A., Marcus, M. D., Levine, M. D., Soulakova, J. N., Courcoulas, A. P., & Wisinski, M. S. (2008). Relationship of psychiatric disorders to 6-month outcomes after gastric bypass. *Surgery for Obesity and Related Diseases*, *4*, 544–549. doi:10.1016/j.soard.2008.03.003

Kalarchian, M. A., Marcus, M. D., Wilson, G. T., Labouvie, E. W., Brolin, R. E., & LaMarca, L. B. (2002). Binge eating among gastric bypass patients at long-term follow-up. *Obesity Surgery*, *12*, 270–275. doi:10.1381/096089202762552494

Karlsson, J., Taft, C., Ryden, A., Sjöström, L., & Sullivan, M. (2007). Ten-year trends in health-related quality of life after surgical and conventional treatment for severe obesity: The SOS intervention study. *International Journal of Obesity*, *31*, 1248–1261. doi:10.1038/sj.ijo.0803573

Khaodhiar, L., McCowen, K. C., & Blackburn, G. L. (1999). Obesity and its comorbid conditions. *Clinical Cornerstone*, *2*, 17–31. doi:10.1016/S1098-3597 (99)90002-9

Klockoff, H., Näslund, I., & Jones, A. W. (2002). Faster absorption of ethanol and higher peak concentration in women after gastric bypass surgery. *British Journal of Clinical Pharmacology*, *54*, 587–591

Kolotkin, R. L., Crosby, R. D., Gress, R. E., Hunt, S. C., Engle, S. G., & Adams, T. D. (2008). Health and health-related quality of life: differences between men and women who seek gastric bypass surgery. *Surgery for Obesity and Related Diseases*, *4*, 651–658. doi:10.1016/j.soard.2008.04.012

Larsen, F., & Torgersen, S. (1989). Personality changes after gastric banding surgery for morbid obesity: A prospective study. *Journal of Psychosomatic Research*, *33*, 323–334. doi:10.1016/0022-3999(89)90023-8

Larsen, J. K., & Geenen, R. (2005). Childhood sexual abuse is not associated with poor outcome after gastric banding for severe obesity. *Obesity Surgery*, *15*, 534–537. doi:10.1381/0960892053723277

Larsen, J. K., Geenen, R., van Ramshorst, B., Brand, N., de Wit, P., Stroebe, W., & van Doornen, L. J. (2003). Psychosocial functioning before and after laparoscopic adjustable gastric banding: A cross-sectional study. *Obesity Surgery*, *13*, 629–636. doi:10.1381/096089203322190871

MacDonald, K. G., Jr., Long, S. D., Swanson, M. S., Brown, B. M., Morris, P., Dohm, G. L., & Pories, W. J. (1997). The gastric bypass operation reduces progression and mortality of non-insulin dependent diabetes mellitus. *Journal of Gastrointestinal Surgery*, *1*, 213–220.

Maggard, M. A., Shugarman, L. R., Suttorp, M., Maglione, M., Sugerman, H. J., Livingston, E. H., & Shekelle, P. G. (2005). Meta-analysis: Surgical treatment of obesity. *Annals of Internal Medicine*, *142*, 547–559.

Mather, A. A., Cox, B. J., Enns, M. W., & Sareen, J. (2009). Associations of obesity with psychiatric disorders and suicidal behaviors in a nationally representative sample. *Journal of Psychosomatic Research*, *66*, 277–285. doi:10.1016/j .jpsychores.2008.09.008

Mechanick, J. I., Kushner, R. F., Sugerman, H. J., Gonzalez-Campoy, J. M., Collazo-Clavell, M. L., . . . Dixon, J. (2008). American Association of Clinical Endocrinologists, The Obesity Society, and American Society for Metabolic & Bariatric Surgery Medical Guidelines for Clinical Practice for the perioperative nutritional, metabolic, and nonsurgical support of the bariatric surgery patient. *Surgery for Obesity and Related Diseases, 4*, S109–S184. doi:10.1016/j.soard.2008.08.009

Millon, T., Antoni, M., Millon, C., Meagher, S., & Grossman, S. (2001). *The Millon Behavioral Medicine Diagnostic (MBMD)*. San Antonio, TX: Pearson Assessments.

Mitchell, J. E., & de Zwaan, M. (2005). *Bariatric surgery: A guide for mental health professionals*. New York, NY: Routledge.

Mitchell, J. E., Lancaster, K. L., Burgard, M. A., Howell, L. M., Krahn, D. D., Crosby, R. D., & Gosnell, B. A. (2001). Long-term follow-up of patients' status after gastric bypass. *Obesity Surgery, 11*, 464–468. doi:10.1381/096089201321209341

National Heart, Lung, and Blood Institute Obesity Education Initiative Expert Panel on the Identification, Evaluation, and Treatment of Obesity in Adults. (1998). *Clinical guidelines on the identification, evaluation, and treatment of overweight and obesity in adults: The evidence report*. Bethesda, MD: National Heart, Lung, and Blood Institute.

Onyike, C. U., Crum, R. M., Lee, H. B., Lyketsos, C. G., & Eaton, W. W. (2003). Is obesity associated with major depression? Results from the Third National Health and Nutrition Examination Survey. *American Journal of Epidemiology, 158*, 1139–1147. doi:10.1093/aje/kwg275

Pine, D. S., Goldstein, R. B., Wolk, S., & Weissman, M. M. (2001). The association between childhood depression and adulthood body mass index. *Pediatrics, 107*, 1049–1056. doi:10.1542/peds.107.5.1049

Pories, W. J., Swanson, M. S., MacDonald, K. G., Long, S. B., Morris, P. G., Brown, B. M., . . . Dolezal, J. M. (1995). Who would have thought it? An operation proves to be the most effective therapy for adult onset diabetes mellitus. *Annals of Surgery, 222*, 339–352. doi:10.1097/00000658-199509000-00011

Puhl, R., & Brownell, K. D. (2001). Bias, discrimination, and obesity. *Obesity Research, 9*, 788–805. doi:10.1038/oby.2001.108

Roberts, R. E., Deleger, S., Strawbridge, W. J., & Kaplan, G. A. (2003). Prospective association between obesity and depression: Evidence from the Alameda County Study. *International Journal of Obesity, 27*, 514–521. doi:10.1038/sj.ijo.0802204

Roberts, R. E., Kaplan, G. A., Shema, S. J., & Strawbridge, W. J. (2000). Are the obese at greater risk for depression? *American Journal of Epidemiology, 152*, 163–170. doi:10.1093/aje/152.2.163

Sarwer, D. B., Cohn, N. I., Gibbons, L. M., Magee, L., Crerand, C. E., Raper, S. E., & Wadden, T. A. (2004). Psychiatric diagnoses and psychiatric treatment among bariatric surgery candidates. *Obesity Surgery, 14*, 1148–1156. doi:10.1381/0960892042386922

Sarwer, D. B., Dilks, R. J., & Spitzer, J. C. (2011). Weight loss and changes in body image. In T. F. Cash & L. Smolak (Eds.), *Body image: A handbook of science, practice, and prevention* (pp. 369–377). New York, NY: Guilford Press.

Sarwer, D. B., Dilks, R. J., & West-Smith, L. (2011). Dietary intake and eating behavior after bariatric surgery: Threats to weight loss maintenance and strategies for success. *Surgery for Obesity and Related Diseases, 7*, 644–651. doi:10.1016/j.soard.2011.06.016

Sarwer, D. B., & Fabricatore, A. N. (2008). Psychiatric considerations of the massive weight loss patient. *Clinics in Plastic Surgery, 35*, 1–10. doi:10.1016/j.cps.2007.08.006

Sarwer, D. B., Lavery, M., & Spitzer, J. C. (2012). A review of the relationships between extreme obesity, quality of life, and sexual function. *Obesity Surgery, 22*, 668–676.

Sarwer, D. B., Wadden, T. A., & Fabricatore, A. N. (2005). Psychosocial and behavioral aspects of bariatric surgery. *Obesity Research, 13*, 639–648.

Sarwer, D. B., Wadden, T. A., Moore, R. H., Eisenberg, M. H., Raper, S. E., & Williams, N. N. (2010). Changes in quality of life and body image after gastric bypass surgery. *Surgery for Obesity and Related Diseases, 6*, 608–614. doi:10.1016/j.soard.2010.07.015

Sjöström, L., Lindroos, A. K., Peltonen, M., Torgerson, J., Bouchard, C., Carlsson, B., . . . Wedel, H.; Swedish Obese Subjects Study Scientific Group. (2004). Lifestyle, diabetes, and cardiovascular risk factors 10 years after bariatric surgery. *The New England Journal of Medicine, 351*, 2683–2693. doi:10.1056/NEJMoa035622

Sjöström, L., Narbro, K., Sjöström, C. D., Karason, K., Larsson, B., Wedel, H., & Carlsson, L. M.; Swedish Obese Subjects Study (2007). Effects of bariatric surgery on mortality in Swedish obese subjects. *The New England Journal of Medicine, 357*, 741–752. doi:10.1056/NEJMoa066254

Sogg, S. (2007). Alcohol misuse after bariatric surgery: Epiphenomenon or "Oprah" phenomenon? *Surgery for Obesity and Related Diseases, 3*, 366–368. doi:10.1016/j.soard.2007.03.004

Stice, E., Presnell, K., Shaw, H., & Rohde, P. (2005). Psychological and behavioral risk factors for obesity onset in adolescent girls: A prospective study. *Journal of Consulting and Clinical Psychology, 73*, 195–202. doi:10.1037/0022-006X.73.2.195

Sturm, R. (2007). Increases in morbid obesity in the USA: 2000–2005. *Public Health, 121*, 492–496. doi:10.1016/j.puhe.2007.01.006

Tindle, H. A., Omalu, B., Courcoulas, A., Marcus, M., Hammers, J., & Kuller, L. H. (2010). Risk of suicide after long-term follow-up from bariatric surgery. *American Journal of Medicine, 123*, 1036–1042. doi:10.1016/j.amjmed.2010.06.016

Wadden, T., Faulconbridge, L., Jones-Corneille, L., Sarwer, D. B., Fabricatore, A. N., Thomas, J. G., . . . Williams, N. N. (2011). Binge eating disorder and the outcome of bariatric surgery at one year: A prospective, observational study. *Obesity, 19*, 1220–1228.

Wadden, T. A., & Foster, G. D. (2006). Weight and Lifestyle Inventory (WALI). *Surgery for Obesity and Related Diseases, 2*, 180–199. doi:10.1016/j.soard.2006.03.017

Wadden, T. A., & Sarwer, D. B. (2006). Behavioral assessment of candidates for bariatric surgery: A patient oriented approach. *Surgery for Obesity and Related Diseases, 2*, 171–179. doi:10.1016/j.soard.2006.03.011

White, M. A., Masheb, R. M., Rothschild, B. S., Burke-Martindale, C. H., & Grilo, C. M. (2007). Do patients' unrealistic expectations have prognostic significance after bariatric surgery? *Obesity Surgery, 17*, 74–81. doi:10.1007/s11695-007-9009-2

van Hout, G. C. M., Boekestein, P., Fortuin, F A. M., Pelle, A. J. M., & van Heck, G. L. (2006). Psychosocial functioning following bariatric surgery. *Obesity Surgery, 16*, 787–794.

Zhao, G., Ford, E. S., Dhingra, S., Li, C., Strine, T. W., Mokdad, A. H. (2009). Depression and anxiety among US adults: Associations with body mass index. *International Journal of Obesity, 33*, 257–266.

4

PAIN CONTROL PROCEDURES: STIMULATORS AND INTRATHECAL PUMPS

ROBERT N. JAMISON AND ROBERT R. EDWARDS

Chronic pain, generally defined as pain persisting for more than 6 months or beyond the normal healing and recovery time, is a costly problem that influences every aspect of a person's quality of life, interfering significantly with sleep, employment, social functioning, and activities of daily living. Patients with chronic pain often report depression, anxiety, irritability, sexual dysfunction, and decreased energy. Family roles are altered, and worries about financial limitations and the consequences of a restricted lifestyle abound (Otis, Cardella, & Kerns, 2004).

Epidemiological studies have documented chronic pain to be an immense international problem (Ehrlich, 2003). Estimates are that one of every three individuals will experience chronic pain at some point in their lifetime. Chronic pain accounts for 21% of emergency department visits and 25% of annual missed workdays. Including both direct and indirect costs, chronic pain imposes the greatest economic burden of any health condition

DOI: 10.1037/14035-005
Presurgical Psychological Screening: Understanding Patients, Improving Outcomes, Andrew R. Block and David B. Sarwer (Editors)

(Ferrari & Russell, 2003). Persistent back pain in particular is one of the principal drivers of these costs, both in the United States (Becker et al., 2010) and internationally (Hoy et al., 2010), with indirect costs (e.g., lost or reduced work productivity) accounting for more than half of this economic burden.

Optimal care of patients requires attention to the breadth of factors that determine the experience of pain and related disability. Physical pathology arising from injury and disease and the patient's general physical status are necessarily the immediate focus of attention, but psychological and social well-being are also important determinants of pain and pain-related disability. Psychological and social issues often complicate the lives of people with both pain that is attributable to physical pathology and pain for which physical pathology cannot be identified despite intensive medical investigation.

Psychological assessment is designed to identify problematic emotional reactions, maladaptive thinking and behavior, and social problems that contribute to pain and disability. When psychosocial issues are identified, treatment can be tailored to address these challenges in the patient's life, thereby improving the likelihood and speed of recovery and aiding the prevention of ongoing or more severe problems. In this chapter, we provide a brief review of strategies for assessing psychological and social factors that predict outcome from an implantable device (e.g., spinal cord stimulator, intrathecal pump) designed to control pain. A case study illustrates some of the issues discussed.

OVERVIEW OF STIMULATION AND INTRATHECAL PUMP THERAPY

The treatment for chronic pain remains a challenge in medicine. The various options include medications, physical therapy, interventional procedures, and behavioral interventions (e.g., relaxation training, cognitive–behavioral therapy). When these methods fail or are ineffective, spinal cord stimulation (SCS) and an intrathecal pump (ITP) are potentially beneficial treatment options for people with severe intractable pain.

SCS with implantable or externalized systems has been available since the 1960s (Shealy, Mortimer, & Reswick, 1967). The theoretical basis of the efficacy of SCS is Melzack and Wall's (1965) gate control theory, which proposes that stimulation of large nerve fibers overrides the transmission of small nerve fibers that transmit pain. SCS is expected to reduce, not eliminate, pain by blocking the conduction of primary nerve pathways (North & Linderoth, 2010). It seems to be most successful in relieving pain in the limbs (e.g., leg, arm). Throughout the years, improvements in SCS systems have allowed for better coverage of painful areas with multiple channels, electrode surfaces with an increased number of contacts, and leads that are shaped to provide varying degrees of coverage. Spinal cord stimulators have had reported success rates ranging from 20% to 70% (Kemler et al., 2000). They have been found to be efficacious for neuropathic pain (Monhemius & Simpson, 2003) and radiculopathy (Hassenbusch, Stanton-Hicks, & Covington, 1995). Recent reviews have noted the rapid increase in the number of implanted SCSs, with annual estimates in the 10,000 to 20,000 range (Sparkes et al., 2010), and some econometric analyses have indicated that SCS may be a cost-effective treatment option, particularly for patients with persistent neuropathic pain syndromes (Simpson, Duenas, Holmes, Papaioannow, & Chilcott, 2009).

Spinal infusion of analgesics, by means of an ITP, has been used since the 1980s (Harbaugh & Reeder, 1984). Spinally administered analgesics were initially used for treatment of cancer pain (Onofrio, Yaksh, & Arnold, 1981), and with the subsequent development of implantable components for continuous intrathecal infusions became an acceptable method to treat patients with intractable cancer pain (Hassenbusch et al., 1990). Basically, this technology consists of implanting a drug delivery device designed for long-term continuous infusion of medication. The pump consists of a collapsible drug reservoir into which the drug is injected; powered by a battery and computer chip, it allows for variable infusion rates and bolus injections through a catheter anchored in the back (Osenbach, 2010). Such infusions for malignant pain have good success rates (defined as a reduction of pain by one third), ranging from 60% to 90% (Onofrio & Yaksh, 1990). Collectively, intrathecal infusion devices have provided pain relief in noncancer pain patients for whom more conservative therapies had failed (Hassenbusch, Stanton-Hicks, Soukup, Covington, & Boland, 1991), and patients with an ITP have demonstrated a reduction in side effects from oral medications, decreased need for oral analgesia, and improvement in their physical assessment (Anderson & Burchiel, 1999). The data have indicated variable success rates for noncancer pain ranging from 25% to 70% (Kumar, Kelly, & Pirlot, 2001; Roberts, Finch, Goucke, & Price, 2001).

Although outcome studies have reported that SCS and ITPs are efficacious in treating chronic pain, decisions for implantation have historically been based on clinical judgment. Recent empirical work, though, has begun to investigate the clinical characteristics that are associated with outcomes for implantable devices. Hassenbusch et al. (1995) compared SCS with intrathecal infusions by measuring postoperation verbal numeric scores and activity levels. The findings suggested that ITPs were useful in reducing bilateral or axial pain (e.g., pain just in the low back), while SCS was better for unilateral radicular symptoms (e.g., pain down one leg stemming from nerve damage in the back). In general, patients considered for an implantable device are often not seen as surgery candidates because of either previous failed surgery or lack of clear pathology accounting for the pain and have failed to respond to conservative approaches and long-term use of oral opioids.

Implantation of these devices, however, is not without risks. Reports of infection or intrathecal inflammatory masses (granulomas) have been documented (Deer, Raso, & Garten, 2007), and the safety of these devices for use with chronic noncancer pain patients is an important consideration. The risks associated with SCS include possible nerve injury, spinal cord puncture, bleeding, and infection. Similar risks also exist for ITPs, including discomfort at the implantation site, as well as possible disconnections, kinking, migration of the catheter, and granulomas that build up at the tip of the catheter. Risks also include increased depression if the device becomes ineffective in reducing pain (Osenbach, 2010). Because of the risks associated with implantation of these devices, as well as their substantial costs, a good deal of emphasis has been placed on patient selection. As noted earlier, some studies have focused on identifying pain phenotypes that are most responsive to implantable therapies (Hassenbusch et al., 1995; Osenbach, 2010); other areas of investigation have included evaluation of psychosocial factors that might predict success or failure of stimulators or pumps. Thus, a careful evaluation of each candidate for an implantable device is judged to be important, and in clinical practice a psychological evaluation is often a recommended or mandatory part of the evaluation process for patients being considered for implantable pain management devices.

REVIEW OF THE LITERATURE ON OUTCOMES

Given the significant interpatient variability in treatment outcomes, it would be of tremendous value, from both a societal and a patient perspective, to identify in advance who is most and least likely to benefit from an implanted device. In general, some risk factors have been identified that correlate with greater risk for pain or poor outcomes from treatment for pain. These risk factors include variables such as pain chronicity, psychological distress, a history of abuse or trauma, poor social support, and significant cognitive deficits (Tunks, Crook, & Weir, 2008). In particular, psychopathology, extreme emotionality, or both have been seen as contraindications for certain therapies (Main & Spanswick, 2000). Outcome studies have highlighted the poor response of patients with psychiatric comorbidity (which is quite prevalent in the context of chronic pain; Fishbain, 1999) to many treatments (Evers, Kraaimaat, Van Reil, & Bijlsma, 2001). For example, spinal pain patients with both anxiety and depression have a 62% worse return-to-work rate than those with no psychopathology (Boersma & Linton, 2005).

Epidemiologic research has suggested a bidirectional association between back pain and emotional distress; pain increases symptoms of depression, and individuals with a preexisting depressive disorder have a disproportionately high risk for developing spine pain (Edwards, Cahalan, Mensing, Smith, & Haythornthwaite, 2011). Similarly, cognitive processes such as maladaptive beliefs and pessimistic expectations are associated with a greater likelihood of developing chronic pain and with poorer functional outcomes among patients with chronic low back pain (Harkins, Price, & Braith, 1989).

Overall, numerous factors are likely to play a role in shaping back pain outcomes after surgical interventions. However, no consensus seems to exist on what factors are the strongest and most consistently predictive of outcomes, and certainly no accepted gold-standard approach exists for screening surgical candidates, although a presurgical psychological evaluation is often recommended on the basis of research on such evaluations with spine patients (Block, Gatchell, Deardorff, & Guyer, 2003; North & Linderoth, 2010).

Using critical appraisal and strategies to limit bias, Celestin, Edwards, and Jamison (2009) carried out a systematic review of the current literature to determine the strength of the evidence for the assumption that careful screening will help to predict pain-related and functional outcomes from lumbar surgery or SCS. Of 753 studies, 25 were identified, of which none were randomized controlled trials and only four met inclusion criteria. The methodological quality of the studies varied, and some important shortcomings were identified. Collectively, however, a statistically significant relationship was found between psychological factors and treatment outcome (e.g., high preimplant levels of distress were prospectively associated with less SCS-related pain relief) in 92.0% of the studies reviewed. In particular, presurgical somatization, depression, anxiety, and poor coping were most useful in helping to predict poor response (i.e., less treatment-related benefit) to lumbar surgery and SCS. Older age and longer pain duration were also predictive of poorer outcome in some studies, and pretreatment physical findings, activity interference, and pain intensity were minimally predictive. Several additional studies have, interestingly, confirmed that younger patients treated earlier in the course of their pain condition derive the most benefit from SCS (Kumar, Rizvi, & Bnurs, 2011), which might suggest that using SCS as a last resort could be a suboptimal management strategy.

Even though Celestin et al. (2009) determined that the empirical evidence that psychological screening before device implantation helps to improve treatment outcomes was insufficient, the results of the review suggested that psychological factors are predictive of outcome of treatment. An even more recent review (Sparkes et al., 2010) of psychosocial characteristics as predictors of outcomes after SCS highlighted the fairly small empirical literature in this area, while noting that depression appears to be the psychosocial factor that is most robustly linked to SCS outcomes. Indeed,

Sparkes et al. (2010) cited a total of six studies suggesting that higher levels of preimplantation depressive symptoms have a negative impact on the efficacy of SCS treatment. However, some studies have suggested that successful SCS implantation that reduces 50% of pain can improve symptoms of depression associated with chronic pain (Jamison et al., 2008).

COMPONENTS OF PSYCHOLOGICAL EVALUATIONS

Generally speaking, the goal of an implanted device for pain is to reduce pain by at least 50%. Other potential positive outcomes from an implanted device for pain include (a) relying less on prescription medication, (b) improving activities of daily living, and (c) returning individuals to productive lifestyles and back to work. A psychological evaluation is designed to help identify the right patient to achieve maximum benefit from an implanted device. In the United States, Medicare and many health insurance companies require implant candidates to have a psychological evaluation. As part of the evaluation, patients need to be informed of the risks as well as the possible benefits of the device and to address realistic expectations. For SCS and ITPs, patients undergo a trial designed to determine the likely efficacy of a permanent implant. For SCS, the trial consists of temporary placement of a stimulator lead for 4 to 10 days, and a successful trial, often required by Medicare and third-party payers, includes a 50% reduction in self-reported pain and overall patient satisfaction. For ITP patients, the trial is often conducted during a brief inpatient stay. It is important to remind patients with an ITP that they need to return periodically to refill their pump and patients with SCS that their time using the device directly affects battery longevity. Showing a model of the device so that the patients can hold it and understand its mechanism of action can be important. Also, open discussion of any concerns about having a device implanted can be useful. Some SCS patients may have some loss of normal sensation, and having future MRIs is generally contraindicated. For any device, future revisions or explants may be necessary in the event of infection or other potentially severe complication.

Psychological evaluations should include the assessment of sensory, affective, cognitive, and behavioral components of the pain experience, expectations of the benefit of an implanted device, and identification of personality and psychosocial factors that can influence treatment outcome (Jamison et al., 2011). The sensory experience is usually best understood through description of the severity, location, and temporal characteristics of chronic pain. Distressing emotional qualities of the experience of pain as well as preexisting emotional dispositions need to be understood, because fear (Vlaeyen & Linton, 2000) and depression (Edwards, Cahalan, et al., 2011) are powerful determinants of the response and emotional reactions to pain, related disability, and care. Patterns of thinking may exacerbate and maintain dysfunctional pain as well as facilitate coping that enhances adjustment during painful flare-ups. The extent to which chronic pain interferes with activities of daily living or contributes to substantial functional impairment varies. Clinicians have long relied on careful appraisal of nonverbal behavior in the course of physical examinations and through observation of patients outside the examining situation, for example, when engaged in spontaneous behavior elsewhere in clinics or in everyday situations. Self-report can also be useful in assessing nonverbal behavior by focusing on overt activity rather than subjective experience, for example, functional capacity or competence and disability in different situations. Finally, family socialization and important life experiences influence both effective and ineffective patterns of attempts to cope with pain. History gathering is typically the primary source of this information. Ethnic and cultural variation and family history of managing pain and illness may be of importance. For example, when significant others in a person's family have had a history of recurrent, persistent, or particularly severe pain, the patient may be disposed to similar patterns (Hermann, Hohmeister, Zohsel, Ebinger, & Flor, 2007).

Of comparable importance are current social contexts. Patients experiencing social distress (e.g., with employers, family members, or others) either directly related (e.g., reduced employment, isolation from the community) or unrelated (e.g., financial distress, difficult relationships) to painful episodes are likely to increase demands on the health care system. Furthermore, the presence of a supportive social environment is associated with lower levels of pain and less physical disability after surgical intervention (Hack et al., 2010).

Although clinicians must be aware of the objectives of referral sources, patients are similarly typically carefully attuned to the expectations and goals of referral agencies and those engaged in the assessment. Patients frustrated with lack of success in treating pain or provision of financial and other support when unable to earn a livelihood bring different concerns to the assessment than patients who are not worried by such situations and expect that the assessment will lead to effective care. Long histories of inadequate care or denial of care are more likely to lead to hostile behavior.

VALIDATED PSYCHOLOGICAL MEASURES

A psychological evaluation should include valid and reliable assessments of subjective pain intensity, mood and personality, activity interference, pain beliefs, and coping. The following categories include some popular assessment tools used to measure these constructs.

Pain Intensity

Because one of the obvious primary goals of an implanted device for chronic pain is to decrease pain intensity, it is important to monitor pain intensity both before and throughout the course of a device trial, using multiple measures. Empirically validated measures include visual analogue scales (Jensen & Karoly, 2001), electronic pain ratings to obtain time-stamped multiple assessments of pain in the patient's natural environment (Jamison et al., 2002; Marceau, Link, Smith, Carolan, & Jamison, 2010), and verbal scales used to describe the quality of pain (e.g., piercing, stabbing, shooting, burning, throbbing; Jamison, Vasterling, & Parris, 1987).

Mood and Personality

Patients with chronic pain often report depression, anxiety, irritability, a history of physical or sexual abuse, or a past history of a mood disorder (Andersson, 1999; Jamison, 1996). As many as one half of patients with chronic pain have a comorbid psychiatric condition, and 35% of patients with chronic back and neck pain have a comorbid depression or anxiety disorder (Von Korff et al., 2005). In surveys of chronic pain clinic populations, 50% to 80% of patients with chronic pain had signs of psychopathology, making this the most prevalent comorbidity among these patients (Kalso, Edwards, Moore, & McQuay, 2004). The measures most commonly used to evaluate personality and emotional distress include the Minnesota Multiphasic Personality Inventory (Hathaway et al., 1989), a restructured form of the Minnesota Multiphasic Personality Inventory—2 (Ben-Porath & Tellegen, 2008), the Symptom Checklist—90—Revised (Derogatis, 1977), the Beck Depression Inventory (Beck, Ward, Mendelson, Mock, & Erbaugh, 1961), and the Hospital Anxiety and Depression Scale (Zigmond & Snaith, 1983).

Functional Capacity and Activity Interference

Most clinicians consider pain reduction meaningless unless it is accompanied by a noticeable change in function. Measures that can be used to assess activity level and function include the Short-Form Health Survey (Ware & Sherbourne, 1992), the West Haven-Yale Multidimensional Pain Inventory (Kerns, Turk, & Rudy, 1985), and the Pain Disability Index (Pollard, 1984).

Pain Beliefs and Coping

Pain perception, beliefs about pain, and coping mechanisms are important in predicting the outcome of treatment and are particularly relevant as predictors for the success of implantable devices. Unrealistic or negative thoughts about an ongoing pain problem may contribute to increased pain and emotional distress, decreased functioning, and greater reliance on medication. Certain chronic pain patients are prone to maladaptive beliefs about their condition that may not be compatible with the physical nature of their pain (DeGood & Shutty, 1992; Jamison, 1996). Several self-report measures assess coping and pain attitudes. The most popular tests used to measure maladaptive beliefs include the Coping Strategies Questionnaire (Rosenstiel & Keefe, 1983), the Pain Management Inventory (Brown, Nicassion, & Wallston, 1989), the Pain Self-Efficacy Questionnaire (Lorig, Chastain, Ung, Shoor, & Holman, 1989), the Survey of Pain Attitudes (Karoly & Jensen, 1987), and the Inventory of Negative Thoughts in Response to Pain (Gil, Williams, Keefe, & Beckham, 1990). Finally, the Pain Catastrophizing Scale (Sullivan & Pivik, 1995) is a well-validated, widely used self-report measure of catastrophic thinking associated with pain (Edwards, Giles, et al., 2011). The construct of catastrophizing incorporates magnification of pain-related symptoms, rumination about pain, feelings of helplessness, and pessimism about pain-related outcomes. Patients who have a high catastrophizing score, who endorse passive coping on the Pain Management Inventory, who demonstrate low self-efficacy regarding their ability to manage their pain on the Pain Self-Efficacy Questionnaire, who describe themselves as disabled by their pain on the Survey of Pain Attitudes, and who report frequent negative thoughts about their pain on the Inventory of Negative Thoughts in Response to Pain are at greatest risk for poor treatment outcome from an implanted device.

Recent studies have also suggested that quantitative sensory testing may be a useful adjunct to psychological evaluation in the assessment of patients under consideration for a stimulator or pump. Quantitative sensory testing involves the administration of standardized noxious stimuli under highly controlled conditions; often, parameters such as pain threshold and tolerance in response to a variety of stimulus modalities are measured as indices of pain sensitivity. Edwards, Wasan, et al. (2011) recently reported that high levels of pain sensitivity may be associated with elevated risk for pain medication misuse, and individual differences in quantitative sensory testing responses may be useful as prognostic indicators in a variety of settings. For example, among patients with neuropathic pain undergoing SCS, the degree of pretrial mechanical allodynia was inversely associated with the amount of pain relief reported by patients (van Eijs et al., 2010). That is, the most mechanosensitive patients reported the least SCS-related analgesic benefit. Functional neuroimaging studies have revealed that SCS functions in part by activating cortical pain-modulatory circuitry (Stancák et al., 2008), and the most preoperatively pain-sensitive individuals may be those whose pain-modulatory systems are the most difficult to engage. Brush-evoked allodynia (hypersensitivity to pain) also predicts outcome of SCS in complex regional pain syndrome Type 1.

CASE STUDY

Mr. Smith is a 47-year-old Caucasian man who was referred for psychological evaluation for consideration of SCS for his chronic back pain.[1] He has a 5-year history of low back and left lower extremity pain related to a work-related incident when he fell down a flight of stairs and fractured his tailbone. He was not seen as a surgery candidate but continued to report intermittent back and leg pain after that incident. He had been a construction worker for 15 years and began working as a salesman at a hardware store when he could no longer lift, bend, or climb ladders. Over time, he began experiencing severe left foot pain, which gradually progressed and interfered with his ability to work. He eventually was not able to work and applied for disability benefits.

He described his pain as a maximum of 10 on a scale ranging from 0 to 10, with an average of 7, and at its best, 5. His pain was worse with prolonged standing, sitting, walking, bending, lifting, or any type of exertion. His pain was better when lying on his right side. He described the pain as constant in nature but varying in intensity on the basis of his activity. His pain was most bothersome over the buttocks and into his left leg.

He reported having severe sleep disturbances and relied on medication for his sleep. He had problems with word retrieval, short-term memory, and concentration and admitted to being very depressed with recurrent worried thoughts, such as "How can I live the rest of my life with this pain?"

Mr. Smith was single, with no children, and lived with his father. He spent time taking care of his dog and cooking for his father. He had a high school education and technical training. Many members of his family had a significant history of alcohol dependence and mood disorder. Mr. Smith reported that he had been detoxed in a psychiatric facility on two occasions in the past and had three serious incidences of medication overdose, including once when he left a suicide note at age 21. He also had a long history of alcohol dependence and occasional cocaine use. He stated that he had been sober for 9 months. He was seeing a counselor and attending Alcoholics Anonymous meetings. He smoked approximately one pack of

---

[1]Details of this case have been altered to protect the patient's identity.

cigarettes a day. His medications included methadone, pregabalin (Lyrica), trazadone, quetiapine (Seroquel), acetaminophen (Tylenol), and ibuprofen as needed.

Mr. Smith was seen in a face-to-face interview along with his father. He ambulated to the interview room with a noticeable limp. He was verbal, alert, and oriented. He sat leaning on the right side and showed significant pain behavior during the interview session. His speech was slightly slurred, and his father stated that this was because of his medication. He did not show signs of significant emotional distress. There was no indication of any psychotic processes, and he denied any current suicidal ideation.

He was asked to complete the Beck Depression Inventory–II, and he scored a 30, which suggested significant depression. He also endorsed a number of neurovegetative symptoms including fatigue, poor appetite, loss of sexual interest, and poor sleep. He admitted to having problems with his temper, having close friends who had problems with alcohol or drugs, having a history of legal problems, and running out of his pain medication early. He was also asked to complete the Coping Strategies Questionnaire and the Pain Catastrophizing Scale, scoring a 32 on the latter, which suggested high levels of catastrophizing about pain. He showed low scores on the Coping Strategies Questionnaire subscales of Distraction and Coping Self-Statements, indicating fairly low levels of adaptive pain-coping skills.

Despite his interest in SCS for his pain, he was informed that he presented with several risk factors that could interfere with his benefiting from an implanted device, including a recent history of substance abuse, smoking cigarettes, and having a significant mood disorder. He also had recurrent negative thoughts and limited perceived support that could further affect the outcome of an implanted device.

Following his evaluation, Mr. Smith's physician was informed that he would not be a good candidate for an implanted device at this time. Instead, he would be better suited to participate in a multidisciplinary pain management approach that would also address improving his mood. Mr. Smith accepted that he needed to do something about managing his pain. He actively participated in physical therapy and individual cognitive therapy to help manage his mood disorder and recurrent negative thinking while being following by his physician for medication management and trigger point injections. He showed improvement in his mood, sleep, activity, and coping. He reduced his reliance on prescription pain medication and was carefully monitored. He did not show any aberrant drug-related behavior. He recognized that he would likely not return to his former place of employment, so he began training to be a codes inspector.

A repeat evaluation showed that despite significant pain (6 of 10), he had made a number of improvements in coping with his pain. He had stopped smoking, was engaged in a regular exercise program, and demonstrated an improvement in his mood and a decrease in recurrent worries as shown by the results of repeated testing. Six months later, he had a successful stimulator trial with a reported average pain rating ranging from 7 to 3 of 10; overall, he reported benefiting from a SCS implant. One-year follow-up showed that Mr. Smith had less pain but had periodic painful flare-ups that were managed with his SCS. He had been working part time as a codes inspector and was coping well with his condition without signs of reduced function, aberrant drug-related behavior, or mood disorder.

FUTURE AREAS OF INVESTIGATION

Electronic diaries have much promise for future psychological assessment of pain patients. They allow for improved communication between patients and providers and may be an efficient means of evaluating and tracking important clinical information related to implanted devices. With the availability of smartphones and pain assessment websites and the ability to capture time-stamped data, more clinicians are using electronic diary data to assess pain, mood, function, and adverse effects of medication. Use of daily electronic pain diaries helps clinicians understand how pain affects patients in their natural environment, known as *ecological momentary assessment*. Electronic diaries allow two-way communication between patients and providers and are an efficient means of evaluating and tracking medication use and associated symptoms (Jamison et al., 2001). Ever-changing technology will include implanted devices that will electronically detect movement, body position, and device usage and will better determine the outcome of a device trial.

The ways in which health care services are offered are changing rapidly. More and more decisions about treatment are made by employees of insurance carriers on the basis of financial resources rather than by heath care professionals on the basis of need. Brief, reliable measures are necessary to establish need for service and to monitor outcome. An increasing need for accountability and efficacy has encouraged the implementation of cost-saving measures and program evaluation.

In light of the attention given to these changes, the economic efficiency of treatment for chronic noncancer pain is worthy of discussion. Although evidence exists for the cost effectiveness of multidisciplinary therapy for chronic pain (Chapman, Jamison, Sanders, Lyman, & Lynch, 2000), such treatment may not meet the criterion of increased benefit with very little cost. Prior classification and reliable phenotyping of patients may help in identifying those individuals who will benefit most from pain therapy. No reported studies have satisfactorily addressed this issue, and outcome data are needed. Documentation of increased function and decreased health care use among certain patients as a result of pain therapy would support the continued use of implanted devices for pain management. Furthermore, a potentially exciting area of future research involves examination of whether preimplantation modification of psychosocial risk factors (e.g., alleviation of depressive symptoms with pharmacotherapy and psychotherapy) can improve the efficacy and cost-effectiveness of SCS treatment. Such findings would have substantial implications for optimizing implantable device therapy and could extend the potential benefits of these procedures to many of the most challenging high-risk chronic pain patients.

REFERENCES

Anderson, V. C., & Burchiel, K. J. (1999). A prospective study of long-term intrathecal morphine in the management of chronic nonmalignant pain. *Neurosurgery, 44,* 289–300. doi:10.1097/00006123-199902000-00026

Andersson, G. B. J. (1999). Epidemiological features of low back pain. *The Lancet, 354,* 581–585. doi:10.1016/S0140-6736(99)01312-4

Beck, A. T., Ward, C. H., Mendelson, M., Mock, J., & Erbaugh, J. (1961). An inventory for measuring depression. *Archives of General Psychiatry, 4,* 561–571. doi:10.1001/archpsyc.1961.01710120031004

Becker, A., Held, H., Redaelli, M., Strauch, K., Chenot, J. F., Leonhardt, C., . . . Donner-Banzhoff, N. (2010). Low back pain in primary care: Costs of care and prediction of future health care utilization. *Spine, 35,* 1714–1720.

Ben-Porath, Y., & Tellegen, A. (2008). *Minnesota Multiphasic Personality Inventory—2 Restructured Form: Technical manual.* Minneapolis: University of Minnesota Press.

Block, A. R., Gatchell, R. J., Deardorff, W. W., & Guyer, R. D. (2003). *The psychology of spine surgery.* Washington, DC: American Psychological Association. doi:10.1037/10613-000

Boersma, K., & Linton, S. J. (2005). Screening to identify patients at risk: Profiles of psychological risk factors for early intervention. *Clinical Journal of Pain, 21,* 38–43. doi:10.1097/00002508-200501000-00005

Brown, G. K., Nicassion, P. M., & Wallston, K. A. (1989). Pain coping strategies and depression in rheumatoid arthritis. *Journal of Consulting and Clinical Psychology, 57,* 652–657. doi:10.1037/0022-006X.57.5.652

Celestin, J., Edwards, R. R., & Jamison, R. N. (2009). Pretreatment psychosocial variables as predictors of outcomes following lumbar surgery and spinal cord stimulation: A systematic review and literature synthesis. *Pain Medicine, 10,* 639–653. doi:10.1111/j.1526-4637.2009.00632.x

Chapman, S. L., Jamison, R. N., Sanders, S. H., Lyman, D. R., & Lynch, N. T. (2000). Perceived treatment helpfulness and cost in chronic pain rehabilitation. *Clinical Journal of Pain, 16,* 169–177. doi:10.1097/00002508-200006000-00011

Deer, T. R., Raso, L. J., & Garten, T. G. (2007). Inflammatory mass of an intrathecal catheter in patients receiving baclofen as a sole agent: A report of two cases and a review of the identification and treatment of the complication. *Pain Medicine, 8,* 259–262. doi:10.1111/j.1526-4637.2006.00150.x

DeGood, D. E., & Shutty, M. S. (1992). Assessment of pain beliefs, coping, and self-efficacy. In D. C. Turk & R. Melzack (Eds.), *Handbook of pain assessment* (pp. 214–)234). New York, NY: Guilford Press.

Derogatis, L. (1977). *SCL–90—R (revised version) administration, scoring, and procedure manual.* Baltimore, MD: Johns Hopkins School of Medicine Press.

Edwards, R. R., Cahalan, C., Mensing, G., Smith, M., & Haythornthwaite, J. A. (2011). Pain, catastrophizing, and depression in the rheumatic diseases. *Nature Reviews Rheumatology, 7,* 216–224. doi:10.1038/nrrheum.2011.2

Edwards, R. R., Giles, J., Bingham, C. O., Campbell, C. M., Haythornwaite, J. A., & Bathon, J. (2010). Moderators of the negative effects of catastrophizing in arthritis. *Pain Medicine, 11,* 591–599.

Edwards, R. R., Wasan, A., Michna, E., Greenbaum, S., Ross, E., & Jamison, R. N. (2011). Elevated pain sensitivity in chronic pain patients at risk for opioid misuse. *Journal of Pain, 12,* 953–963. doi:10.1016/j.jpain.2011.02.357

Ehrlich, G. E. (2003). Back pain. *Journal of Rheumatology, 67*(Suppl.), 26–31.

Evers, A. W. M., Kraaimaat, F. W., Van Reil, P. L. C. M., & Bijlsma, J. W. J. (2001). Cognitive, behavioral and physiological reactivity to pain as a predictor of long-term pain in rheumatoid arthritis patients. *Pain, 93,* 139–146. doi:10.1016/S0304-3959(01)00303-7

Ferrari, R., & Russell, A. S. (2003). Regional musculoskeletal conditions: Neck pain. *Best Practice & Research Clinical Rheumatology, 17,* 57–70. doi:10.1016/S1521-6942(02)00097-9

Fishbain, D. A. (1999). Approaches to treatment decisions for psychiatric comorbidity in the management of the chronic pain patient. *Medical Clinics of North America, 83,* 737–760. doi:10.1016/S0025-7125(05)70132-2

Gil, K., Williams, D. A., Keefe, F. J., & Beckham, J. C. (1990). The relationship of negative thoughts to pain and psychological distress. *Behavior Therapy, 21,* 349–362. doi:10.1016/S0005-7894(05)80336-3

Hack, T. F., Kwan, W. B., Thomas-Maclean, R. L., Towers, A., Miedema, B., Tilley, A., & Chateau, D. (2010). Predictors of arm morbidity following breast cancer surgery. *Psycho-Oncology, 19,* 1205–1212. doi:10.1002/pon.1685

Harbaugh, R. E., & Reeder, T. M. (1984). Continuous drug delivery by an implantable pump. *American Journal of Hospice Care, 1,* 17–20. doi:10.1177/104990918400100215

Harkins, S. W., Price, D. D., & Braith, J. (1989). Effects of extraversion and neuroticism on experimental pain, clinical pain, and illness behavior. *Pain, 36*, 209–218. doi:10.1016/0304-3959(89)90025-0

Hassenbusch, S. J., Pillay, P. K., Magdinec, M., Currie, K., Bay, J. W., Covington, E. C., & Tomaszewski, M. Z. (1990). Constant infusion of morphine for intractable cancer pain using an implanted pump. *Journal of Neurosurgery, 73*, 405–409. doi:10.3171/jns.1990.73.3.0405

Hassenbusch, S. J., Stanton-Hicks, M., & Covington, E. C. (1995). Spinal cord stimulation versus spinal infusion for low back and leg pain. *Acta Neurochirurgica, 64*(Suppl.), 109–115. doi:10.1007/978-3-7091-9419-5_24

Hassenbusch, S. J., Stanton-Hicks, M. D., Soukup, J., Covington, E. C., & Boland, M. B. (1991). Sufentanil citrate and morphine/bupivacaine as alternative agents in chronic epidural infusions for intractable non-cancer pain. *Neurosurgery, 29*, 76–81. doi:10.1227/00006123-199107000-00013

Hathaway, S. R., McKinley, J. C., Butcher, J. N., Dahlstrom, W. G., Graham, J. R., & Tellegen, A. (1989). *Minnesota Multiphasic Personality Inventory—2: Manual for administration.* Minneapolis: University of Minnesota Press.

Hermann, C., Hohmeister, J., Zohsel, K., Ebinger, F., & Flor, H. (2007). The assessment of pain coping and pain-related cognitions in children and adolescents: Current methods and further development. *Journal of Pain, 8*, 802–813. doi:10.1016/j.jpain.2007.05.010

Hoy, D., March, L., Brooks, P., Woolf, A., Blyth, F., Vos, T., & Buchbinder, R. (2010). Measuring the global burden of low back pain. *Best Practice & Research Clinical Rheumatology, 24*, 155–165. doi:10.1016/j.berh.2009.11.002

Jamison, R. N. (1996). *Mastering chronic pain: A professional's guide to behavioral treatment.* Sarasota, FL: Professional Resource Press.

Jamison, R. N., Gracely, R. H., Raymond, S. A., Levine, J. G., Marino, B., Herrmann, T. J., . . . Katz, N. P. (2002). Comparative study of electronic vs. paper VAS ratings: A randomized, crossover trial using healthy volunteers. *Pain, 99*, 341–347. doi:10.1016/S0304-3959(02)00178-1

Jamison, R. N., Raymond, S. A., Levine, J. G., Slawsby, E. A., Nedeljkovic, S. S., & Katz, N. P. (2001). Electronic diaries for monitoring chronic pain: 1-year validation study. *Pain, 91*, 277–285. doi:10.1016/S0304-3959(00)00450-4

Jamison, R. N., Vasterling, J. J., & Parris, W. C. (1987). Use of sensory descriptors in assessing chronic pain patients. *Journal of Psychosomatic Research, 31*, 647–652. doi:10.1016/0022-3999(87)90044-4

Jamison, R. N., Washington, T. A., Fanciullo, G. J., Ross, E. L., McHugo, G. J., & Baird, J. C. (2008). Do implantable devices improve mood? Comparisons of chronic pain patients with or without an implantable device. *Neuromodulation, 11*, 260–266.

Jamison, R. N., Washington, T. A., Padma, G., Fanciullo, G. J., Arscott, J. R., McHugo, G. J., . . . Baird, J. C. (2011). Reliability of a preliminary 3-D pain mapping program. *Pain Medicine, 12*, 344–351. doi:10.1111/j.1526-4637.2010.01049.x

Jensen, M. P., & Karoly, P. (1991). Motivation and expectancy factor in symptom perception: A laboratory study of the placebo effect. *Psychosomatic Medicine*, *53*, 144–152.

Jensen, M. P., & Karoly, P. (2001). Self-report scales and procedures for assessing pain in adults. In D. C. Turk & R. Melzack (Eds.), *Handbook of pain assessment* (2nd ed., pp. 15–34). New York, NY: Guilford Press.

Kalso, E., Edwards, J. E., Moore, R. A., & McQuay, H. J. (2004). Opioids in chronic non-cancer pain: Systematic review of efficacy and safety. *Pain*, *112*, 372–380. doi:10.1016/j.pain.2004.09.019

Karoly, P., & Jensen, M. P. (1987). *Multimethod assessment of chronic pain*. New York, NY: Pergamon Press.

Kemler, M. A., Barendse, G. A. M., van Kleef, M., de Vet, H. C. W., Rijks, C. P. M., Furnée, C. A., & van den Wildenberg, F. A. J. M. (2000). Spinal cord stimulation in patients with chronic reflex sympathetic dystrophy. *New England Journal of Medicine*, *343*, 618–624. doi:10.1056/NEJM200008313430904

Kerns, R. D., Turk, D. C., & Rudy, T. E. (1985). The West Haven-Yale Multidimensional Pain Inventory (WHYMPI). *Pain*, *23*, 345–356. doi:10.1016/0304-3959(85)90004-1

Kumar, K., Kelly, M., & Pirlot, T. (2001). Continuous intrathecal morphine treatment for chronic pain of nonmalignant etiology: Long-term benefits and efficacy. *Surgical Neurology*, *55*, 79–86. doi:10.1016/S0090-3019(01)00353-6

Kumar, K., Rizvi, S., & Bnurs, S. B. (2011). Spinal cord stimulation is effective in management of complex regional pain syndrome I: Fact or fiction. *Neurosurgery*, *69*, 566–578. doi:10.1227/NEU.0b013e3182181e60

Lorig, K., Chastain, R. L., Ung, E., Shoor, S., & Holman, H. R. (1989). Development and evaluation of a scale to measure perceived self-efficacy in people with arthritis. *Arthritis and Rheumatism*, *32*, 37–44. doi:10.1002/anr.1780320107

Main, C. J., & Spanswick, C. C. (2000). *Pain management: An interdisciplinary approach*. New York, NY: Churchill Livingstone.

Marceau, L. D., Link, C. L., Smith, L. D., Carolan, S. J., & Jamison, R. N. (2010). In-clinic use of electronic pain diaries: Barriers of implementation among pain physicians. *Journal of Pain and Symptom Management*, *40*, 391–404. doi:10.1016/j.jpainsymman.2009.12.021

Melzack, R., & Wall, P. D. (1965). Pain mechanisms: A new theory. *Science*, *150*, 971–979. doi:10.1126/science.150.3699.971

Monhemius, R., & Simpson, B. A. (2003). Efficacy of spinal cord stimulation for neuropathic pain: assessment by abstinence. *European Journal of Pain*, *7*, 513–519. doi:10.1016/S1090-3801(03)00023-5

North, R. B., & Linderoth, B. (2010). Spinal cord stimulation. In S. M. Fishman, J. C. Ballantyne, & J. P. Rathmell (Eds.), *Bonica's management of pain* (4th ed., pp. 1379–1392). Philadelphia, PA: Lippincott Williams & Wilkins.

Onofrio, B. M., & Yaksh, T. L. (1990). Long-term pain relief produced by intrathecal morphine infusion in 53 patients. *Journal of Neurosurgery, 72,* 200–209. doi:10.3171/jns.1990.72.2.0200

Onofrio, B. M., Yaksh, T. L., & Arnold, P. G. (1981). Continuous low-dose intrathecal morphine administration in the treatment of chronic pain of malignant origin. *Mayo Clinic Proceedings, 56,* 516–520.

Osenbach, R. K. (2010). Intrathecal drug delivery in the management of pain. In S. M. Fishman, J. C. Ballantyne, & J. P. Rathmell (Eds.), *Bonica's management of pain* (4th ed., pp. 1437–1458). Philadelphia, PA: Lippincott Williams & Wilkins.

Otis, J. D., Cardella, L. A., & Kerns, R. D. (2004). The influence of family and culture on pain. In R. H. Dworkin & W. S. Breitbart (Eds.), *Psychosocial aspects of pain: A handbook for health care providers* (pp. 29–45). Seattle, WA: IASP Press.

Pollard, C. A. (1984). Preliminary validity study of the Pain Disability Index. *Perceptual and Motor Skills, 59,* 974. doi:10.2466/pms.1984.59.3.974

Roberts, L. J., Finch, P. M., Goucke, C. R., & Price, L. M. (2001). Outcome of intrathecal opioids in chronic non-cancer pain. *European Journal of Pain, 5,* 353–361. doi:10.1053/eujp.2001.0255

Rosenstiel, A. K., & Keefe, F. J. (1983). The use of coping strategies in chronic low back pain patients: Relationship to patient characteristics and current adjustment. *Pain, 17,* 33–44. doi:10.1016/0304-3959(83)90125-2

Shealy, C. N., Mortimer, J. T., & Reswick, J. B. (1967). Electrical inhibition of pain by stimulation of dorsa columns: Preliminary clinical report. *Anesthesia and Analgesia, 46,* 489–491. doi:10.1213/00000539-196707000-00025

Simpson, E. L., Duenas, A., Holmes, M. W., Papaioannow, D., & Chilcott, J. (2009). Spinal cord stimulation for chronic pain of neuropathic or ischaemic origin: Systematic review and economic evaluation. *Health Technology Assessment, 13*(17), iii, ix–x, 1–154.

Sparkes, E., Raphael, J. H., Duarte, R. V., LeMarchand, K., Jackson, C., & Ashford, R. L. (2010). A systematic literature review of psychological characteristics as determinants of outcome for spinal cord stimulation therapy. *Pain, 150,* 284–289. doi:10.1016/j.pain.2010.05.001

Stancák, A., Kozák, J., Vrba, I., Tintěra, J., Vrána, J., Polácek, H., & Stancák, M. (2008). Functional magnetic resonance imaging of cerebral activation during spinal cord stimulation in failed back surgery syndrome patients. *European Journal of Pain, 12,* 137–148. doi:10.1016/j.ejpain.2007.03.003

Sullivan, M. J., & Pivik, J. (1995). The Pain Catastrophizing Scale: Development and validation. *Psychological Assessment, 7,* 524–532. doi:10.1037/1040-3590.7.4.524

Tunks, E. R., Crook, J., & Weir, R. (2008). Epidemiology of chronic pain with psychological comorbidity: Prevalence, risk, course, and prognosis. *Canadian Journal of Psychiatry, 53,* 224–234.

Van Eijs, F., Smits, H., Geurts, J. W., Kessels, A. G. H., Kemler, M. A., van Kleef, M., . . . Faber, C. G. (2010). Brush-evoked allodynia also predicts outcome of spinal cord stimulation in complex regional pain syndrome type I. *European Journal of Pain, 14*, 164–169. doi:10.1016/j.ejpain.2009.10.009

Vlaeyen, J. W., & Linton, S. J. (2000). Fear-avoidance and its consequences in chronic musculoskeletal pain: A state of the art. *Pain, 85*, 317–332. doi:10.1016/S0304-3959(99)00242-0

Von Korff, M., Crane, P., Lane, M., Miglioretti, G. L., Simon, G., Saunders, K., . . . Kessler, R. (2005). Chronic spinal pain and physical-mental comorbidity in the United States: results from the National Comorbidity Survey Replication. *Pain, 113*, 331–339. doi:10.1016/j.pain.2004.11.010

Ware, J. E., & Sherbourne, C. D. (1992). The MOS 36-item short-form health survey (SF-36). I. Conceptual framework and item selection. *Medical Care, 30*, 473–483. doi:10.1097/00005650-199206000-00002

Zigmond, A. S., & Snaith, R. P. (1983). The Hospital Anxiety and Depression Scale. *Acta Psychiatrica Scandinavica, 67*, 361–370. doi:10.1111/j.1600-0447.1983.tb09716.x

5

BONE MARROW
AND STEM CELL TRANSPLANT

JANE E. AUSTIN AND CHRISTINE RINI

Bone marrow and stem cell transplantation, also known as *hematopoietic stem cell transplant* (HSCT), is an aggressive treatment used for hematological cancers and other disorders. Despite advances that have improved survival rates, it remains a risky treatment associated with physical and psychological challenges as well as considerable early mortality and morbidity (Copelan, 2006; Pasquini & Wang, 2010). Not only do transplant recipients face a rigorous conditioning regimen involving high-dose chemotherapy (possibly with total body irradiation), painful side effects, lengthy hospitalization, and social isolation due to immunosuppression, but during the protracted recovery they also face the possibility of further physical complications, such as organ toxicity, infections, and graft-versus-host disease.

Understandably, transplant recipients also report psychological distress. For many recipients, distress is highest at admission and during hospitalization, subsequently diminishing over time (Fife et al., 2000); however,

DOI: 10.1037/14035-006
Presurgical Psychological Screening: Understanding Patients, Improving Outcomes, Andrew R. Block and
David B. Sarwer (Editors)

research has indicated that more than 40% of recipients experience clinical or subclinical distress as many as 10 years posttransplant (Mosher, Redd, Rini, Burkhalter, & DuHamel, 2009). Other adverse psychosocial effects of HSCT include delayed return to work, sexual dysfunction, body image concerns, sleep disturbance, fatigue, and relationship issues (Andrykowski et al., 1999).

Yet adverse effects of transplant vary across recipients. Medical risk factors that help explain this variability are increasingly well understood. In addition, a small body of research has identified psychosocial factors linked to survival, quality of life, and psychological adjustment. These medical and psychosocial risk factors are primary targets for pretransplant screening, which is typically undertaken in this population to reduce mortality and morbidity (e.g., by identifying patients who require prophylactic medical treatment and supplementary psychosocial services). Although seemingly less common, screening can sometimes identify reasons to disqualify a patient from proceeding with transplant. Screening in HSCT is less well characterized than screening in other medical areas, and the roles of mental health professionals in these settings also vary greatly. Mental health professionals may screen all candidates before transplant and serve as an integral part of medical team consultations throughout the process. Conversely, some sites employ mental health professionals to field referrals from the medical team only when psychological concerns become apparent. As we discuss, the high degree of variability across treatment centers highlights the need to establish empirically based best practices.

In this chapter, our primary focus is on psychosocial research and its implications for screening. First, we review the reasons for pretransplant psychosocial screening. Next, we describe the medical and psychosocial aspects of transplant and outline risk factors for poor outcomes. We then discuss the importance of developing goals to guide assessment strategies. Finally, we conclude with approaches to assessment, including relevant instruments, a case study highlighting the application of several important prescreening concepts, and a discussion of challenges, recommendations, and future directions.

NEED FOR SCREENING IN HEMATOPOIETIC STEM CELL TRANSPLANT

Because HSCT is often the last-chance treatment option, psychological prescreening for HSCT rarely involves the question of whether a patient will go forward with transplant, except in extreme cases such as addiction, active psychosis, absence of caregiving resources, or suicidal ideation. For instance, one survey of HSCT physicians, social workers, and nurses provided various patient scenarios and then collected information on whether the transplant process should proceed (Foster et al., 2006). Findings revealed some agreement not to proceed when active suicidal ideation, substance abuse, history of noncompliance, lack of social support, or dementia was present. However, actual clinical decisions appear to be made on a case-by-case basis considering the severity of a patient's situation, often with the recommendation to seek care to remedy the issue at hand rather than outright refusal. Potentially problematic conditions identified with screening, therefore, are more likely to be viewed as red flags than as an indication to discontinue the transplant procedure.

Transplant site requirements appear to have a high degree of variability, and no standardized protocol exists (Hamadani, Craig, Awan, & Devine, 2010). Yet the fact that many or perhaps most transplant centers include psychosocial factors in their pretransplant screening protocols may demonstrate general recognition that psychosocial screening can be beneficial for understanding a patient's strengths and vulnerabilities. Most notably, findings can help the transplant team anticipate and address challenges to help reduce adverse patient outcomes.

A primary reason to conduct psychosocial screening is that it enables at-risk transplant recipients to be referred for services that can mitigate their specific areas of risk. For instance, although patients' psychological distress can have a negative impact on medical adherence (Kennard et al., 2004) and quality of life (Andrykowski et al., 1999), it may be successfully treated through psychological interventions, medication, or both (e.g., Holland et al., 2010). Although a detailed review of psychological interventions is beyond the scope of this chapter, a variety of approaches to address these difficulties are discussed. Interventions involving patient education, coping strategies such as relaxation training and cognitive–behavioral techniques, support groups, and psychotherapy have shown benefit for oncology patients, although reviews of interventions have cautioned that more evidence-based studies are needed to determine effectiveness (e.g., Fawzy, 1999; Lepore & Coyne; 2006; Stanton, 2006).

PHYSICAL AND PSYCHOSOCIAL ASPECTS OF HEMATOPOEITIC STEM CELL TRANSPLANT

Understanding the physical and psychosocial challenges many HSCT recipients face over time may help guide pretransplant screening so that clinicians can foresee problems and address risks. Thus, screening may focus on problems that could arise in the relatively near term (e.g., determining eligibility for transplant or uncovering risks that affect impending procedures and short-term outcomes). It could also prove useful in anticipating longer term sequelae of HSCT. Psychosocial research exploring HSCT-related emotional distress and quality-of-life concerns (physical, social roles, and relationships) is discussed later. Of note is the fact that the physical challenges of HSCT are likely to be emotionally distressing to transplant recipients, and conversely, psychosocial problems could also cause poor physical outcomes.

Physical Demands of Transplant and Recovery

HSCT is performed when problems with bone marrow functioning occur, as is the case with various hematological cancers (e.g., leukemias, multiple myeloma, non-Hodgkin's lymphoma), some solid tumors, metabolic disorders, and other diseases. Its use has been increasing steadily for years (Gratwohl et al., 2007, 2010), and that trend is expected to continue as advances allow it to be used in new patient populations. Transplant recipients may go through a myeloablative transplant process whereby high doses of chemotherapy are used to destroy the disease before transplantation of stem cells, sometimes accompanied by total body irradiation. Because of the high-intensity preparative regimen, the immune system is also destroyed, and strict precautions are necessary to prevent infection. Alternatively, nonmyeloablative or reduced-intensity transplants may be appropriate for individuals who are unable to tolerate high doses of chemotherapy or radiation or whose diseases may be treated with a less rigorous approach.

For some diseases, it is possible for transplant recipients to donate their own cells before the preparative regimen (autologous transplant), whereas other diseases require stem cell donation from others (allogeneic transplant). After the preparative regimen, often involving iatrogenic effects such as nausea and painful mouth sores, stem cells are infused directly into the bloodstream, after which they begin the process of normalizing blood cell counts. The first 100 days are generally considered to be crucial; during this time, immune functioning is reestablished, and physical complications must be closely monitored. Hospitalized patients are placed in isolation to prevent infection until their blood counts return to appropriate levels, which may take several weeks or longer. Recovery of immune functioning may take as long as 2 years.

Complications of HSCT include mucositis, hepatic veno-occlusive disease, infections, organ toxicity, lung injury, or—for allogeneic transplant recipients—graft-versus-host disease, a complication that occurs when transplanted functional immune cells recognize the recipient's tissues as foreign and mount an immunologic attack on them. Estimated survival rates vary widely depending on many factors. However, for the most common applications of HSCT, 100-day mortality rates range from approximately 3% to 20% for autologous transplant and 5% to 45% for allogeneic transplant (Copelan,

2006). Infection is a primary cause of death in 15% to 20% of allogeneic transplant recipients and approximately 8% of autologous transplant recipients (Tomblyn, Gea-Banacloche, Szabolcs, & Boeckh, 2010). Other common causes of death include graft-versus-host-disease for allogeneic transplant recipients and disease relapse for autologous transplant recipients.

On their return home, transplant recipients must take primary responsibility for a variety of activities vital to their recovery. Details of self-care depend on diagnosis and type of transplant, but transplant recipients typically need to manage side effects, monitor physical symptoms, adhere to multiple drug regimens with complex dosing schedules, complete scheduled medical follow-up, get vaccinations, and make protective behavioral changes related to diet and food preparation, physical activity, dental and oral care, hand and body hygiene, social contacts, home and pet care, and leisure activities. As they face these challenges, they may also be coping with neurologic and cognitive deficits (e.g., memory, information processing, attention) and fatigue (Syrjala, Dikmen, Langer, Roth-Roemer, & Abrams, 2004). Transplant recipients may also face problems with relapse, diminished fertility, cataracts, sexual dysfunction, secondary cancers, and cardiovascular complications. Depending on disease type and stage, age, and pretransplant physical condition, physical symptoms may resolve over time or continue to be problematic over the course of the patient's lifetime.

Psychosocial Aspects of Hematopoietic Stem Cell Transplant

Several studies have provided an increasingly clear picture of the toll HSCT exacts on recipients' psychological well-being and quality of life. Although the psychological impact of HSCT appears to diminish for many after the 1-year point (Syrjala, Chapko, Vitaliano, Cummings, & Sullivan, 1993), others experience enduring effects even several years posttransplant. Levels of distress and individual concerns vary depending on the current challenges with which HSCT patients are faced and various risk factors. Patterns or clusters of difficulties also seem to emerge depending on the phase of treatment and recovery. An understanding of psychosocial concerns over time informs the clinician's selection of appropriate assessment instruments and the development of interventions focused on salient concerns.

Psychological Challenges Over Time

Pretransplant evaluations of well-being consistently identify high levels of anxiety, which may involve both existential and practical concerns and reflect distress about the underlying diagnosis as well as the impending transplant. Before transplant, patients face fear of dying, possible side effects of treatment, and an uncertain course of recovery (Prieto et al., 2005). Consenting to the transplant procedure is distressing (Dermatis & Lesko, 1991) as patients contemplate the seriousness of their disease and its treatment and prepare to make decisions (Andrykowski, 1994). Vying for the patient's emotional attention are new challenges revolving around understanding the details of a sometimes complicated medical diagnosis and treatment along with concerns about practical issues such as health insurance, making work and financial arrangements for several weeks or months, extensive pretransplant workups, and delegating family responsibilities. Concerns about child care and the well-being of family members are often stressful. Because fertility is adversely affected by treatment, decisions about family planning can be important for patients who are in their childbearing years. In addition, patient and caregiver not uncommonly relocate to distant transplant centers for needed care, creating the potential for yet another layer of stress in leaving support systems and learning to navigate an unfamiliar terrain.

For allogeneic transplant patients, the process of finding a donor match may be challenging. If a family member is not a good match, patients must access bone marrow transplant registries and sometimes appeal to communities through marrow drives. Family dynamics may come into play with potential donors, such as familial conflict if a family member does not consent to donate or guilt if donation does not lead to a cure.

During the preparatory phase, physical and emotional symptoms increase as the myleoablative process progresses and as patients adjust to being isolated from friends and family. Once patients have received the infusion of stem cells, a stressful waiting period occurs in which blood counts are regularly measured to see how well the graft is working. When the immune system is functioning sufficiently, patients make the transition to a prolonged period of being at home (or in temporary housing near the treatment center) but still needing continuous medical attention and extensive preventive precautions. Self-care can be a source of stress for some, as is leaving the reassurance of a medical environment where help is readily at hand. Compliance in HSCT is understudied, but there is reason to believe that some patients' compliance falls short of ideal levels, increasing their risk for complications such as infection. Others may become highly anxious as they attempt to apply every detail of complex self-care requirements. The social isolation that began with hospitalization still exists to some extent because patients must avoid crowds, and isolation can affect potentially beneficial relationships.

One to 3 years posttransplant, recipients may find that symptoms lessen over time while they slowly return to a semblance of normality. Posttransplant concerns involving employment, finances and insurance, close relationships, physical health, and planning for the future tend to increase over time. McQuellon et al. (1998) surmised that as physical symptoms decrease,

HSCT patients have more psychological energy to devote to dealing with other aspects of their lives, allowing these concerns to rise to the forefront. Return to work and other normal life activities may occur more slowly than anticipated. Andrykowski et al. (1999) noted additional adjustment issues that can occur during this period, including body image, fatigue, sleep problems, sexual functioning, and lingering cognitive issues. Patients also report wrestling with issues such as personal control, loneliness, existential concerns, and the impact of caregiving on important relationships.

Emotional Impact of HSCT

Symptoms of anxiety and depression are common among HSCT recipients throughout the transplant process, with high levels of distress having been found in 5% to more than 40% of transplant recipients (Mosher et al., 2009). Psychiatric diagnoses were noted in Prieto et al.'s (2002) evaluation of HSCT patients, including adjustment disorder (27.7%), mood disorders (14.1%), and anxiety disorders (8.2%). One longitudinal study reported that distress was at its highest before transplant and remained high for the next 3 months (Syrjala et al., 2004), and another study by Baker, Marcellus, Zabora, Polland, and Jodrey (1997) found that approximately one third of 437 people being evaluated for transplant reported symptoms of depression (13% mild, 13% moderate, and 5% severe). Research has indicated that even though anxiety levels tend to go down just after transplant, depressive symptomatology tends to increase (Prieto et al., 2005).

This does not mean, however, that all transplant recipients' distress is resolved after a brief time. Looking at a longer time frame, 79% of recipients in Syrjala et al.'s (2004) study continued to report distress at 1 year, 42% at 3 years, and 13% at 5 years posttransplant. Although medical factors may affect distress—patients with more physical symptoms (e.g., pain, graft-versus-host disease) reported higher levels of distress (Fife et al., 2000)—it is interesting to note that in Syrjala et al.'s study, recipients were mostly physically recovered at the 1-year point. Existential issues and loneliness continue to be concerns for some over time (Rusiewicz et al., 2008), and posttraumatic stress disorder is estimated to occur in 9% to 15% of HSCT recipients (Mosher et al., 2009).

Social Roles and Relationships Affected by HSCT

It is not surprising that social roles and relationships are affected by HSCT—it is an intense treatment with a lengthy recovery requiring extensive reliance on others for care and support. Recipients' employment is usually put on hold because of transplant, with multiple potential adverse effects (e.g., reduction in income, contact with possible support providers, and opportunities to engage in valued roles). One prospective study (McQuellon et al., 1998) noted that the percentages of recipients reporting job concerns at discharge, 100 days, and 12 months were 19%, 22%, and 43%, respectively. A prospective longitudinal study following recipients from pretransplant through 5 years posttransplant found that of those with outside work history, only 20% had returned to work after 1 year. This number increased to 34% at 5 years (Syrjala et al., 2004). Recipients without recurring malignancies who had a prior work or school history returned at a higher rate (84% at 5 years posttransplant). Overall, return to work was much slower than actual physical recovery.

Social relationships are also affected by isolation and infection control guidelines (e.g., not going to crowded places such as movie theaters). Indeed, one study (Baker et al., 1997) noted significant negative effects on social relationships and roles at 6 months (62%) and even 12 months (48%) after discharge. Close relationships are often stressed because of the changes in roles and the burden that HSCT exacts on both the recipient and the caregiver (Andrykowski et al., 2005). The quality of these relationships is important for a variety of reasons, one of which is that they are associated with adjustment to transplant (Frick et al., 2006; Syrjala et al., 2004). Not unlike recipients' experiences, caregiver distress is highest at the beginning of treatment (Foxall & Gaston-Johansson, 1996), which can affect the ability for effective care provision. Recipients with lower perceived social support before transplant have been found to have more depressive symptoms posttransplant (Jenks Kettmann & Altmaier, 2008).

PRETRANSPLANT SCREENING: RISK FACTORS, GOALS, APPROACHES, AND ASSESSMENTS

When developing a screening protocol for HSCT patients, several areas should be considered, including patient risk factors, the institution's specific goals for screening, which approach to screening is appropriate for the given resources, and which assessments would best meet the stated goals. We begin the following section by examining research that highlights patient risk factors for poor outcomes and then include a discussion of the importance of identifying goals on the basis of both patient need and the institution's available resources. This understanding provides a starting point from which to discern the approaches and types of assessments that can most effectively serve HSCT patients at a particular site.

Risk Factors

Although the interaction of medical and psychosocial factors appears to be a complex one, research has given us a glimpse into risk factors that can assist us in identifying those who may be particularly susceptible to problems after HSCT. General medical and sociodemographic factors point to factors associated with greater vulnerability for poor outcomes, including disease status (Andrykowski et al., 1995), smoking and addiction (Hoodin, Kalbfleisch, Thornton, & Ratanatharathorn, 2004; Prieto et al., 2006), poorer pre-HSCT physical functioning (Loberiza et al., 2002; Prieto et al., 2006), lower level of education (Andrykowski et al., 1995; Heinonen et al., 2001), not being married (Hoodin et al., 2004; Syrjala et al., 1993), poorer social support (Sryjala, Dikmen, Langer, Roth-Roemer, & Abrams, 2004), and a history of psychiatric disorders (Prieto et al., 2006). Conversely, those who are more optimistic (Baker et al., 1997), more self-controlled (Fife et al., 2000), more compliant with medical treatment, better adjusted, and less depressed pretransplant tend to report fewer posttransplant psychosocial concerns (Hoodin et al., 2004). Also interesting to note is that research has linked psychosocial issues with risk of mortality, although the literature is mixed (e.g., Andrykowski, Brady, & Henslee-Downey, 1994; Colón, Callies, Popkin, & McGlave, 1991; Loberiza et al., 2002; Molassiotis, van den Akker, & Boughton, 1997).

Pretransplant psychological maladjustment has been shown to be a risk factor for future problems. Although some variation in incidence of pretransplant depression and anxiety has been reported in the literature, the overall implications are clinically important, particularly as research on their predictive value and utility in guiding early interventions increases. The importance of identifying pretransplant depression in HSCT patients is illustrated in one study in which pretransplant depression accounted for 25% of the variance in depression at a 1-year follow-up (Jenks Kettmann & Altmaier, 2008), along with another finding that pretransplant HSCT distress is correlated with posttransplant distress (Lee et al., 2005). Overall, several studies have indicated that pretransplant psychological functioning is predictive of posttransplant functioning (e.g., Broers, Kaptein, Le Cessie, Fibbe, & Hengeveld, 2000; Fife et al., 2000; Hoodin et al., 2004; Lee et al., 2005; Syrjala et al., 1993) with self-reports of both physical and psychological functioning being more predictive of recovery than even factors such as age or disease stage and type (Andorsky, Loberiza, & Lee, 2006).

Research has pointed to greater vulnerability for poor outcomes among HSCT recipients who have lower levels of education (e.g., Heinonen et al., 2001), which, in turn, implicates health literacy. Health literacy, along with the necessary social support (i.e., the availability of others who can help them understand and apply information), is an important factor to consider when assessing risk because it contributes to deficits in self-care after HSCT. Difficulties with understanding place about 30% of allogeneic HSCT recipients at risk for poor outcomes (Foster et al., 2009). Medication nonadherence ranges from 32% to 58%, with distressed HSCT patients being less adherent than nondistressed patients (Lee et al., 2005). Patients with adequate information and the ability to apply it are better prepared to adhere to self-care regimens and respond appropriately to symptoms, and they are also less distressed (Epstein & Street, 2007; Kahn, 2007). Finally, related to literacy is research indicating that HSCT patients whose presurgery expectations are in line with what actually transpires seem to have less distress than those who have unfulfilled expectations of where they believe they should be (Andrykowski et al., 1995).

Goals of Hematopoietic Stem Cell Transplant Prescreening

Given the nature of HSCT, screening goals tend to focus on identifying and managing psychosocial problems in transplant candidates to ensure the best possible psychosocial and medical outcomes. The mechanisms for achieving these goals, however, appear to depend largely on an institution's resources (e.g., the number of transplant team members available to identify and treat psychosocial concerns) but may also be influenced by the identified need for expanded research in this area. Assessments and procedures vary greatly across sites (Hamadani et al., 2010). For some sites, the goal of prescreening may be to determine eligibility for the transplant procedure itself with the objective of addressing areas of concern (e.g., addiction, lack of social support) to get the patient back on track for transplant. Some sites screen only those with obvious high-risk factors, whereas others conduct routine screening with all potential candidates. Some transplant centers focus on the more immediate concern of supporting patients through the transplant and subsequent hospitalization, and others have the goal of continuing to follow up with patients after discharge. Considering that recent medical advancements in HSCT have improved survival rates among this population and that many experience distress even years after transplant, prescreening may serve as an important starting point for long-term psychosocial care.

A variety of assessments have shown promise in clinical utility, and specific screening goals will guide the selection of appropriate assessment instruments. Prescreening for exclusionary criteria for transplant (e.g., substance abuse, psychosis) dictates use of certain measures, whereas screening for general distress or quality-of-life concerns suggests the use of others. Overall, when considering the goals of assessment, several questions may be posed: Is assessment used solely to determine eligibility for transplant or will it serve as a baseline by which to measure future functioning and provide interventions? Will all patients with some need receive care, or are resources allocated to those with the most distress? How often will assessments be scheduled, and at what time points? Which measures will best meet the set goals? What intervention resources are available, and how does screening guide the delivery of these interventions? Simply stated, specific goals will inform the assessment plan and must be considered carefully to make effective use of available resources.

Approaches to Hematopoietic Stem Cell Transplant Prescreening

Prescreening for HSCT may take place at the physician's office or, more commonly, on admission to the hospital, and it may initially be conducted by medical staff or mental health care professionals. Many transplant units employ clinicians to guide prescreening efforts, although some rely on referrals to psychosocial services by medical staff. However, underrecognition of psychosocial distress is not uncommon and is potentially the result of a lack of time, training, and willingness to inquire about psychosocial problems (Merckaert et al., 2008); the unwillingness of the patient to discuss these concerns; or both. The use of standardized assessments can prove helpful in referring patients to appropriate psychosocial services, and research exploring various approaches to using assessments may serve as a model for those developing a prescreening process. Given the limited research on HSCT prescreening, some assessment models used in general cancer populations can be helpful in guiding the development of HSCT screening efforts.

One example is a stepped approach (Bonacchi et al., 2010) to evaluating the psychosocial needs of cancer patients and determining appropriate treatment recommendations. The first step of this evaluation involves an initial meeting between the clinician and the patient that combines a short, nonstructured clinical interview in conjunction with brief questionnaires completed by the patient. The clinical interview focuses on patients' awareness and experience of their illness, an assessment of illness-related distress levels, past and current psychopathology, and psychosocial support, including family support and other social resources. A second phase of assessment takes place if the clinician, on reviewing results of the initial assessment, deems additional evaluation necessary or if a patient requested assistance. This step includes another clinical interview and the administration of additional measures along with referrals for consultation (e.g., psychiatric, couples or family). Referral for intervention is made after team consultation with the evaluating clinicians and ranges from brief, supportive therapy to psychiatric or pharmacological evaluation or possibly longer term support. An evaluation of this approach found benefit in using both interviews and questionnaires together rather than assessment based solely on an interview or self-reports because using only one approach may not capture all those in need. This stepped approach involved assessing every patient admitted to the cancer unit, which, although ideal, may not be feasible for some sites.

Keeping in mind that resources at some sites may be scarce and that patients may find a battery of assessments burdensome, another approach that may be more cost-effective and efficient involves the use of a brief screening measure. Jacobsen et al. (2005) explored how a single-item measure of distress (the Distress Thermometer; DT) compared with longer, more commonly used instruments: the Hospital Anxiety and Depression Scale and the 18-Item Brief Symptom Inventory. Their findings confirmed that the DT fared well in identifying clinically significant distress compared with both the Hospital Anxiety and Depression Scale and 18-Item Brief Symptom Inventory. The DT was used with a problem checklist that provided details regarding the specific areas of patient concern, which, in turn, could guide the provision of psychosocial services. The DT has also been validated in the HSCT population (Ransom, Jacobsen, & Booth-Jones, 2006). Although one short assessment tool cannot take the place of a more comprehensive battery and clinical interview, it can certainly prove to be a more efficient and acceptable approach for initial and repeated assessments of patient distress.

Assessments

Selection of measures and the development of assessment protocols should be based on specific goals with consideration of patient burden and instrument validity and reliability. Although some studies have examined assessed factors and outcomes for many measures, additional research is certainly needed for screening to be most useful in guiding delivery of services. The following assessments have been used with HSCT and cancer patients in research settings, clinical settings, or both.

Clinical Interviews

Areas to explore in a clinical interview include psychiatric history, substance use or abuse, mental status, psychosocial and family history, history of trauma, and cultural beliefs and current concerns. Specific illness-related areas of inquiry are also helpful in determining the patient's status, such as health behaviors, prior history of illness and coping, adherence to treatment recommendations, and understanding of the diagnosis and treatment options. Alternatively, standardized instruments may be used to detail information that would be gathered in a clinical interview, such as the Patient Health Questionnaire (Jacobs, Jacobsen, Donovan, & Booth-Jones, 2001; Spitzer, Kroenke, & Williams, 1999) and the Transplant Evaluation Rating Scale (Twillman, Manetto, Wellisch, & Wolcott, 1993). The Patient Health Questionnaire is a brief (15-item), self-administered instrument that assesses five common types of mood disorder: anxiety, depression, eating, somatoform, and alcohol abuse. The Transplant Evaluation Rating Scale is a clinician-administered instrument that assesses 10 areas of psychosocial functioning: Axis I and II disorders, substance use and abuse, health behaviors, compliance, quality of family and social support, history of coping, coping with disease and treatment, quality of affect, and both current and past mental status. The Transplant Evaluation Rating Scale has been validated for use with HSCT patients; it demonstrates good clinical utility and can be used to categorize patients by level of need, with Level 1 indicating that the patient is at lower risk of having transplant-related difficulties and Level 3 indicating the highest level of risk.

Because the patient will rely heavily on his or her caregiver during the transplant process, interviewing the primary caregiver is also helpful in determining possible issues that may arise. A caregiver who does not have the ability to cope effectively with the strain of supporting the transplant patient may be at risk for burnout, which may subsequently affect the patient's quality of life (Molassiotis et al., 1997). Evaluating factors such as current mental health status, coping, social support, ability to provide caregiving (e.g., competing demands), and an understanding of the disease and treatment are all important considerations.

HSCT-Specific Assessments

One measure specific to HSCT is the Functional Assessment of Cancer Therapy—Bone Marrow Transplant (McQuellon et al., 1997), which combines the Functional Assessment of Cancer Therapy with 12 additional items geared to the HSCT patient. Psychosocial domains assessed include physical, social and family, emotional, and functional well-being as well as the patient–physician relationship. This self-administered measurement contains 47 items and takes approximately 10 minutes to complete.

Cancer- and Illness-Specific Assessments

Because HSCT patients have a wide range of quality-of-life issues, the Functional Living Index—Cancer (Schipper, Clinch, & McMurray, 1984) offers a brief way to assess a patient's physical functioning, psychological functioning, current well-being, gastrointestinal symptoms, and social functioning. This self-administered 22-item measure uses a Likert-scale format for each item.

The Hospital Anxiety and Depression Scale (Zigmond & Snaith, 1983) is a widely used measure that provides a brief assessment of illness-related anxiety and depression. It is unique in that it assesses anxiety and depression solely on the basis of psychological issues and excludes somatic items that are prevalent in many patients but may not be indicative of emotional functioning. This 14-item measure can be administered easily in a variety of settings and provides cutoff scores for clinical, subclinical, and nonclinical levels of both anxiety and depression.

Distress, Depression, and Anxiety

Several valid and reliable assessments of distress, depression, and anxiety are commonly used in a wide range of settings and have also proven to be valuable in this population, including the Center for Epidemiologic Studies Depression Scale (Radloff, 1977), the Beck Depression Inventory—II (Beck, Steer, & Brown, 1996), and the Brief Symptom Inventory—18 (Derogatis, 2000). In addition, the DT (Roth et al., 1998) used with a problem checklist appears to successfully exclude those without distress but is limited in discerning heightened distress, which could lead to a higher number of referrals for patients who may not necessarily need support.

Substance Use

Substance use among HSCT patients has not been widely studied to date; however, the physical sequelae of substance use disorders have an impact on the patient's medical status, and issues such as compliance, social support, and impaired decision making and judgment may increase the risk for morbidity and affect survival (Battaglioli et al., 2006; Chang et al., 1997). Stagno et al. (2008) recommended assessment using the Transplant Evaluation Rating Scale or the Alcohol Use Disorders Identification Test (Reinert & Allen, 2002); a brief, self- or clinician-administered scale; or another substance use scale when substance use is suspected with referral to specialists for treatment when needed.

Neuropsychological Assessments

Whenever possible, neuropsychological testing that assesses memory, psychomotor skills, and executive functioning should be included as a baseline point. Neuropsychological assessment is a helpful tool because cognitive impairment resulting from chemotherapy and other medication can change over time and may also affect assessments of anxiety and depression. The Functional Assessment of Cancer Therapy—Cognition scale (Jacobs, Jacobsen, Booth-Jones, Wagner, & Anasetti, 2007) is a fairly brief (50-item) self-administered instrument that has been used with HSCT patients and provides information on perceived cognitive abilities and impairment, impairment perceived by others, and the impact on quality of life. The Mini-Mental State Examination (Folstein, Folstein, McHugh, & Fanjiang, 2000) is a clinician-administered instrument used to assess cognition with items on attention, orientation, recall, visuospatial construction, and language.

Effective communication between the patient and medical staff regarding the goals of assessment can prove to be beneficial in understanding results and implementing interventions. As is the case in the general population, a stigma regarding psychological issues continues to be problematic for some HSCT patients; however, with education these barriers can often be overcome. The National Comprehensive Cancer Network (2003) specifically recommended using the term *distress* rather than other terms such as *depression* to minimize stigmatization that may affect willingness to participate in assessment and treatment. In addition, explaining that distress is not uncommon in HSCT and that it can be managed effectively helps to normalize the experience for the patient. Finally, when the medical team is educated about the psychosocial issues recipients often face, how to identify symptoms and situations requiring attention, and the psychosocial services available at their sites, they can then serve as important referral sources for their patients.

CASE STUDY

Although some transplant candidates display clear symptoms of psychosocial distress, others may not initially appear to be particularly vulnerable. The latter is true in the case of R. T.,[1] a 37-year-old Caucasian woman who was referred for an autologous transplant after a diagnosis of a hematological malignancy. She and her husband arrived for a consultation with the oncologist and transplant nurse to discuss the transplant procedure and to go over questions and concerns. Before the meeting, R. T. had reviewed material online about her disease and came prepared with questions. She carefully made notes during the meeting and often stopped to reassure and sometimes joke with her husband, who appeared to be anxious but involved. At the conclusion of the meeting, R. T. seemed satisfied with the information and scheduled an appointment for the following week for a routine pretransplant examination and tests. Overall, R. T. presented as a self-assured and well-prepared patient with a supportive spouse who understood the transplant process.

At the next visit, the nurse made a point of asking R. T. how she was doing because she seemed anxious and uncharacteristically disorganized. R. T. commented that she was okay and that she "just wanted to hurry up and get this over with." The nurse, sensing that more might be going on, gave her the DT and the Problem Checklist to complete along with the standard medical forms. She was surprised that R. T. had rated her distress at 8 out of 10 and endorsed each item under Emotional Concerns (depression, nervousness, fears, sadness, worry, and anger) along with concerns about child care and dealing with family and partner. The nurse immediately referred R. T. to psychosocial services.

A psychologist met with R. T., and the evaluation revealed no prior history of psychiatric disorders or substance use. Before diagnosis, she noted

---

[1]Details of this case have been altered to protect the patient's identity.

that she had a generally happy and fulfilled life, with a successful career as the manager of an accounting department, and she was an avid cyclist. When asked about the concerns she had listed regarding her family, R. T. began to cry. Her distress revolved largely around her children, for whom she was the primary caregiver. She had never spent a night away from the girls and felt as though she was failing them with the impending separation. R. T. noted that her husband did not know how to care for them and that they would all surely be traumatized by the separation. She felt that everyone, including her husband, would fall apart. She also admitted that her dedication in putting her family first had been detrimental to her own well-being. R. T. had been experiencing symptoms a full 10 months before visiting her doctor, rationalizing that she did not have the time to get checked and that all mothers felt tired. She had also given up cycling and maintaining connections with close friends as she focused on her family.

The evaluation uncovered several areas of concern for R. T., including risk of increased anxiety and depression during her separation from her family, because she would be unable to care for them and worried about their reactions to being without her. Whereas she understood that the recovery process would take time, R. T.'s expectations of her ability to rebound and get back to her routine were unrealistic, which could also contribute to distress. Potential lack of adherence to the complex self-care routine was of concern, particularly because she had a history of neglecting herself physically in deference to her family's needs. Finally, social support would need to be addressed. Although she noted supportive friends and family, R. T. was a self-described "independent go-getter" and perfectionist who had difficulty asking for help and, in fact, had not even told her extended family about her transplant.

The psychologist then met with R. T. and her husband to evaluate their plans for dealing with R. T.'s treatment and family needs. Her husband had initially intended to take off only 3 weeks from work at R. T.'s insistence. R. T. had also planned on keeping in constant contact with her husband to direct the girls' daily activities by phone. Facing the fact that this was not a realistic arrangement, R. T. continued to struggle with giving up control but found reassurance in planning for her absence. She reluctantly contacted her sister in another state, who readily agreed to stay with the girls during R. T.'s hospitalization. R. T. created a schedule for her family and busied herself with writing special notes to send them while she was away. This, along with planning meals for them before hospitalization, helped her to feel as though she would have a continued presence in her girls' lives. R. T.'s husband also set up video conferencing on their home computer. A meeting with a child psychologist proved helpful in learning how to explain to the children what was going on. After frank discussion, R. T. and her husband decided to include close friends and family in various caregiving activities such as shopping and providing transportation. Although R. T.'s prognosis was good because of her age and stage of disease, her fear of death and the subsequent fate of her children was a constant source of distress for her, and she found great comfort in writing out a detailed will outlining the care of her children.

In sum, screening identified (a) the potential for R. T. to be noncompliant with self-care and unresponsive to physical symptoms and limitations, (b) the potential for poor psychological adjustment during and after transplant because of anxieties and unrealistic expectations, and (c) an unwillingness to mobilize and use social support that could reduce practical and emotional strains. Although R. T. had moments of feeling anxious and depressed, her pretransplant planning proved helpful throughout hospitalization and her return home.

Although only the DT and Problem Checklist were used in this case study, they proved to be sufficient for flagging potential issues for this particular patient. The clinician's knowledge of the importance of addressing both the practical side of the transplant process, through a problem-solving approach, and the emotional aspects, through supportive counseling, were sufficient to alleviate current anxiety and prevent further distress. Certainly, if this level of intervention failed to address clinical concerns, additional evaluation and services may have been required.

CHALLENGES, RECOMMENDATIONS, AND FUTURE DIRECTIONS

Although pretransplant screening among HSCT populations is pivotal in ensuring the identification of distress and the provision of adequate psychosocial care, its implementation poses several challenges. First, accurate identification of distress requires using validated assessments at various time points throughout each patient's treatment and recovery experience. Inherent in this process is finding a balance between gathering information and patient burden. Completing several measures at a time when one is feeling overwhelmed may be too much to ask of some patients. Administering brief, sound measures that adequately detect distress levels and specific areas of concern would allow for targeted interventions at appropriate times. The effectiveness of this approach was clearly demonstrated in the case study of R. T., in which the DT and Problem Checklist were used to evaluate her status and subsequently greatly contributed to her positive recovery. The use of computerized or touch-screen technology would be one way to ease patient burden and provide immediate scoring results that could be placed in patients' charts for treatment planning. Research has supported the transition to this technology, and patients have found it preferable or easy to use (McLachlan et al., 2001; Velikova et al., 1999). In addition, computer-assisted technology, such as that being developed within the Patient-Reported Outcomes Measurement Information System initiative sponsored by the National Institutes of Health (n.d.), minimizes the number of questions asked depending on patient responses. This system reduces burden while also providing reliable and valid standardized measures.

Second, the lack of specific guidelines regarding psychosocial screening for transplant candidates may be in part because HSCT has fewer large, multisite research studies than other types of cancer. Comparing results of studies that use different measures at different time points is problematic in clearly understanding the impact of HSCT. In turn, funding for psychosocial screening and intervention resources may be dependent on such research demonstrating the feasibility of investing in resources based on improved outcomes. The National Comprehensive Cancer Network (2003) has recommended that every cancer patient be provided with a thorough clinical evaluation of distress before treatment with additional follow-up at all stages of disease along with appropriate treatment. Continued, rigorous research that addresses the impact of HSCT on recipients from diagnosis through long-term survival will serve as a foundation to guide assessment and the development of successful interventions at all stages of the HSCT experience.

REFERENCES

Andorsky, D. J., Loberiza, F. R., & Lee, S. J. (2006). Pre-transplantation physical and mental functioning is strongly associated with self-reported recovery from stem cell transplantation. *Bone Marrow Transplantation, 37,* 889–895. doi:10.1038/sj.bmt.1705347

Andrykowski, M. A. (1994). Psychosocial factors predictive of survival after allogeneic bone marrow transplantation for leukemia. *Psychosomatic Medicine, 56,* 432–439.

Andrykowski, M. A., Bishop, M. M., Hahn, E. A., Cella, D. F., Beaumont, M. J., Brady, M. M., . . . Wingard, J. R. (2005). Long-term health-related quality of life, growth, and spiritual well-being after hematopoietic stem-cell transplantation. *Journal of Clinical Oncology, 23,* 599–608. doi:10.1200/JCO.2005.03.189

Andrykowski, M. A., Brady, M. J., & Henslee-Downey, P. J. (1994). Psychosocial factors predictive of survival after allogeneic bone marrow transplantation for leukemia. *Psychosomatic Medicine, 56,* 432–439.

Andrykowski, M. A., Bruehl, S., Brady, M. J., & Henslee-Downey, P. J. (1995). Physical and psychosocial status of adults one-year after bone marrow transplantation: A prospective study. *Bone Marrow Transplantation, 15,* 837–844.

Andrykowski, M. A., Cordova, M. J., Hann, D. M., Jacobsen, P. B., Fields, K. K., & Phillips, G. (1999). Patients' psychosocial concerns following stem cell transplantation. *Bone Marrow Transplantation, 24,* 1121–1129. doi:10.1038/sj.bmt.1702022

Baker, F., Marcellus, D., Zabora, J., Polland, A., & Jodrey, D. (1997). Psychological distress among adult patients being evaluated for bone marrow transplantation. *Psychosomatics, 38,* 10–19. doi:10.1016/S0033-3182(97)71498-1

Battaglioli, T., Gorini, G., Seniori Constantini, A., Crosignani, P., Miligi, L., Nanni, O., . . . Vineis, P. (2006). Cigarette smoking and alcohol consumption as determinants of survival in non-Hodgkin's lymphoma: A population-based study. *Annals of Oncology, 17,* 1283–1289. doi:10.1093/annonc/mdl096

Beck, A. T., Steer, R. A., & Brown, G. K. (1996). *BDI–II manual: Beck Depression Inventory* (2nd ed.). San Antonio, TX: Psychological Corporation.

Bonacchi, A., Rossi, A., Bellotti, L., Franco, S., Toccafondi, A., Miccinesi, G., & Rosselli, M. (2010). Assessment of psychological distress in cancer patients: A pivotal role for clinical interview. *Psycho-Oncology, 19,* 1294–1302. doi:10.1002/pon.1693

Broers, S., Kaptein, A. A., Le Cessie, S., Fibbe, W., & Hengeveld, M. W. (2000). Psychological functioning and quality of life following bone marrow transplantation: A 3-year follow-up study. *Journal of Psychosomatic Research, 48,* 11–21. doi:10.1016/S0022-3999(99)00059-8

Chang, G., Antin, J., Orav, E. J., Randall, U., McGarigle, C., & Behr, H. M. (1997). Substance abuse and bone marrow transplant. *American Journal of Drug and Alcohol Abuse, 23,* 301–308. doi:10.3109/00952999709040948

Colón, E. A., Callies, A. L., Popkin, M. K., & McGlave, P. B. (1991). Depressed mood and other variables related to bone marrow transplantation survival in acute leukemia. *Psychosomatics, 32,* 420–425. doi:10.1016/S0033-3182(91)72045-8

Copelan, E. A. (2006). Hematopoietic stem cell transplantation. *New England Journal of Medicine, 354,* 1813–1826. doi:10.1056/NEJMra052638

Dermatis, H., & Lesko, L. M. (1991). Psychosocial correlates of physician-patient communication at time of informed consent for bone marrow transplantation. *Cancer Investigation, 9,* 621–628. doi:10.3109/07357909109039873

Derogatis, L. R. (2000). *Brief Symptom Inventory (BSI) 18: Administration, scoring and procedures manual.* Minneapolis, MN: NCS Pearson.

Epstein, R. M., & Street, R. L., Jr. (2007). *Patient-centered communication in cancer care: Promoting healing and reducing suffering* (NIH Pub. No. 07-6225). Bethesda, MD: National Cancer Institute.

Fawzy, F. I. (1999). Psychosocial interventions for patients with cancer: What works and what doesn't. *European Journal of Cancer, 35,* 1559–1564. doi:10.1016/S0959-8049(99)00191-4

Fife, B. L., Huster, G. A., Cornetta, K. G., Kennedy, V. N., Akard, L. P., & Broun, E. R. (2000). Longitudinal study of adaptation to the stress of bone marrow transplantation. *Journal of Clinical Oncology, 18,* 1539–1549.

Folstein, M. F., Folstein, S. E., McHugh, P. R., & Fanjiang, G. F. (2000). *Mini-Mental State Examination: User's guide*. Lutz, FL: Psychological Assessment Resources.

Foster, L. W., McLellan, L., Rybicki, L., Dabney, J., Visnosky, M., & Bolwell, B. (2009). Utility of the Psychosocial Assessment of Candidates for Transplantation (PACT) scale in allogeneic BMT. *Bone Marrow Transplantation, 44*, 375–380. doi:10.1038/bmt.2009.37

Foster, L. W., McLellan, L. J., Rybicki, L. A., Dabney, J., Welsh, E., & Bolwell, B. J. (2006). Allogeneic BMT and patient eligibility based on psychosocial criteria: A survey of BMT professionals. *Bone Marrow Transplantation, 37*, 223–228. doi:10.1038/sj.bmt.1705219

Foxall, M. J., & Gaston-Johansson, F. (1996). Burden and health outcomes of family caregivers of hospitalized bone marrow transplant patients. *Journal of Advanced Nursing, 24*, 915–923. doi:10.1111/j.1365-2648.1996.tb02926.x

Frick, E., Ramm, G., Bumeder, I., Schulz-Kindermann, F., Tyroller, M., Fischer, N., & Hasenbring, M. (2006). Social support and quality of life of patients prior to stem cell or bone marrow transplantation. *British Journal of Health Psychology, 11*, 451–462. doi:10.1348/135910705X53849

Gratwohl, A., Baldomero, H., Schwendener, A., Gratwohl, M., Apperley, J., Niederwieser, D., & Frauendorfer, K; Joint Accreditation Committee of the International Society for Cellular Therapy; European Group for Blood and Marrow Transplantation; and European Leukemia Net. (2007). Predictability of hematopoietic stem cell transplantation rates. *Haematologica, 92*, 1679–1686. doi:10.3324/haematol.11260

Gratwohl, A., Schwendener, A., Baldomero, H., Gratwohl, M., Apperley, J., Niederwieser, D., & Frauendorfer, K. (2010). Changes in the use of hematopoietic stem cell transplantation: A model for diffusion of medical technology. *Haematologica, 95*, 637–643. doi:10.3324/haematol.2009.015586

Hamadani, M., Craig, M., Awan, F. T., & Devine, S. M. (2010). How we approach patient evaluation for hematopoietic stem cell transplantation. *Bone Marrow Transplantation, 45*, 1259–1268. doi:10.1038/bmt.2010.94

Heinonen, H., Volin, L., Uutela, A., Zevon, M., Barrick, C., & Ruutu, T. (2001). Quality of life and factors related to perceived satisfaction with quality of life after allogeneic bone marrow transplantation. *Annals of Hematology, 80*, 137–143. doi:10.1007/s002770000249

Holland, J. C., Breibart, W. S., Jacobsen, P. B., Lederberg, M. S., Loscalzo, M. J., & McCorkle, R. (Eds.). (2010). *Psycho-Oncology* (2nd ed.). New York, NY: Oxford University Press.

Hoodin, F., Kalbfleisch, K. R., Thornton, J., & Ratanatharathorn, V. (2004). Psychosocial influences on 305 adults' survival after bone marrow transplantation: Depression, smoking, and behavioral self-regulation. *Journal of Psychosomatic Research, 57*, 145–154. doi:10.1016/S0022-3999(03)00599-3

Jacobs, S. R., Jacobsen, P. B., Booth-Jones, M., Wagner, L. I., & Anasetti, C. (2007). Evaluation of the Functional Assessment of Cancer Therapy Cognitive Scale with hematopoietic stem cell transplant patients. *Journal of Pain and Symptom Management, 33*, 13–23.

Jacobs, S. R., Jacobsen, P. B., Donovan, K., & Booth-Jones, M. (2001). Utility of the Patient Health Questionnaire-9 (PHQ-9) in identifying depression among hematopoietic stem cell transplant patients. *Annals of Behavioral Medicine, 33*(Suppl.), S056. doi:10.1016/j.jpainsymman.2006.06.011

Jacobsen, P. B. (2007). Screening for psychological distress in cancer patients: Challenges and opportunities. *Journal of Clinical Oncology, 25*, 4526–4527. doi:10.1200/JCO.2007.13.1367

Jacobsen, P. B., Donovan, K. A., Trask, P. C., Fleishman, S. B., Zabora, J., Baker, F., & Holland, J. C. (2005). Screening for psychologic distress in ambulatory cancer patients: A multicenter evaluation of the Distress Thermometer. *Cancer, 103*, 1494–1502. doi:10.1002/cncr.20940

Jenks Kettmann, J. D., & Altmaier, E. M. (2008). Depression among bone marrow transplant patients. *Journal of Health Psychology, 13*, 39–46. doi:10.1177/1359105307084310

Kahn, K. L. (2007). Patient centered experiences in breast cancer predicting long-term adherence to tamoxifen use. *Medical Care, 45*, 431–439. doi:10.1097/01.mlr.0000257193.10760.7f

Kennard, B. D., Smith, S. M., Olvera, R., Bawdon, R. E., O hAilin, A., Lewis, C. P., & Winick, N. J. (2004). Nonadherence in adolescent oncology patients: Preliminary data on psychological risk factors and relationships to outcome. *Journal of Clinical Psychology in Medical Settings, 11*, 30–39. doi:10.1023/B:JOCS.0000016267.21912.74

Lee, S. J., Loberiza, F. R., Antin, J. H., Kirkpatrick, T., Prokop, L., Alvea, E. P., . . . Soiffer, R. J. (2005). Routine screening for psychosocial distress following hematopoietic stem cell transplantation. *Bone Marrow Transplantation, 35*, 77–83. doi:10.1038/sj.bmt.1704709

Lepore, S. J., & Coyne, J. C. (2006). Psychological interventions for distress in cancer patients: A review of reviews. *Annals of Behavioral Medicine, 32*, 85–92. doi:10.1207/s15324796abm3202_2

Loberiza, F. R., Rizzo, J. D., Bredeson, C. N., Antin, J. H., Horowitz, M. M., Weeks, J. C., & Lee, S. J. (2002). Association of depressive syndrome and early deaths among patients after stem-cell transplantation for malignant diseases. *Journal of Clinical Oncology, 20*, 2118–2126. doi:10.1200/JCO.2002.08.757

McLachlan, S. A., Allenby, A., Matthews, J., Wirth, A., Kissane, D., Bishop, M., . . . Zalcberg, J. (2001). Randomized trial of coordinated psychosocial interventions based on patient self-assessments versus standard care to improve the psychosocial functioning of patients with cancer. *Journal of Clinical Oncology, 19*, 4117–4125.

McQuellon, R. P., Russell, G. B., Cella, D. F., Craven, B. L., Brady, M., Bonomi, A., & Hurd, D. D. (1997). Quality of life measurement in bone marrow transplantation: Development of the Functional Assessment of Cancer Therapy-Bone

Marrow Transplant (FACT-BMT) scale. *Bone Marrow Transplantation, 19*, 357–368. doi:10.1038/sj.bmt.1700672

McQuellon, R. P., Russell, G. B., Rambo, T. D., Craven, B. L., Radford, J., Perry, J. J., . . . Hurd, D. D. (1998). Quality of life and psychological distress of bone marrow transplant recipients: The "time trajectory" to recovery over the first year. *Bone Marrow Transplantation, 21*, 477–486. doi:10.1038/sj.bmt.1701115

Merckaert, I., Libert, Y., Delvaux, N., Marchal, S., Boniver, J., Etienne, A.-M., . . . Razavi, D. (2008). Factors influencing physicians' detection of cancer patients' and relatives' distress: Can a communication skills training program improve physicians' detection? *Psycho-Oncology, 17*, 260–269. doi:10.1002/pon.1233

Molassiotis, A., van den Akker, O. B., & Boughton, B. J. (1997). Perceived social support, family environment and psychosocial recovery in bone marrow transplant long-term survivors. *Social Science & Medicine, 44*, 317–325. doi:10.1016/S0277-9536(96)00101-3

Mosher, C. E., Redd, W. H., Rini, C. M., Burkhalter, J. E., & DuHamel, K. N. (2009). Physical, psychological, and social sequelae following hematopoietic stem cell transplantation: A review of the literature. *Psycho-Oncology, 18*, 113–127. doi:10.1002/pon.1399

National Comprehensive Cancer Network. (2003). Distress management clinical practice guidelines in oncology. *Journal of the National Comprehensive Cancer Network, 1*, 344.

National Institutes of Health. (n.d.). *PROMIS: Patient-Reported Outcomes Measurement Information System.* Retrieved from http://www.nihpromis.org/

Pasquini, M. C., & Wang, Z. (2010). *Current use and outcome of hematopoietic stem cell transplantation: CIBMTR Summary Slides, 2010.* Retrieved from http://www.cibmtr.org

Prieto, J. M., Atala, J., Blanch, J., Carreras, E., Rovira, M., Cirera, E., & Gasto, C. (2005). Patient-rated emotional and physical functioning among hematologic cancer patients during hospitalization for stem-cell transplantation. *Bone Marrow Transplantation, 35*, 307–314.

Prieto, J. M., Blanch, J., Atala, J., Carreras, E., Rovira, M., Cirera, E., & Gasto, C. (2006). Stem cell transplantation: Risk factors for psychiatric morbidity. *European Journal of Cancer, 42*, 514–520. doi:10.1016/j.ejca.2005.07.037

Radloff, L. S. (1977). The CES-D Scale: A self-report depression scale for research in the general population. *Applied Psychological Measurement, 1*, 385–401. doi:10.1177/014662167700100306

Ransom, S., Jacobsen, P. B., & Booth-Jones, M. (2006). Validation of the distress thermometer with bone marrow transplant patients. *Psycho-Oncology, 15*, 604–612. doi:10.1002/pon.993

Reinert, D. F., & Allen, J. P. (2002). The Alcohol Use Disorders Identification Test (AUDIT): A review of recent research. *Alcoholism: Clinical and Experimental Research, 26*, 272–279. doi:10.1111/j.1530-0277.2002.tb02534.x

Roth, A. J., Kornblith, A. B., Batel-Copel, L., Peabody, E., Scher, H. I., & Holland, J. C. (1998). Rapid screening for psychologic distress in men with prostate carcinoma: A pilot study. *Cancer, 82,* 1904–1908. doi:10.1002/(SICI)1097-0142(19980515)82:10<1904::AID-CNCR13>3.0.CO;2-X

Rusiewicz, A., DuHamel, K. N., Burkhalter, J., Ostroff, J., Winkel, G., Scigliano, E., . . . Redd, W. (2008). Psychological distress in long-term survivors of hematopoietic stem cell transplantation. *Psycho-Oncology, 17,* 329–337. doi:10.1002/pon.1221

Schipper, H., Clinch, J., & McMurray, A. (1984). Measuring the quality of life of cancer patients: The Functional Living Index-Cancer: Development and validation. *Journal of Clinical Oncology, 2,* 472–483.

Spitzer, R. L., Kroenke, K., & Williams, J. B. W. (1999). Validation and utility of a self-report version of PRIME-MD: The PHQ Primary Care Study. *JAMA, 282,* 1737–1744. doi:10.1001/jama.282.18.1737

Stagno, S. J., Busby, K., Shapiro, A., & Kotz, M. M. (2008). Patients at risk: Addressing addiction in patients undergoing hematopoietic SCT. *Bone Marrow Transplantation, 42,* 221–226. doi:10.1038/bmt.2008.211

Stanton, A. L. (2006). Psychosocial concerns and interventions for cancer survivors. *Journal of Clinical Oncology, 24,* 5132–5137. doi:10.1200/JCO.2006.06.8775

Syrjala, K. L., Chapko, M. K., Vitaliano, P. P., Cummings, C., & Sullivan, K. M. (1993). Recovery after allogeneic marrow transplantation: Prospective study of predictors of long-term physical and psychosocial functioning. *Bone Marrow Transplantation, 11,* 319–327.

Syrjala, K. L., Dikmen, S., Langer, S. L., Roth-Roemer, S., & Abrams, J. R. (2004). Neuropsychologic changes from before transplantation to 1 year in patients receiving myeloablative allogeneic hematopoietic cell transplant. *Blood, 104,* 3386–3392. doi:10.1182/blood-2004-03-1155

Tomblyn, M., Gea-Banacloche, J., Szabolcs, P., & Boeckh, M. (2010). Infection and immune reconstitution working committee. *Center for International Blood and Marrow Transplant Research Newsletter, 16*(2), 2.

Twillman, R. K., Manetto, C., Wellisch, D. K., & Wolcott, D. L. (1993). The Transplant Evaluation Rating Scale: A revision of the psychosocial levels system for evaluating organ transplant candidates. *Psychosomatics, 34,* 144–153. doi:10.1016/S0033-3182(93)71905-2

Velikova, G., Wright, E. P., Smith, A. B., Cull, A., Gould, D., Forman, T., & Selby, P. J. (1999). Automated collection of quality-of-life data: A comparison of paper and computer touch-screen questionnaires. *Journal of Clinical Oncology, 1,* 998–1007.

Zigmond, A. S., & Snaith, R. P. (1983). The Hospital Anxiety and Depression Scale. *Acta Psychiatrica Scandinavica, 67,* 361–370. doi:10.1111/j.1600-0447.1983.tb09716.x

6

DEEP BRAIN STIMULATION FOR PARKINSON'S DISEASE

SARAH K. LAGEMAN, MELODY MICKENS, THERESE VERKERKE, AND KATHRYN HOLLOWAY

Parkinson's disease (PD), the second most prevalent neurodegenerative disease in the United States, is a disease of the central nervous system characterized by impairments in motor skills, cognition, and other functions. A prevalence study of PD in 2005 (Dorsey et al., 2007) estimated that more than 4 million people worldwide were affected by the disease, and this number will likely double by 2030. The average age of onset is 60; however, individuals have been diagnosed as early as age 18. Motor symptoms are the hallmark of the disease and include tremor, rigidity, bradykinesia (i.e., slowness of movement), and postural instability. However, in recent years increasing attention has been focused on nonmotor symptoms of PD, given their prevalence and significant impact on quality of life (QOL). Nonmotor symptoms of PD include gastrointestinal, urinary, sexual function, cardiovascular, neurocognitive, psychiatric, mood, sleep disorder, and other symptoms (Chaudhuri et al.,

DOI: 10.1037/14035-007
Presurgical Psychological Screening: Understanding Patients, Improving Outcomes, Andrew R. Block and David B. Sarwer (Editors)
Copyright © 2013 by the American Psychological Association. All rights reserved.

2010). With regard to psychological and neuropsychological symptoms, the neurobehavioral changes observed in PD are well characterized and include slowness of thought, deficits in visuospatial processing, working memory, learning and recall, executive dysfunction, and mood disturbance (Bondi & Tröster, 1997; Tröster & Fields, 2008).

The psychological and neuropsychological symptoms of PD likely emanate from underlying brain pathology. Brain pathology studies have revealed that individuals presenting with PD symptoms have already been affected at the neuronal level by the disease for several decades. Braak, Ghebremedhin, Rub, Bratzke, and Del Tredici (2004) proposed a six-stage neuropathology of PD in which the disease progressively involves different areas of the autonomic, limbic, and somatomotor systems of the brain. Clinical symptoms typically emerge in Stages 3 to 4 when the substantia nigra and other regions of the midbrain and forebrain develop pathology. Three clinicopathological phenotypes of PD have been proposed, which differ with regard to age and timing of symptom onset and severity of cognitive impairment (Halliday & McCann, 2010). These phenotypes are categorized as (a) dementia with Lewy bodies (i.e., dementia-dominant syndrome with onset of cognitive symptoms at the same time or within a year of PD symptom onset and core features of cognitive fluctuations, visual hallucinations [VHs], and motor symptoms of PD), (b) PD with dementia (i.e., dementia onset more than 1 year after onset of PD symptoms), and (c) idiopathic PD (i.e., dementia onset in the very late stage of the disease, after approximately 10–15 years). Only the idiopathic PD phenotype is described as conforming to the Braak et al. six-stage neuropathological model of PD. Thus, although some disagreement about clinicopathological phenotypes and pathological progression exists in the field, PD is widely accepted as an incurable, progressive neurodegenerative disorder. Most cases of PD are thought to have a multifactorial etiology, and interested readers are referred to recent reviews of PD etiology for more in-depth discussion (Morley & Hurtig, 2010; Wirdefeldt, Adami, Cole, Trichopoulos, & Mandel, 2011).

Although no cure for PD currently exists, research efforts are focused on development of neuroprotection or disease-modifying drugs. Currently, deep brain stimulation (DBS) and pharmacotherapy can provide considerable symptom management. In the late 1960s, the emergence of dopamine agonist therapy for PD represented a turning point in clinical care, and today levodopa (L-dopa) still represents the first-line treatment approach for PD motor symptoms; however, most patients ultimately develop uncomfortable side effects from the drug, such as involuntary movements (i.e., dyskinesia) and abrupt on-and-off fluctuations (i.e., symptom fluctuations associated with L-dopa medication wearing off). DBS is a surgical procedure involving implantation of an electrode in various sites in the brain, followed by paced electrical stimulation, that can provide lasting motor symptom relief (Morley & Hurtig, 2010).

Over the past decade, DBS has evolved from an emerging last-resort treatment for advanced, L-dopa–resistant PD to an increasingly accepted surgical option to alleviate the primary motor symptoms of the disorder: dyskinesias and on–off fluctuations (Kleiner-Fisman et al., 2006). The ideal DBS candidate is young, mentally and physically healthy, and responsive to L-dopa but has medication-refractory tremor, motor fluctuations, or dyskinesia. Although few individuals with PD are ideal candidates on all of these parameters, many benefit from surgery, and currently between 10% and 15% of PD patients are believed to be appropriate candidates for DBS (Morley & Hurtig, 2010). Emerging DBS research is focused on optimally tailoring surgical targets for specific symptoms and exploration of how nonmotor symptoms of the disease influence DBS outcomes, given the significant contribution of nonmotor symptoms to QOL (Chaudhuri et al., 2006; Lang et al., 2006).

Although a review of DBS electrode placement outcomes is beyond the scope of this chapter, a brief review of recent randomized controlled trial (RCT) studies illustrates how psychological and neuropsychological factors are now dominant outcome measures in this field and are currently being used to optimize DBS surgical parameters. Common DBS electrode placement areas include the globus pallidus interna (Gpi) or subthalamic nucleus (STN) to treat on–off symptoms or dyskinesias and the ventral intermediate nucleus of the thalamus to treat tremor. Researchers have speculated that placement of electrodes differentially affects DBS outcomes, particularly mood and cognition, but studies have had inconsistent findings, and methodological issues have limited conclusions. A recent multicenter RCT compared bilateral Gpi and STN stimulation in 299 patients. At the 2-year follow-up, patients in both study groups had similar minor decreases on measures of neurocognitive function (Follett et al., 2010). The only differences between the groups consisted of a greater decline in the processing speed index in the STN DBS subgroup and improved depression in the Gpi DBS subgroup, but worsening of depression in the STN DBS subgroup, as measured by self-ratings on the Beck Depression Inventory—II. Similarly, an RCT compared unilateral Gpi and STN DBS among a sample of patients with PD, and no significant differences in mood or motor symptoms were detected. However, patients receiving STN DBS showed greater deterioration in letter verbal fluency and an increased likelihood of adverse events than those who received Gpi DBS but greater reductions in medication usage (Okun et al., 2009). Despite these trade-offs, STN continues to be the target of DBS for the vast majority of patients with PD (Kleiner-Fisman et al., 2006). In the future, researchers hope to develop procedures for determining which neural target best suits individual patient treatment needs, but this work is still in its infancy, and more RCTs are needed. For the purposes of this chapter, we discuss predictors and outcomes of DBS in general rather than by electrode placement site.

In this chapter, we offer specific recommendations for appropriate psychosocial and neuropsychological screening of DBS-eligible patients with PD based on a review of the established literature that examined motor, cognitive, and psychiatric symptoms as both predictors and outcome variables in DBS for PD. We discuss studies of both predictors and outcome variables because they directly inform presurgical screening methods. We also highlight newer research that demonstrates that psychiatric conditions, social functioning, and personality traits are important to assess in both preoperative screening for DBS and postoperative follow-up. Although DBS remains a treatment for the motor symptoms of PD, researchers are increasingly recognizing that nonmotor symptoms and psychosocial issues contribute to surgical outcomes in important ways. As a result, we recommend that best clinical practice should include multiple follow-up visits with thorough evaluation of psychiatric, social, and cognitive functioning. We end this chapter by offering recommendations for future research in this area.

PRESURGICAL SCREENING AND OUTCOMES OF DEEP BRAIN STIMULATION SURGERY IN PEOPLE WITH PARKINSON'S DISEASE

As noted earlier, although DBS was initially considered a last-resort treatment for advanced, L-dopa–resistant PD, it is now an increasingly accepted surgical option to alleviate the primary motor symptoms of the disorder as well as dyskinesias and on–off fluctuations (Kleiner-Fisman et al., 2006). Indeed, DBS has been demonstrated to be an effective therapy for motor disability. Thus, assessment of patients' motor symptoms remains essential in the presurgical screening process.

Motor Symptoms

Screening of a patient's presurgical on-response to L-dopa medication is critical in determining DBS candidacy because preoperative responsiveness to dopaminergic medication remains the best predictor of success with DBS. A convincing body of empirical literature has supported the use of DBS to treat motor symptoms, on–off fluctuations, and dyskinesia in patients with PD. A recent meta-analysis of DBS outcomes reported a mean improvement rate of 52% in motor scores on the Unified Parkinson's Disease Rating Scale (UPDRS; Kleiner-Fisman et al., 2006). Significant reductions in dyskinesia, daily off periods, and L-dopa equivalent dose were also common benefits gained from DBS. In general, the surgery resulted in average improvements equivalent to a patient's best on-response to L-dopa. Patient QOL and activities of daily living (ADLs) also tended to improve postoperatively; however, these advances were typically limited to physical aspects of functioning, such as mobility.

Cognition

Second to motor symptoms, cognitive functioning and neuropsychological status have received substantial empirical attention in the PD DBS literature as both presurgical screening tests and postoperative outcome measures. Evaluation of cognitive functioning is currently considered standard practice in prescreening for DBS in PD (Okun, Fernandez, Rodriguez, & Foote, 2007); however, comprehensiveness of neurocognitive testing varies widely.

Role of Neuropsychological Screening in Deep Brain Stimulation

Neuropsychologists who are members of DBS teams are called on to evaluate neurocognitive and psychological functioning in potential candidates and provide treatment recommendations as needed (Fields & Tröster, 2000; Okun et al., 2007). Attention to both psychological and neurocognitive issues is essential in this population given the prevalence of psychiatric symptoms and neurobehavioral changes often observed in people with PD. In the prescreening phase of DBS, emphasis is placed on identification of psychological or neurocognitive conditions that are frequently considered contraindications to DBS (e.g., dementia, severe depression, anxiety).

Dementia Screening

Although PD is associated with a pattern of frontal–subcortical dysfunction as well as visuospatial processing deficits (Bondi & Tröster, 1997; Tröster & Fields, 2008), these symptoms are not contraindications to DBS unless severe cognitive dysfunction, in the form of dementia, is present. *Dementia*, as defined by the *Diagnostic and Statistical Manual of Mental Disorders* (4th ed., text rev.; *DSM–IV–TR*; American Psychiatric Association, 2000), is significant impairment and decline in cognitive functioning, including memory and at least one other area, as well as impairment in ADLs. Dementia is commonly operationally defined as more than 2 standard deviations below published norms, corrected for age and education. Global evaluations of cognitive functioning, such as the Mini-Mental State Examination (MMSE) and the Dementia Rating Scale—2, are commonly used to screen for dementia (Lang et al., 2006). Although cut-scores on screening tests can be used as heuristic guides, clinical interpretation of scores in the context of individuals' educational and psychosocial backgrounds and consideration of changes in ADLs are important factors to consider when evaluating for dementia.

Dementia is frequently considered grounds for exclusion from receiving DBS because individuals with dementia historically experience poor postoperative recovery and have often been described as rapidly declining postsurgery, resulting in limited benefit from the surgery. For example, lower preoperative scores on the MMSE are associated with extended hospital stays post-DBS, and declines on the MMSE from pre- to postsurgery predicted longer hospital stays, indicating that lower cognitive functioning at baseline is related to greater declines and increased risk of postoperative complications (Mikos et al., 2010). Although motor symptom improvements have been observed in individuals with dementia who received DBS, the stimulators may be turned off postsurgery in response to declining cognitive function to limit risk for self-injury (e.g., falls). Given the significant risks and cost associated with DBS, knowing whether dementia is present is critical for the DBS team to avoid unnecessary complications and to educate the patient and the family about realistic outcomes.

Unfortunately, there are case examples of individuals who have not completed neuropsychological evaluation before surgery and in whom dementia was not detected preoperatively. In the absence of presurgery baseline data, when cognitive decline is observed postsurgery, the empirical evidence to make statements about the etiology of the cognitive decline is limited. In contrast, circumstances also occur when a patient with dementia may benefit from DBS, as described in the following vignette:

> Case 1 is a 68-year-old man with a 5-year history of PD, which was severely disabling.[1] Although he had significant difficulties with walking, his most significant complaint was bilateral rest tremor. His family noted mild memory difficulties, but a cognitive screening test revealed significant cognitive impairment (MMSE = 20/30). During his evaluation for DBS surgery, his UPDRS score was found to be 55, which indicated severe motor symptoms, including 3+ tremor bilaterally, and neuropsychological testing documented dementia (Dementia Rating Scale—2 = 88/144). In talking with the family further to identify why they were unaware of his severe dementia, they said that they had attributed his lack of response to questions to the motor problems of PD.
>
> Therefore, the patient was not offered Gpi or STN DBS to treat all the features of PD because it was contraindicated by the severe dementia. However, he was offered ventral intermediate nucleus DBS for treatment of his severe tremor to improve his QOL. He underwent unilateral ventral intermediate nucleus DBS with an 80% reduction in his tremor.

---

[1]Details of the cases in this chapter have been altered to protect each patient's identity.

Repeat testing postoperatively showed no worsening in his cognition and a minor improvement in his memory with discontinuation of some of his medications (Dementia Rating Scale—2 = 105/144). The patient and his family felt the DBS was of significant benefit. The second hemisphere was subsequently implanted with a similar result.

As this case demonstrates, presurgical neuropsychological evaluation is critical to identify dementia if present, to appropriately evaluate the risks and benefits associated with DBS, and to create a baseline for comparison purposes in the event that the DBS team determines DBS to be appropriate for the candidate.

Neuropsychological Screening

Neuropsychological screening of all potential DBS candidates, regardless of dementia risk, is recommended because it facilitates evaluation of DBS outcomes. Across multiple review papers and meta-analyses, the most consistent post-DBS outcome related to cognition is reduced verbal fluency (Lang et al., 2006; Parsons, Rogers, Braaten, Woods, & Tröster, 2006; Voon, Kubu, Krack, Houeto, & Tröster, 2006). However, the verbal fluency findings are identified using standardized neuropsychological testing procedures, and the daily life implications of these declines are unknown. Research has demonstrated less consistent findings with regard to reductions in verbal memory, conditional associative learning, visuospatial memory, processing speed, and some domains of executive functioning (Parsons et al., 2006; Voon et al., 2006; Witt et al., 2008). Given these findings, presurgical neuropsychological evaluation is recommended to include assessment of these domains at a minimum.

Interested readers are encouraged to review several recent articles for additional details regarding neuropsychological profiles and screening measures commonly used in DBS evaluations (Lang et al., 2006; Okun et al., 2007). Although no single recommended neuropsychological battery for DBS evaluations exists, several movement disorder research groups have proposed the use of specific instruments in this population, and agreement on the inclusion of specific measures is likely in the future as this research develops (Lang et al., 2006).

Psychiatric Issues

Despite being a primary neurologic disorder, people with PD can develop many psychiatric symptoms because of dopamine dysfunction and involvement of frontal–subcortical circuitry. Individuals diagnosed with PD often report clinically significant symptoms of anxiety, depression, apathy, VHs, and impulsivity, and indeed some psychological symptoms are likely to be present in almost all candidates for DBS. Elevated rates of depression and anxiety presurgery may reflect long-standing premorbid conditions, new symptoms associated with neurochemical changes, and maladaptive adjustments to role changes and symptoms associated with PD. Underscoring the importance of recognizing and treating these conditions, research has demonstrated a consistent correlation between psychiatric symptoms and decreased QOL and increased caregiver distress, disability, and motor and cognitive impairments in patients with PD (Weintraub & Stern, 2005). Because of the negative outcomes associated with comorbid psychiatric disorders, researchers, clinicians, and health care providers have begun focusing on the presentation and treatment of psychopathology among patients with PD to optimize surgery success. Research has demonstrated that premorbid symptoms are not likely to change postoperatively and may in fact worsen, warranting close follow-up evaluation and care by the DBS team.

The available treatment options for individuals with PD and comorbid psychiatric or psychological problems are limited. Studies examining treatment practices have demonstrated that most physicians and, in some cases, psychiatrists who treat these disorders prescribe antidepressants and anxiolytics as the first line of treatment (Palanci, Marsh, & Pontone, 2011). Although psychotherapy is another effective treatment option for depression and anxiety, therapy is less often used either alone or as an adjunct to pharmacotherapy (Weintraub & Stern, 2005).

Depression

As many as 40% of patients with PD will report experiencing clinically significant symptoms of depression at some point during the course of the illness (Reijnders, Ehrt, Weber, Aarsland, & Leentjens, 2008). Patients with PD who report a history of depression before receiving a diagnosis of PD are more likely to report severe symptoms of depression. Weintraub and Stern (2005) observed the following negative outcomes in patients with PD and depression: lower QOL ratings on self-report measures, increased progression of motor and cognitive impairment, and increased distress ratings among caregivers of patients with PD and depression. Despite these negative outcomes and an increasing need to quickly identify patients at risk for or currently experiencing depression, research has demonstrated that health care providers struggle with diagnosing and treating depression in patients with PD (Oehlberg et al., 2008; Shulman, Taback, Rabinstein, & Weiner, 2002).

Depression Screening and Treatment. Presurgical screening for depression in all DBS candidates with PD is recommended given the high prevalence of depression and potential for suicide risk. A literature review revealed that health care providers and clinicians have several instruments available to them for assessing depressive symptomatology. Self-report scales used in

PD include the Beck Depression Inventory—Second Edition, Center for Epidemiologic Studies Depression Scale—Revised, Geriatric Depression Scale, Inventory of Depressive Symptoms Self-Report, and Patient Health Questionnaire—9. Clinician-rated scales include the Hamilton Depression Rating Scale, the Harvard Department of Psychiatry/National Depression Screening Day Scale, Inventory of Depressive Symptoms Clinician-Rated, Montgomery–Åsberg Depression Rating Scale, and unstructured and structured interviews based on *DSM–IV–TR* criteria. A recent study comparing nine depression scales found that all scales studied, except the UPDRS—Part I, were valid screens when PD-specific cutoff scores were used (Williams et al., 2012).

Despite valid screening tools, health care providers may not accurately diagnose depression among patients with PD. In a study of neurologists assessing patients with PD for psychiatric disorders, Shulman et al. (2002) reported a concordance rate of 35% for depression diagnoses among this population. Researchers have noted that diagnosing depression in patients with PD is challenging because many PD-related nonmotor symptoms overlap with symptoms of depression (Oehlberg et al., 2008).

To improve detection of depression, use of both a diagnostic clinical interview and standardized self-report measures is recommended to facilitate disclosure and discussion of symptoms. Collateral information from a caregiver can be particularly helpful to obtain information regarding the functional impact of mood issues and chronology of symptoms. Furthermore, effective treatments for depression and anxiety should occur presurgically so that patients are functioning optimally before surgery and have maximum coping resources available to manage the stressors associated with brain surgery. Treatment goals for presurgical DBS candidates for depression and anxiety include (a) reduction of symptoms into a mild to moderate range of severity, with absence of suicidal ideation, and (b) stability of symptoms for several months while on medications, engaged in psychotherapy, or both.

Psychopharmacotherapy Treatments. The Movement Disorder Society recently published an evidence-based medicine review of treatments for nonmotor symptoms of PD (Seppi et al., 2011). The only pharmacological treatment designated as efficacious for the management of depressive symptoms was pramipexole, and likely efficacious treatments included the tricyclic antidepressants nortriptyline and desipramine. Insufficient evidence was found for the tricyclic antidepressant amitriptyline, all SSRIs reviewed (i.e., paroxetine, citalopram, sertraline, and fluoxetine), the newer antidepressants atomoxetine and nefazodone, pergolide, omega-3 fatty acids, and repetitive transcranial magnetic stimulation. Patients can experience difficulties tolerating anticholinergic and noradrenergic side effects of various antidepressants, and adverse event profiles of pharmacological treatments also need to be considered with patients' unique medical histories. Many patients also express concerns about taking an additional medication (Oehlberg et al., 2008). Together, these factors present challenges to both patients and health care providers alike because of their impact on medication compliance.

Psychotherapeutic Interventions. Psychotherapeutic interventions are efficacious in the treatment of patients with PD diagnosed with depression (Dobkin et al., 2011; Weintraub & Stern, 2005). Patients receiving both cognitive–behavioral therapy and problem-solving therapy interventions reported lower depression scores on measures such as the Beck Depression Inventory—2 and the Hamilton Depression Rating Scale posttreatment (Dobkin et al., 2011). In a qualitative study, patients with PD reported a preference for psychotherapy because of the reduced chance of negative side effects (Oehlberg et al., 2008). However, many of the psychotherapeutic interventions for depression continue to be underused in this population. Studies have indicated that underuse may be related to the stigma associated with seeking mental health treatment (Oehlberg et al., 2008) as well as physician overreliance on medication as a first line of treatment (Weintraub et al., 2005).

Establishing relationships with mental health professionals before surgery not only provides presurgical treatment but also facilitates access to care postoperatively if needed. In a number of patients who have undergone DBS, sudden onset of depressive symptomatology postoperatively has been reported, as demonstrated in the following example.

> Case 2 is a 65-year-old woman with 10-year history of PD who alternated between off periods with freezing of gait (off-medication UPDRS = 30) and on periods with dyskinesias (on-medication UPDRS = 15) most of the day. Neuropsychological testing revealed good cognition, with test scores all within expected ranges (MMSE = 30/30) and no evidence of depression. Bilateral STN stimulators were placed in surgery using microelectrode recording and test stimulation for efficacy and side effects. In routine programming appointments 1 and 2 months postsurgery, her program settings were changed to maximize efficacy while minimizing side effects, which for her consisted of right leg dragging. After the 2-month programming appointment, the patient returned to the clinic 2 weeks later complaining of sadness. The stimulator was switched off, and she described feeling instant relief. She was programmed at a higher contact, and a month later reported doing well with no further depression. One year later, the patient complained of depression again. The stimulator was switched off, but no change in her emotional state occurred. On further inquiry, the patient explained that she had recently lost two family members to cancer. Her depression lingered, and her primary care

physician prescribed an antidepressant. Three months later, she returned to the clinic feeling well; her depression had resolved, and she required only minimal voltage adjustment to optimize her gait.

This case highlights the need for continued coordinated care postoperatively from the DBS team. Some symptoms of depression or anxiety may be stimulator related, whereas others may be reactions to psychosocial stressors, best addressed by psychotherapy, medications, or both.

Depression Postoperative Issues. The role of psychiatric symptoms in DBS outcomes has been well researched and well summarized in two review articles (Lang et al., 2006; Voon et al., 2006). Depression and apathy have received the most research attention, whereas less is known about anxiety, hypomania, psychosis, disinhibition, and suicidality. Although mixed findings have been reported, a general trend has emerged in considering psychiatric predictors and outcomes of DBS. The thrust of the empirical evidence has suggested that preoperative psychiatric symptoms are likely to either remain consistent or worsen postoperatively (Lang et al., 2006; Thobois et al., 2010). In other words, DBS should not be entertained as a therapeutic option to treat psychiatric symptoms associated with PD, and furthermore, the increased stress associated with brain surgery may exacerbate preexisting psychological issues.

In addition to the surgery-as-life-stressor hypothesis, several researchers have posited that reductions in dopamine agonist therapy after DBS can lead to psychiatric changes associated with dopamine agonist withdrawal syndrome (Kirsch-Darrow et al., 2011; Thobois et al., 2010; Voon et al., 2006). Researchers have defined dopamine agonist withdrawal syndrome as a group of physical and psychological symptoms (e.g., anxiety, depression, insomnia, pain, orthostatic hypotension, drug cravings) that emerge in a dose-dependent manner as a consequence of reductions in dopamine agonist medication usage (Thobois et al., 2010). One recent PET imaging study revealed that patients who develop psychiatric symptoms after DBS may have increased neuronal susceptibility to dopamine agonist withdrawal syndrome, which emerges postoperatively after L-dopa reductions (Thobois et al., 2010). Further research is needed to disentangle the biological, social, and psychological processes involved in the acquisition and progression of psychiatric symptoms pre- and post-DBS surgery.

Anxiety

As with depression, approximately 40% to 49% of patients with PD report symptoms of anxiety at some point during the course of the illness, exceeding the reported rate of anxiety in the general population (Pontone et al., 2009; Walsh & Bennett, 2001). Although prevalence rates are unknown, researchers have reported that patients with PD and anxiety often report symptoms of generalized anxiety disorder, social phobia, panic disorder, and medication-induced anxiety symptoms (Pontone et al., 2009; Walsh & Bennett, 2001). Although the pathophysiology of increased anxiety in PD is not known, onset generally occurs after diagnosis, and researchers have hypothesized that development of anxiety may be a psychological response to physical symptoms or related to neurochemical changes in PD (Walsh & Bennett, 2001). As with many chronically ill populations, comorbid symptoms of anxiety are associated with negative physical and emotional health outcomes, including increased insomnia, poorer quality of sleep, and higher levels of depression (Walsh & Bennett, 2001).

Anxiety Screening and Treatment. Presurgical screening of anxiety in all DBS candidates with PD is recommended, given the high prevalence of anxiety and poor DBS outcomes associated with severe anxiety. A literature review indicated that when assessing symptoms of anxiety in patients with PD clinicians often use diagnostic clinical interview and evaluation of *DSM–IV–TR* criteria in addition to the following standardized self-report measures: Anxiety Status Inventory, Beck Anxiety Inventory, Hamilton Anxiety Rating Scale, Hospital Anxiety and Depression Scale, the Neuropsychiatric Inventory—Anxiety subscale, the Spielberger State–Trait Anxiety Inventory, and the Zung Self-Rating Anxiety Scale. A Movement Disorder Society Task Force critique (Leentjens et al., 2008a) of anxiety symptom rating scales in samples with PD found that all anxiety scales reviewed were missing clinimetric information and noted a critical need for validation studies. A more recent validation study (Leentjens et al., 2011) of the Beck Anxiety Inventory, Hamilton Anxiety Rating Scale, and Hospital Anxiety and Depression Scale among patients with PD found these scales to be acceptable regarding their clinimetric properties but noted construct validity limitations and suggested the design of a new anxiety scale for use with people with PD. In the absence of a PD-specific anxiety scale, anxiety screening with one of the validated anxiety scales in conjunction with a diagnostic clinical interview are recommended.

Individuals with severe anxiety are typically considered poor candidates for DBS because of difficulties tolerating postoperative activation and programming procedures. As a result, presurgical screening for all patients, and treatments as necessary, are critical to optimize patients' candidacy for DBS. Patients with mild anxiety that has minimal functional impact on their daily activities will likely not require ongoing therapy, but establishment of a connection with the psychologist can be helpful if treatment is needed postoperatively. Patients with more moderate to severe anxiety will require treatment before candidacy for DBS can be considered, given the difficulty these patients tend to have with postoperative programming. If symptoms lessen with treatment, patients may become candidates for DBS; however, severe treatment-resistant anxiety is generally a contraindication to DBS because of the postoperative programming issues. Discussion of postoperative procedures may be especially helpful to educate patients about expectations of their role and involvement in necessary continued programming procedures with the DBS team. DBS outcome studies have only recently examined depression outcomes, and anxiety symptoms remain to be systematically examined.

Psychopharmacotherapy Treatments. Despite the prevalence of anxiety in patients with PD, there is a dearth of studies examining the treatment of this disorder. Health care providers typically prescribe benzodiazepines, SSRIs, SNRIs, and in some cases antipsychotic medications or tricyclic antidepressants. In a survey of neurologists, Palanci et al. (2011) reported that all of the doctors who reported treating anxiety used pharmacological treatments and that none referred their patients to psychotherapy in addition to or in place of pharmacotherapy.

Psychotherapeutic Interventions. Current research on the psychotherapeutic treatment of anxiety in PD is in its very early stages. Cognitive–behavioral therapy, relaxation techniques, and mindfulness-based stress reduction have been demonstrated to be beneficial for individuals with other chronic illness and in older adults, suggesting that these interventions may benefit patients with comorbid PD and anxiety (Cimpean & Drake, 2011).

Apathy

Although apathy has traditionally been characterized as a component of depression, this symptom has been recognized as a significant issue in PD that can occur with and without symptoms of depression (Kirsch-Darrow, Fernandez, Marsiske, Okun, & Bowers, 2006). Because of its prevalence and distinctive features, there has been a movement to create diagnostic criteria for an apathy syndrome. Apathy is a nonmotor symptom of PD that is characterized by diminished motivation, decreased interest, flat affect, reduced effort, and reduced productivity (Kirsch-Darrow et al., 2006). Prevalence estimates have revealed that 17% to 70% of patients with PD report experiencing some symptoms of apathy during the course of the illness (Starkstein, Ingram, Garau, & Mizrahi, 2005). Reports of apathy have been correlated with increased cognitive dysfunction, decreased QOL, and difficulties in ADLs.

Apathy Screening and Treatment. Presurgical screening of apathy in all DBS candidates with PD is recommended given the high prevalence of apathy. Currently, health care providers must rely on self-report data from one of the various apathy scales (e.g., Apathy Evaluation Scale, Apathy Scale, Apathy Inventory, Item 4 on the UPDRS, Item 7 on the Neuropsychiatric Inventory and the Lille Apathy Rating Scale). A Movement Disorder Society Task Force evaluation of apathy scales used in PD samples found that the Apathy Scale and Item 4 of the UPDRS were classified as recommended to assess apathy;

however, the Task Force suggested use of Item 4 of the UPDRS only as a screening measure given limited reliability associated with using a single item measure (Leentjens et al., 2008b). Despite numerous measures, many clinicians and health care providers struggle to differentiate between apathy as a unique entity in PD and apathy as a traditional symptom of depression (e.g., anhedonia). More research is needed to help health care providers verify whether apathy truly represents a unique syndrome in PD and, if so, to develop diagnostic criteria and improved assessments and treatments specific to apathy in PD.

Presently, the treatment options for apathy in individuals with PD are limited. Available treatment options include the use of methylphenidate, a stimulant medication, which has shown some efficacy in preliminary trials (Chatterjee & Kahn, 2002).

Apathy Postoperative Issues. Unfortunately, apathy often continues to be a problematic symptom with few specific treatment recommendations for individuals with PD post-DBS. Development of new-onset postoperative apathy symptoms, as well as abulia and anomia, are rare but possible and very serious complications of DBS. These phenomena necessitate follow-up care by a multidisciplinary treatment team.

Other Psychiatric Conditions

Most literature on PD-related psychiatric conditions has focused on depression, anxiety, and apathy; however, VHs, impulsivity, and impulse control disorders can also be observed in PD. Although the literature regarding VHs and impulsivity in PD is more limited than that on depression in PD, study of these conditions is increasing given their impact on QOL; highlights from the literature are provided below.

Visual Hallucinations

Between 6% and 60% of patients with PD report experiencing VHs at some point during the course of the illness, and although neuropathology of VHs is likely multifactorial, combined L-dopa–dopamine agonist therapy appears to play a role in presentation of VHs (Ibarretxe-Bilbao, Junque, Marti, & Tolosa, 2011). VHs typically occur later in the course of the disease and can occur even in patients without dementia. They are typically associated with increased impairment in the following cognitive domains: verbal fluency, verbal and visual memory, language comprehension, and visuospatial perception. Additionally, VHs have been associated with lower scores on the MMSE and higher scores on self-report measures of depression.

Fujimoto (2009) described using a five-step process to manage VHs consisting of eliminating multiple medications, reducing anti-Parkinsonian drugs (e.g., anti-cholinergic medications, dopamine agonists, L-dopa), followed by treatment with mianserin hydrochloride and supplementation with atypical antipsychotics if necessary and consideration of modified electroconvulsive therapy as a last resort. Groundbreaking research on the use of nonpharmacological treatments for VHs has demonstrated that PD patients with VHs often report the use of cognitive strategies (e.g., distraction) and interactive techniques (e.g., talking to someone) as ways to cope with the hallucinations (Diederich, Pieri, & Goetz, 2003).

Impulsivity and Impulse Control Disorders

Pontone, Williams, Bassett, and Marsh (2006) described impulsivity and impulse control disorders (ICDs) as impairment or distress resulting from an inability to inhibit detrimental behaviors. Behaviors associated with ICDs include pathological gambling, compulsive sexual behaviors, excessive spending, and binge eating (Voon et al., 2011). A multicenter study of patients with PD demonstrated that those with ICDs reported functional impairment, symptoms of depression, higher levels of state and trait anxiety, and increased levels of novelty seeking, impulsivity, and obsessive–compulsive symptoms (Voon et al., 2011). The data from this multicenter investigation also indicated that at least one ICD was prevalent in 13.5% of patients with PD. Pharmacological and medical interventions such as dopamine agonist treatment and DBS have been associated with increased reports of impulsivity and ICDs (Weintraub et al., 2010).

As with treating VHs, research findings have demonstrated that modification of dopamine agonists and L-dopa therapy are useful in the treatment of ICDs and impulsivity in patients with PD (Galpern & Stacy, 2007). Additional therapies include the use of antidepressants, STN DBS among patients taking high doses of dopamine replacement therapy, and a combination of reduced dopamine agonist therapy, antidepressants, group therapy or individual psychotherapy, and behavioral modification (e.g., monitoring of spending; Galpern & Stacy, 2007).

Deep Brain Stimulation as a Treatment for Psychological and Psychiatric Symptoms in Parkinson's Disease

As described earlier, DBS is a specific treatment to target motor symptoms producing the best L-dopa response; however, the research to evaluate its efficacy as a treatment for psychological and psychiatric symptoms in PD has been limited. Presently, STN DBS has demonstrated some efficacy in the treatment of ICDs (Galpern & Stacy, 2007), but little to no data exist on its effectiveness in treating other psychological and psychiatric disorders in patients with PD. By contrast, much of the literature has demonstrated that after DBS, patients with PD may experience the onset of psychological and psychiatric symptoms such as anxiety, psychosis, depression, and VHs or preexisting psychiatric symptoms may worsen after the procedure and medication changes (Lang et al., 2006; Thobois et al., 2010). Moreover, the negative outcomes associated with psychological and psychiatric symptoms that patients with PD may experience and the likelihood that these symptoms may be exacerbated after DBS demonstrate the need for psychological screening, intervention, and treatment pre- and post-DBS.

Psychosocial Factors

Increased recognition of the nonmotor symptoms of PD has spawned interest in the implications of these factors for patients seeking DBS surgery (Lang et al., 2006). More than a decade ago, researchers using a PD-specific QOL measure (the Parkinson's Disease Questionnaire—39) discovered that patients undergoing DBS surgery reported experiencing improvements in a variety of important areas, including nonmotor symptoms such as cognitive functioning, communication problems, and perceived social stigma (Straits-Tröster et al., 2000). Interestingly, similar gains were not made on the Problems in Social Relationships subscale of the questionnaire, suggesting that psychosocial outcomes of DBS are not universally positive. Since this preliminary investigation of nonmotor outcomes in DBS, research on the topic has blossomed. Two comprehensive reviews have reported that psychosocial factors such as age, gender, psychiatric status, social support, access to care, expectations, and individual motivation are relevant when determining appropriateness of DBS treatment for patients with PD (Lang et al., 2006; Voon et al., 2006).

Age

Although advanced age is often cited as a risk factor for surgical complications, the issue is confounded by age-related comorbidities such as the onset of dementia and L-dopa–resistant symptoms. In one longitudinal investigation (Ory-Magne et al., 2007), older preoperative age predicted increased risk of apathy and depression symptoms, more frequent incidence of surgical complications (e.g., hemorrhage, death), reductions in self-reported cognition, and fewer gains in QOL than for younger patients, but no significant differences for motor outcomes. Similarly, in a multicenter RCT of best medical therapy versus DBS surgery in 255 patients with PD, no differences in motor outcomes were noted in patients older than age 70 compared with patients younger than age 70, but older patients were reported to experience a higher rate of adverse events (Weaver et al., 2009). Despite these more pessimistic findings for older patients, a review of preoperative issues recommended that advanced age should not, on its own, exclude an otherwise suitable patient from receiving DBS (Lang et al., 2006).

Gender

As with age, gender differences have been detected in response to DBS. Similarly, however, the research has supported awareness of increased risk factors and differential outcomes rather than consideration of gender as exclusionary criteria. PD presentation and progression have previously been established to differ by gender (Accolla et al., 2007). Specifically, women are more prone to difficulty with ADLs, psychiatric symptoms, and nonmotor problems in general, whereas men tend to experience a more rapid progression of motor symptoms with more varied symptoms including hypophonia, apathy, postural disturbances, and hypersalivation. Differences have also been observed in responsiveness to L-dopa. Not surprisingly, because of higher body mass, male patients with PD typically require higher doses of L-dopa; however, somewhat counterintuitively, female patients are more affected by L-dopa–induced dyskinesias. Given these existing differences in PD symptomatology, gender differences in DBS outcomes are not unexpected; however, few studies have examined these differences. In one recent study, female patients with PD who underwent DBS experienced less relief of bradykinesia symptoms and slightly greater improvement in ADLs than matched male patients (Accolla et al., 2007). More research is needed to examine these differences in the context of DBS outcomes.

Social Roles

In an effort to better understand the psychosocial mechanisms at play among patients with PD who receive DBS, several research teams have performed qualitative studies, involving detailed interviews with patients, caregivers, and health care providers. The major themes, outlined in a recent review article (Bell, Maxwell, McAndrews, Sadikot, & Racine, 2011), that have emerged from these investigations include the role of social support, ethical issues related to access to care and ability to comply with follow-up, and upheavals in patient identity after potentially life-changing surgery. Many researchers have emphasized that the intensive nature of DBS follow-up requires that patients be able to identify a supportive person who can attend doctors' meetings and assist with care management postoperatively (Bell et al., 2011). At some care centers, lack of a supportive other, residence far from the center, lack of consistent transportation, or insufficient insurance coverage can be exclusionary criteria for DBS treatment (Bell et al., 2011; Lang et al., 2006).

Finally, although DBS motor outcomes are usually positive, social relationships and a patient's sense of self may deteriorate postoperatively. Researchers believe that multiple factors may contribute to increased marital discord and patient loss of identity after DBS (Schüpbach & Agid, 2008). Health care providers have reported that unrealistic expectations on the part of patients and caregivers alike may lead to disappointment when patients do not experience a miraculous recovery postoperatively. However, sudden and dramatic improvements in motor function may disrupt entrenched caregiver–care recipient relationship dynamics. Likewise, many individuals who experienced rapid changes in disease status have reported a forced normalization and a loss of their sick role identity. As a result of living with an often debilitating chronic illness for many years, individuals with PD may have suffered losses in social or occupational skills, placing them at a disadvantage when they are expected to reenter the workforce or assume increased self-care responsibilities after DBS. Researchers studying these issues have emphasized that psychosocial prescreening and increased education will help to ensure that patients and support people have realistic expectations regarding DBS outcomes and access to needed postoperative care (Bell et al., 2011; Lang et al., 2006; Okun et al., 2007).

CONCLUSION

Prescreening for and postsurgical follow-up of DBS require a multidisciplinary team of neurosurgeons, neurologists, neuropsychologists, geriatric psychiatrists, and nurses to provide optimal care. Many preexisting psychological symptoms may not improve postsurgery and may potentially worsen. Thus, follow-up evaluation and continued care are critical for optimal outcomes for individuals with DBS. The neuropsychologist is a vital member of this team, given the complex interaction of neurocognitive and psychological symptoms and phenomena that may present in this population. Geriatric psychiatrists are also critical, and often underrepresented, members of the team and are especially important in long-term follow-up care and management of medications.

As highlighted by the cases included in this chapter, baseline neuropsychological evaluation of functioning is critical to identify dementia, provide an individual postoperative comparison, and optimize surgical outcomes. Follow-up care by a multidisciplinary team is also essential to manage postoperative medication changes for both new-onset symptoms and altered management of established symptoms post-DBS. Within the treatment team, clear identification of team members who will screen for the development of depression and ICDs is particularly important.

Several areas of critical need exist in the research literature and include development and optimization of effective pharmacological and psychological treatments for apathy, anxiety, and other ICDs in PD. Further development of cognitive–behavioral therapies tailored to treat the psychological and cognitive symptoms frequently experienced by individuals with PD hold great promise for this growing population and warrant further investigation. The complexity of DBS presurgical screening and postsurgical follow-up illustrates the multidimensional nature of PD and highlights the importance of monitoring psychosocial, cognitive, and psychiatric factors throughout the surgical treatment process.

REFERENCES

Accolla, E., Caputo, E., Cogiamanian, F., Tamma, F., Mrakic-Sposta, S., Marceglia, S., . . . Priori, A. (2007). Gender differences in patients with Parkinson's disease treated with subthalamic deep brain stimulation. *Movement Disorders, 22,* 1150–1156. doi:10.1002/mds.21520

American Psychiatric Association. (2000). *Diagnostic and statistical manual of mental disorders* (4th ed., text rev.). Washington, DC: Author.

Bell, E., Maxwell, B., McAndrews, M. P., Sadikot, A. F., & Racine, E. (2011). A review of social and relational aspects of deep brain stimulation in Parkinson's disease informed by healthcare provider experiences. *Parkinson's Disease, 2011,* Article 871874. doi:10.4061/2011/871874

Bondi, M. W., & Tröster, A. I. (1997). Parkinson's disease: Neurobehavioral consequences of basal ganglia dysfunction. In P. D. Nussbaum (Ed.), *Handbook of neuropsychology and aging* (pp. 216–245). New York, NY: Plenum Press.

Braak, H., Ghebremedhin, E., Rub, U., Bratzke, H., & Del Tredici, K. (2004). Stages in the development of Parkinson's disease-related pathology. *Cell and Tissue Research, 318,* 121–134. doi:10.1007/s00441-004-0956-9

Chatterjee, A., & Kahn, S. (2002). Methylphenidate treats apathy in Parkinson's disease. *Journal of Neuropsychiatry and Clinical Neurosciences, 14,* 461–462. doi:10.1176/appi.neuropsych.14.4.461

Chaudhuri, K. R., Martinez-Martin, P., Schapira, A. H., Stocchi, F., Sethi, K., Odin, P., . . . Olanow, C. W. (2006). International multicenter pilot study of the first comprehensive self-completed nonmotor symptoms questionnaire for Parkinson's disease: The NMSQuest study. *Movement Disorders, 21,* 916–923. doi:10.1002/mds.20844

Chaudhuri, K. R., Prieto-Jurcynska, C., Naidu, Y., Mitra, T., Frades-Payo, B., Tluk, S., . . . Martinez-Martin, P. (2010). The nondeclaration of nonmotor symptoms of Parkinson's disease to health care professionals: An international study using the nonmotor symptoms questionnaire. *Movement Disorders, 25,* 704–709. doi:10.1002/mds.22868

Cimpean, D., & Drake, R. E. (2011). Treating co-morbid chronic medical conditions and anxiety/depression. *Epidemiology and Psychiatric Sciences, 20,* 141–150. doi:10.1017/S2045796011000345

Diederich, N. J., Pieri, V., & Goetz, C. G. (2003). Coping strategies for visual hallucinations in Parkinson's disease. *Movement Disorders, 18,* 831–832. doi:10.1002/mds.10450

Dobkin, R. D., Menza, M., Allen, L. A., Gara, M. A., Mark, M. H., Tiu, J., . . . Friedman, J. (2011). Cognitive-behavioral therapy for depression in Parkinson's disease: A randomized, controlled trial. *American Journal of Psychiatry, 168,* 1066–1074. doi:10.1176/appi.ajp.2011.10111669

Dorsey, E. R., Constantinescu, R., Thompson, J. P., Biglan, K. M., Holloway, R. G., Kieburtz, K., . . . Tanner, C. M. (2007). Projected number of people with Parkinson disease in the most populous nations, 2005 through 2030. *Neurology, 68,* 384–386. doi:10.1212/01.wnl.0000247740.47667.03

Fields, J. A., & Tröster, A. I. (2000). Cognitive outcomes after deep brain stimulation for Parkinson's disease: A review of initial studies and recommendations for future research. *Brain and Cognition, 42,* 268–293. doi:10.1006/brcg.1999.1104

Follett, K. A., Weaver, F. M., Stern, M., Hur, K., Harris, C. L., Luo, P., . . . Reda, D. J.; CSP 468 Study Group. (2010). Pallidal versus subthalamic deep-brain stimulation for Parkinson's disease. *The New England Journal of Medicine, 362,* 2077–2091. doi:10.1056/NEJMoa0907083

Fujimoto, K. (2009). Management of non-motor complications in Parkinson's disease. *Journal of Neurology, 256*(Suppl. 3), 299–305. doi:10.1007/s00415-009-5245-9

Galpern, W. R., & Stacy, M. (2007). Management of impulse control disorders in Parkinson's disease. *Current Treatment Options in Neurology, 9,* 189–197. doi:10.1007/BF02938408

Halliday, G. M., & McCann, H. (2010). The progression of pathology in Parkinson's disease. *Annals of the New York Academy of Sciences, 1184,* 188–195. doi:10.1111/j.1749-6632.2009.05118.x

Ibarretxe-Bilbao, N., Junque, C., Marti, M. J., & Tolosa, E. (2011). Cerebral basis of visual hallucinations in Parkinson's disease: Structural and functional MRI studies. *Journal of the Neurological Sciences, 310,* 79–81. doi:10.1016/j.jns.2011.06.019

Kirsch-Darrow, L., Fernandez, H. H., Marsiske, M., Okun, M. S., & Bowers, D. (2006). Dissociating apathy and depression in Parkinson disease. *Neurology, 67,* 33–38. doi:10.1212/01.wnl.0000230572.07791.22

Kirsch-Darrow, L., Zahodne, L. B., Marsiske, M., Okun, M. S., Foote, K. D., & Bowers, D. (2011). The trajectory of apathy after deep brain stimulation: From pre-surgery to 6 months post-surgery in Parkinson's disease. *Parkinsonism & Related Disorders, 17,* 182–188. doi:10.1016/j.parkreldis.2010.12.011

Kleiner-Fisman, G., Herzog, J., Fisman, D. N., Tamma, F., Lyons, K. E., Pahwa, R., . . . Deuschl, G. (2006). Subthalamic nucleus deep brain stimulation: Summary and meta-analysis of outcomes. *Movement Disorders, 21*(Suppl. 14), S290–S304. doi:10.1002/mds.20962

Lang, A. E., Houeto, J. L., Krack, P., Kubu, C., Lyons, K. E., Moro, E., . . . Voon, V. (2006). Deep brain stimulation: Preoperative issues. *Movement Disorders, 21*(Suppl. 14), S171–S196. doi:10.1002/mds.20955

Leentjens, A. F. G., Dujardin, K., Marsh, L., Martinez-Martin, P., Richard, I. H., Starkstein, S. E., . . . Goetz, C. G. (2008a). Anxiety rating scales in Parkinson's disease: Critique and recommendations. *Movement Disorders, 23*, 2015–2025. doi:10.1002/mds.22233

Leentjens, A. F. G., Dujardin, K., Marsh, L., Martinez-Martin, P., Richard, I. H., Starkstein, S. E., . . . Goetz, C. G. (2008b). Apathy and anhedonia rating scales in Parkinson's disease: Critique and recommendations. *Movement Disorders, 23*, 2004–2014. doi:10.1002/mds.22229

Leentjens, A. F. G., Dujardin, K., Marsh, L., Richard, I. H., Starkstein, S. E., & Martinez-Martin, P. (2011). Anxiety rating scales in Parkinson's disease: A validation study of the Hamilton Anxiety Rating Scale, the Beck Anxiety Inventory, and the Hospital Anxiety and Depression Scale. *Movement Disorders, 26*, 407–415. doi:10.1002/mds.23184; 10.1002/mds.23184

Mikos, A., Pavon, J., Bowers, D., Foote, K. D., Resnick, A. S., Fernandez, H. H., . . . Okun, M. S. (2010). Factors related to extended hospital stays following deep brain stimulation for Parkinson's disease. *Parkinsonism & Related Disorders, 16*, 324–328. doi:10.1016/j.parkreldis.2010.02.002

Morley, J. F., & Hurtig, H. I. (2010). Current understanding and management of Parkinson's disease: Five new things. *Neurology, 75*(18, Suppl. 1), S9–S15. doi:10.1212/WNL.0b013e3181fb3628

Oehlberg, K., Barg, F. K., Brown, G. K., Taraborelli, D., Stern, M. B., & Weintraub, D. (2008). Attitudes regarding the etiology and treatment of depression in Parkinson's disease: A qualitative study. *Journal of Geriatric Psychiatry and Neurology, 21*, 123–132. doi:10.1177/0891988708316862

Okun, M. S., Fernandez, H. H., Rodriguez, R. L., & Foote, K. D. (2007). Identifying candidates for deep brain stimulation in Parkinson's disease: The role of the primary care physician. *Geriatrics, 62*, 18–24.

Okun, M. S., Fernandez, H. H., Wu, S. S., Kirsch-Darrow, L., Bowers, D., Bova, F., . . . Foote, K. D. (2009). Cognition and mood in Parkinson's disease in subthalamic nucleus versus globus pallidus interna deep brain stimulation: The COMPARE trial. *Annals of Neurology, 65*, 586–595. doi:10.1002/ana.21596

Ory-Magne, F., Brefel-Courbon, C., Simonetta-Moreau, M., Fabre, N., Lotterie, J. A., Chaynes, P., . . . Rascol, O. (2007). Does ageing influence deep brain stimulation outcomes in Parkinson's disease? *Movement Disorders, 22*, 1457–1463. doi:10.1002/mds.21547

Palanci, J., Marsh, L., & Pontone, G. M. (2011). Gaps in treatment for anxiety in Parkinson disease. *American Journal of Geriatric Psychiatry, 19*, 907–908. doi:10.1097/JGP.0b013e318227fa37

Parsons, T. D., Rogers, S. A., Braaten, A. J., Woods, S. P., & Tröster, A. I. (2006). Cognitive sequelae of subthalamic nucleus deep brain stimulation in Parkinson's disease: A meta-analysis. *Lancet Neurology, 5,* 578–588. doi:10.1016/S1474-4422(06)70475-6

Pontone, G. M., Williams, J. R., Anderson, K. E., Chase, G., Goldstein, S. A., Grill, S., . . . Marsh, L. (2009). Prevalence of anxiety disorders and anxiety subtypes in patients with Parkinson's disease. *Movement Disorders, 24,* 1333–1338. doi:10.1002/mds.22611

Pontone, G. M., Williams, J. R., Bassett, S., & Marsh, L. (2006). Clinical features associated with impulse control disorders in Parkinson's disease. *Neurology, 67,* 1258–1261. doi:10.1212/01.wnl.0000238401.76928.45

Reijnders, J. S., Ehrt, U., Weber, W. E., Aarsland, D., & Leentjens, A. F. (2008). A systematic review of prevalence studies of depression in Parkinson's disease. *Movement Disorders, 23,* 183–189. doi:10.1002/mds.21803

Schüpbach, W. M., & Agid, Y. (2008). Psychosocial adjustment after deep brain stimulation in Parkinson's disease. *Nature Clinical Practice. Neurology, 4,* 58–59. doi:10.1038/ncpneuro0714

Seppi, K., Weintraub, D., Coelho, M., Perez-Lloret, S., Fox, S. H., Katzenschlager, R., . . . Sampaio, C. (2011). The Movement Disorder Society evidence-based medicine review update: Treatments for the non-motor symptoms of Parkinson's disease. *Movement Disorders, 26*(Suppl. 3), S42–S80. doi:10.1002/mds.23884

Shulman, L. M., Taback, R. L., Rabinstein, A. A., & Weiner, W. J. (2002). Non-recognition of depression and other non-motor symptoms in Parkinson's disease. *Parkinsonism & Related Disorders, 8,* 193–197. doi:10.1016/S1353-8020(01)00015-3

Starkstein, S. E., Ingram, L., Garau, M. L., & Mizrahi, R. (2005). On the overlap between apathy and depression in dementia. *Journal of Neurology, Neurosurgery & Psychiatry, 76,* 1070–1074. doi:10.1136/jnnp.2004.052795

Straits-Tröster, K., Fields, J. A., Wilkinson, S. B., Pahwa, R., Lyons, K. E., Koller, W. C., & Tröster, A. I. (2000). Health-related quality of life in Parkinson's disease after pallidotomy and deep brain stimulation. *Brain and Cognition, 42,* 399–416. doi:10.1006/brcg.1999.1112

Thobois, S., Ardouin, C., Lhommee, E., Klinger, H., Lagrange, C., Xie, J., . . . Krack, P. (2010). Non-motor dopamine withdrawal syndrome after surgery for Parkinson's disease: Predictors and underlying mesolimbic denervation. *Brain: A Journal of Neurology, 133,* 1111–1127. doi:10.1093/brain/awq032

Tröster, A. I., & Fields, J. A. (2008). Parkinson's disease, progressive supranuclear palsy, corticobasal degeneration and related disorders of the frontostriatal system. In J. E. Morgan & J. H. Ricker (Ed.), *Textbook of clinical neuropsychology* (pp. 536–577). New York, NY: Psychology Press.

Voon, V., Kubu, C., Krack, P., Houeto, J. L., & Tröster, A. I. (2006). Deep brain stimulation: Neuropsychological and neuropsychiatric issues. *Movement Disorders, 21*(Suppl. 14), S305–S327. doi:10.1002/mds.20963

Voon, V., Sohr, M., Lang, A. E., Potenza, M. N., Siderowf, A. D., Whetteckey, J., . . . Stacy, M. (2011). Impulse control disorders in Parkinson disease: A multicenter case-control study. *Annals of Neurology, 69,* 986–996. doi: 10.1002/ana.22356; 10.1002/ana.22356

Walsh, K., & Bennett, G. (2001). Recognizing psychiatric and cognitive complications in Parkinson's disease: Impulse control disorders and related behaviors. *Postgraduate Medicine, 77,* 89–93. doi:10.1136/pmj.77.904.89

Weaver, F. M., Follett, K., Stern, M., Hur, K., Harris, C., Marks, W. J., Jr., . . . Huang, G. D.; CSP 468 Study Group. (2009). Bilateral deep brain stimulation vs best medical therapy for patients with advanced Parkinson disease: A randomized controlled trial. *JAMA, 301,* 63–73. doi:10.1001/jama.2008.929

Weintraub, D., Koester, J., Potenza, M. N., Siderowf, A. D., Stacy, M., Voon, V., . . . Lang, A. E. (2010). Impulse control disorders in Parkinson's disease: A cross-sectional study of 3090 patients. *Archives of Neurology, 67,* 589–595. doi:10.1001/archneurol. 2010.65

Weintraub, D., Morales, K. H., Moberg, P. J., Bilker, W. B., Balderston, C., Duda, J. E., . . . Stern, M. B. (2005). Antidepressant studies in Parkinson's disease: A review and meta-analysis. *Movement Disorders, 20,* 1161–1169. doi:10.1002/ mds.20555

Weintraub, D., & Stern, M. B. (2005). Psychiatric complications in Parkinson disease. *American Journal of Geriatric Psychiatry, 13,* 844–851. doi:10.1176/appi. ajgp.13.10.844

Williams, J. R., Hirsch, E. S., Anderson, K., Bush, A. L., Goldstein, S. R., Grill, S., . . . Marsh, L. (2012). A comparison of nine scales to detect depression in Parkinson disease: Which scale to use? *Neurology, 78,* 998–1006. doi:10.1212/ WNL.0b013e31824d587f

Wirdefeldt, K., Adami, H. O., Cole, P., Trichopoulos, D., & Mandel, J. (2011). Epidemiology and etiology of Parkinson's disease: A review of the evidence. *European Journal of Epidemiology, 26*(Suppl. 1), 1–58. doi:10.1007/s10654-011-9581-6

Witt, K., Daniels, C., Reiff, J., Krack, P., Volkmann, J., Pinsker, M. O., . . . Deuschl, G. (2008). Neuropsychological and psychiatric changes after deep brain stimulation for Parkinson's disease: A randomised, multicentre study. *Lancet Neurology, 7,* 605–614. doi:10.1016/S1474-4422(08)70114-5

7

TEMPOROMANDIBULAR DISORDER–RELATED ORAL SURGERY

SARAH E. FRALEY, ERIC SWANHOLM, ANNA W. STOWELL,
AND ROBERT J. GATCHEL

If you don't know where you are going, you are likely to end up some-
where else.

—Yogi Berra, New York Yankees great

The symptoms of temporomandibular disorders (TMDs) include pain and
limited jaw opening of the temporomandibular joint (TMJ) and masticatory
musculature pain. Other common TMD symptoms include orofacial pain,
joint grinding, clicks or popping, pain on masticatory muscle palpation, and
limited mandibular movement. Diagnosis of TMD typically involves the
identification of degenerative changes of the TMJ and disc displacements,
muscle disorders, or internal derangements. Although the etiology of TMD
is not yet clear, proposed causal factors may include the physical structure of
the mouth and musculature, and psychosocial factors (Wright et al., 2004).
Additionally, stress-related clenching and grinding, poor muscle discrimination, and unconscious bracing of the orofacial musculature may also contribute
to the etiology of TMD. Other potential contributors include functional and
structural issues in the TMJ, such as trauma, internal derangement, mechanical
displacement, or osteoarthritis (Gatchel, Potter, Hinds, & Ingram, 2011).

DOI: 10.1037/14035-008
Presurgical Psychological Screening: Understanding Patients, Improving Outcomes, Andrew R. Block and
David B. Sarwer (Editors)

TMDs are highly prevalent in the United States, with an estimated 7% to 15% of individuals experiencing symptoms at any given moment (Leresche, 1997) and a lifetime prevalence rate of 75% (American Academy of Orofacial Pain, 2004). Of the estimated 20 million adults who annually report TMD-related pain symptoms, approximately 25% (5.3 million) seek some form of related treatment (Drangsholt & LeResche, 1999). Separate research has estimated that only 5% to 10% of those with existing TMD symptoms require medical treatment (American Academy of Orofacial Pain, 2004). Of those individuals with reported TMD symptoms, the estimated treatment costs for those who require traditional medical intervention compared with the costs for those who do not raise concerns about treatment cost burdens and the need to identify other factors that may be influencing symptom development or maintenance. The annual cost associated with TMD-related treatment in the United States is significant, with estimates reaching $4 billion (Stowell, Gatchel, & Wildenstein, 2007). Thus, the process of identifying factors that affect patients' symptom development and treatment needs is integral to providing effective and comprehensive treatment recommendations.

The model that providers and their staff use in the decision-making process plays a significant role in the range of potential interventions for patients with TMD symptoms. Broadly, the traditional biomedical model conceptualizes patient complaints in strict terms of tissue damage, associated pain, and medically based intervention. However, pain, especially when it becomes chronic, can rarely be understood by merely the linear, nociceptive pathways. Health care professionals are usually unable to identify pathophysiological mechanisms underlying persistent pain complaints because of the absence of documentable isomorphic relationships between pathology and pain. Rather, pain is now appropriately viewed as a biopsychosocial process, the result of a complex and dynamic interaction among physiological, psychological, and social factors that perpetuates, and may even worsen, the clinical presentation (Gatchel, 2005; Turk & Monarch, 2002). Basically, taking a pure biomedical approach to pain is akin to the quotation that opened this chapter: If you are uncertain or incorrect as to where you are going (in terms of the best way to reduce pain), then you will likely not be successful in reaching the desired goal.

Surgical intervention is one of many treatment options available to patients with TMDs. In fact, it is one of the most common options, along with medications, splints, and interocclusal appliances, yet it is also one of the most costly. Surgical interventions for TMD range from less invasive outpatient procedures (e.g., arthrocentesis, arthroscopy) to more intensive inpatient procedures (e.g., arthroplasty, disc repositioning, discectomy, full TMJ replacement; Dimitroulis, 2005). As outpatient procedures, arthrocentesis (i.e., a "wash out" of excess scar tissue using sterile solution delivered via subcutaneous injection proximal to the affected TMJ) and arthroscopy (i.e., removal of scar tissue via insertion of a scope into the TMJ) typically require the least amount of recovery time and overall patient burden (Dimitroulis, 2005; Reston & Turkelson, 2003). Common inpatient procedures for TMD include disc repositioning, discectomy (i.e., removal of damaged cartilage disc in the TMJ), arthroplasty (i.e., removal or replacement of the affected area of the TMJ with tissue or bone grafts), and total TMJ replacement (i.e., removal and replacement of the TMJ with prosthetic); as a group, these procedures require more recovery time (i.e., weeks to months, potentially) and carry greater overall patient burden (Dimitroulis, 2005; Dolwick, 2007; Reston & Turkelson, 2003).

Because of the significant expense associated with surgery and the frequency of its use, candidates' readiness should be an important factor in the decision to proceed with surgery. Unfortunately, because of the high probability of positive short-term outcomes, such as increased function and decreased pain, the choice to proceed with surgery is typically made without significant regard to other factors (Dimitroulis, 2005). However, clinical research has found that several specific psychosocial factors can significantly affect a patient's outcomes after TMD-related surgery (Dworkin & LeResche, 1992). In light of this, case selection for TMD-related surgical intervention should be based on both traditional selection criteria (e.g., failure of nonsurgical therapies, diagnostic accuracy, TMJ symptoms) and salient psychosocial factors (Dimitroulis, 2005). In particular, the need for surgery should be determined by the patient's degree of disability in conjunction with his or her therapeutic response to nonsurgical treatment modalities.

Efforts to study TMD in recent years have moved toward examining a multidimensional model of pain that accounts not only for the physiological variables of the disorder but also the psychosocial variables involved. A patient with pain has a biological problem (activation of pain pathways, whether or not the etiology is known) that may have psychosocial precipitants and responses (e.g., depression, anxiety) and appraisals (thoughts and beliefs about the pain; Klasser & Greene, 2009; Turner & Dworkin, 2004). Additionally, the pain may have behavioral consequences for the patient, such as placing limits on certain activities or interactions with others (Gatchel, Peng, Peters, Fuchs, & Turk, 2007). This situation occurs within a social framework, which includes interpersonal relationships with families, friends, coworkers, and health care providers and how these individuals respond to the patient in pain. The longer the patient's pain persists, the more opportunity these psychosocial factors have to be involved in the pain and subsequent disability (Gatchel et al., 2007). By examining the patient's pain experience from a biopsychosocial perspective, the health care provider will see that the dynamic interactions among the biological, psychosocial, behavioral, social, cultural, and environmental factors all contribute to the patient's suffering and disability.

Indeed, a review of the current literature pertaining to the biopsychosocial approach to chronic pain (discussed more thoroughly in the next section of this chapter) has overwhelmingly demonstrated that mood state can modulate reports of pain, as well as tolerance for pain, at the acute stage (Fernandez & Turk, 1992; Gatchel et al., 2007). Specifically, anxiety level has been shown to influence not just pain severity but also complications after surgery and number of days hospitalized (de Groot et al., 1997; Gatchel et al., 2007). Similarly, level of depression has been observed to be related to chronic pain (Gatchel, 2005), with as many as 50% of chronic pain patients having a depressive disorder (Dersh, Gatchel, Mayer, Polatin, & Temple, 2006; Gatchel et al., 2007). Whether the onset of depression or anxiety occurred before or after the onset of pain, the psychosocial costs incurred by patients with chronic pain can certainly affect emotional functioning in detrimental ways. For instance, patients who are unable to work because of their pain and are faced with increased medical expenses, as well as patients who have difficulty performing activities of daily living, may become fearful and demoralized, especially if an inadequate social support system is in place (Gatchel et al., 2007). Research has demonstrated that patients' appraisals of the pain's effect on their lives (as described earlier) and appraisals of their ability to exert control over their pain and their lives are the two driving factors that appear to mediate chronic pain (Gatchel et al., 2007; Rudy, Kerns, & Turk, 1988; Turk, Okifuji, & Scharff, 1995). Furthermore, Tan, Jensen, Robinson-Whelen, Thornby, and Monga (2002) demonstrated that perceived control over the effects of pain is more strongly related to better adjustment and less disability than perceived control over the pain itself. Thus, surgeons should be cautious when determining surgical candidacy because surgery can provide a quick fix and afford some temporary relief for the patient, whereas other dynamics related to psychosocial adjustment have a significant impact on the patient's long-term physical and mental health and perhaps interfere with the recovery process.

BIOPSYCHOSOCIAL CONCEPTUALIZATION OF PATIENTS WITH TEMPOROMANDIBULAR JOINT DISORDER

Several lines of research have demonstrated how the biopsychosocial model may be appropriately applied to the assessment and treatment of patients with TMD (Gatchel & Dersh, 2002). Patients with TMD vary greatly in levels of pain and pain-related disability and distress, and physical findings do not appear to solely account for these differences (Ohrbach & Dworkin,

1998; Rudy, Turk, Zaki, & Curtin, 1989; Sessle, Bryant, & Dionne, 1995; Turner & Dworkin, 2004). Evidence has also suggested that a strong relationship exists between psychosocial disturbances and physical disorders among medical patients in general but among patients with TMD in particular (Auerbach, Laskin, Frantsve, & Orr, 2001; Gatchel, Garofalo, Ellis, & Holt, 1996; Kinney, Gatchel, Ellis, & Holt, 1992; Wright et al., 2004). In addition, indicators of psychosocial dysfunction are associated with more severe symptoms and worse treatment outcomes for patients with TMD (Turner & Dworkin, 2004). Such variables also better predict the patient's risk of progression from acute TMD (i.e., symptoms persisting for less than 6 months) to chronic TMD (i.e., symptoms persisting for more than 6 months). Over the course of many studies, Gatchel et al. (1996) assessed differences between people with acute and chronic TMD and then devised a model to predict which individuals with acute TMD were at risk for progressing from acute to chronic TMD. Primary predictor variables that were identified across these studies included pain rating, coping style, and presence of psychopathology (Edwards, Gatchel, Adams, & Stowell, 2006; Epker, Gatchel, & Ellis, 1999; Gatchel & Dersh, 2002; Gatchel et al., 1996; Wright et al., 2004). Next, we review each of these variables and its association with TMD.

Pain Ratings

Epker et al. (1999) identified that, when comparing people with chronic TMD with those having acute TMD, subjects in the chronic group reported significantly greater pain intensity and impairments in functioning, as measured by the Graded Chronic Pain Scale (Von Korff, Dworkin, & LeResche, 1990). The Graded Chronic Pain Scale is a set of seven self-report items that assess both pain intensity and pain-related disability; responses are scored to classify respondents into one of five pain–disability grades of increasing severity. Another self-report measure of greater pain intensity, the Characteristic Pain Intensity, has also been found to be a significant predictor of the continuation of TMD-related pain symptoms beyond the acute stage (Garofalo, Gatchel, Wesley, & Ellis, 1998; Wright et al., 2004).

Coping Style

Compared with a population of patients without TMD, patients with chronic TMD exhibit greater prevalence of dysfunctional coping styles on the Multidimensional Pain Inventory (Epker & Gatchel, 2000; Rudy et al., 1989). Epker et al. (1999) found that, compared with a group with acute TMD, subjects in the chronic group frequently displayed a dysfunctional Multidimensional Pain Inventory profile, whereas subjects in the acute group tended to be "adaptive copers." Not surprisingly, patients with a dysfunctional coping style typically display higher levels of affective distress and greater pain-related interference in their lives than patients who are adaptive copers (Epker et al., 1999). Dahlström, Widmark, and Carlsson (1997) reported that the Multi-dimensional Pain Inventory dysfunctional profile also predicted treatment failure in patients with orofacial pain (Dahlström et al., 1997).

Psychopathology

Studies that have used structured interviews for the assessment of psycho-pathology have reported a higher prevalence of clinical disorders among patients with chronic TMD than among patients without TMD (Gatchel et al., 1996; Wright et al., 2004). Gatchel et al. (1996) found that patients with chronic TMD differed significantly with regard to several biopsycho-social variables. Using the Structured Clinical Interview for the *Diagnostic and Statistical Manual of Mental Disorders III–R* (SCID-I), Gatchel et al. (1996) found that patients in the chronic group met criteria for more overall current disorders and, specifically, for more current anxiety disorders, current mood disorders, current somatization disorders, lifetime mood disorders, and life-time anxiety disorders. Self-reports of depressive symptoms, as measured by the Beck Depression Inventory (Beck, Steer, Ball, & Ranieri, 1996), were also significantly greater for subjects in the chronic group than for subjects in the nonchronic group.

SCREENING FOR SURGICAL READINESS

Given the multiple financial and psychosocial costs associated with length of chronicity, it is evident that intervention before the onset of chro-nicity could yield more benefits to prevent, or at least significantly reduce, the negative factors associated with chronic TMD. Moreover, dysfunctional psychosocial factors, such as depression or drug abuse, ongoing pain-related litigation or disability claims, may affect adherence or response to a treatment plan. Patients with identified psychosocial influences that affect their level of pain and disability are unlikely to benefit substantially from biomedical treat-ment alone. Because of this, health care providers would be well advised to screen for such psychosocial factors before determining the appropriate treat-ment intervention. Turner and Dworkin (2004) proposed a screening process for "yellow flags," or indicators that psychosocial factors may be significantly affecting the patient's pain experience. These indicators include disability, symptoms of psychosocial disorders, and prolonged or excessive use of opiates, benzodiazepines, alcohol, or other drugs. In light of the aforementioned strong psychosocial overlay of symptoms within this disorder, prescreening for yellow flags in surgical candidates has significant advantages. Moreover, even if the patient is at high risk for chronicity and the surgeon is reluctant to delay surgery, screening for psychosocial variables would still be helpful to alert the treatment staff, as well as individuals involved in the patient's care and recovery, of potential postsurgical problems.

Assessment of Risk Factors Involved in Presurgical Screening

Given that assessment of risk for poor surgical outcome is important, being familiar with the most common, well-researched, and clinically useful measures to make such a determination is necessary. Several self-report measures have been used to assess the psychosocial risk factors described thus far, including pain-related disability measures, quality-of-life measures, substance use measures, psychiatric symptom measures, and coping style measures. At a 1992 conference at the National Institute of Dental Research, the multiaxial research diagnostic criteria for temporomandibular disorders (RDC–TMD) model was brought forth for use in assessing patients in terms of the disorder's physical and psychosocial characteristics (Dworkin & LeResche, 1992; Garofalo et al., 1998). As the most widely accepted model for accurately diagnosing TMD, the RDC–TMD model provides a method to systematically demarcate the clinical subtypes of the disorder, using a physical disease axis (Axis I) and a psychological–psychosocial axis (Axis II; Garofalo et al., 1998). Axis I identifies physical characteristics of TMD as assessed by facial and jaw measurements (mandibular range of motion and TMJ sounds) and palpation of masticatory muscles (Dworkin et al., 1992). Axis I clinical TMD diagnoses are divided into three groups: Group 1, muscle disorders; Group 2, disc displacements; and Group 3, other types of joint conditions (arthralgia, osteoarthritis, and arthritis) in the right, left, or both joints (Garofalo et al., 1998).

RDC–TMD Axis II assesses psychosocial status and pain-related disability, characteristic pain intensity, depression, nonspecific physical symptoms, and limitations in mandibular functioning (Dworkin & LeResche, 1992; Garofalo et al., 1998). Assessments include the Graded Chronic Pain Scale, subscales of the Symptom Checklist–90—Revised, and the Limitations Related to Mandibular Functioning scale. Relevant measures from RDC–TMD and other sources are discussed in the following sections (see Table 7.1).

Pain and Pain-Related Disability

The Characteristic Pain Intensity is a multifactor pain rating that uses current pain ratings and ratings of both the average and the worst pain over the past 3 months. The Characteristic Pain Intensity rating is calculated

TABLE 7.1
Psychosocial Risk Factors and Associated Self-Report Measures

Psychosocial factors and instruments	Instrument overview	Results interpretation
Pain and pain-related disability		
Graded Chronic Pain Scale (Dworkin & LeResche, 1992)	An index of Axis II RDC–TMD that indicates the extent to which pain is perceived by the patient and the degree to which the pain is disabling	This measure can be used to qualitatively augment other evaluation data. Higher levels of pain-related disability have been associated with greater psychosocial dysfunction.
Characteristic Pain Inventory (Dworkin & LeResche, 1992)	A rating calculated as the mean of the patient's report of current pain, worst pain in the past 3 months, and mean pain in the past 3 months multiplied by 100	Higher scores on the Characteristic Pain Inventory are associated with greater incidence of anxiety and somatoform disorders. Higher scores are also associated with increased likelihood of future chronicity.
Quality of life		
Short Form–36 (Ware & Sherbourne, 1992)	A widely used 36-item quality-of-life measure that assesses a range of scales (e.g., Physical Functioning, Role—Physical, Bodily Pain, General Health, Vitality, Social Functioning, Role—Emotional, Mental Health) and provides two quality-of-life summary scores (Physical and Mental Health)	A significant score on the Mental Health summary score may warrant additional psychosocial assessment. For this summary score, the relevant individual domain scores include the Mental Health scale, the Role—Emotional scale, and the Social Functioning scale.
Substance use		
Alcohol Use Disorders Identification Test—Consumption (Bush et al., 1998)	A three-item screen used for potential alcohol abuse or dependence	A score of 3 or more or self-report of drinking six drinks or more on one occasion in the past year indicates need for further assessment.
Two-Item Conjoint Screen (Brown, Leonard, Saunders, & Papasouliotis, 2001)	Two-item screen for alcohol and drug abuse	One or more positive response indicates need for further assessment.
Pain Medication Questionnaire (Buelow, Haggard, & Gatchel, 2009)	23-item screen for potential pain medication misuse (each item scored on a 5-point scale)	A score of more than 30 indicates high risk.

TABLE 7.1
Psychosocial Risk Factors and Associated Self-Report Measures *(Continued)*

Psychosocial factors and instruments	Instrument overview	Results interpretation
Psychiatric symptoms		
Patient Health Questionnaire (Spitzer, Williams, Kroenke, Hornyak, & McMurray, 2000)	Screens for eight major psychiatric disorders: major depression, panic disorder, anxiety disorder, bulimia nervosa, binge-eating disorder, alcohol abuse or dependence, somatoform disorder	Positive screen outcome indicates need for referral to mental health care professional for further assessment.
Beck Depression Inventory—II (Beck, Steer, Ball, & Ranieri, 1996)	Used to assess symptom severity, but not to diagnose major depression	Score of 2–3 on the Suicidal Ideation scale or a total score higher than 20 indicates need for referral to mental health care professional for further assessment.
Coping style: dysfunctional coping, interpersonal distress, somatization		
Multidimensional Pain Inventory (Kerns, Turk, & Rudy, 1985)	12 scales assessing pain impact (severity and interference), responses of others, activities; three coping-style subgroups: interpersonally distressed, adaptive, and dysfunctional	Patients categorized in the interpersonally distressed and dysfunctional coping style groups will likely need interdisciplinary treatment.
Symptom Checklist— 90 Somatization scale (Derogatis & Unger, 2010)	Screening tool included in RDC–TMD; assesses tendency to report non-specific physical symptoms as causing difficulties; categorizes patients into normal, moderate, or severe symptom levels	Patients with severe levels should be referred to a mental health care provider. Patients with moderate levels should be monitored and reevaluated within 1 year.

Note. RDC–TMD = research diagnostic criteria for temporomandibular disorders.

as the mean of the patient's report of current pain, worst pain in the past 3 months, and mean pain in the past 3 months, multiplied by 100 (Dworkin & LeResche, 1992). As a component of Axis II of the RDC–TMD (Dworkin & LeResche, 1992), clinical research has found pain intensity to be associated with incidence of both anxiety and somatoform disorders, as well as greater risk for developing pain chronicity (Wright et al., 2004). Note that Axis II of the RDC–TMD (Dworkin & LeResche, 1992) is not the same as Axis II of the *Diagnostic and Statistical Manual of Mental Disorders* (4th ed., text rev.; American Psychiatric Association, 2000). As a measure of patients' pain-related disability, the Graded Chronic Pain Scale has often been used in clinical research with patients with TMD (Dworkin & LeResche, 1992; Von Korff, Dworkin, Fricton, & Orbach, 1992). The Graded Chronic Pain Scale is also an Axis II index of the RDC–TMD that indicates the extent to which the patient perceives pain and the degree to which the pain is disabling (Dworkin & LeResche, 1992). Disability measures are combined with Characteristic Pain Intensity to classify the Graded Chronic Pain Scale of TMD patients as functional, which is associated with low disability and either low or high pain intensity, or dysfunctional, which is associated with high disability and high pain intensity (Garofalo et al., 1998).

Quality of Life

The Short Form–36 (Ware & Sherbourne, 1992) is a widely used measure for assessing health-related quality of life for patients in medical settings. Its 36 items yield a range of quality-of-life–related domains, including Physical Functioning, Role—Physical, Bodily Pain, General Health, Vitality, Social Functioning, Role—Emotional, and Mental Health. Furthermore, this measure yields summary quality-of-life scores for two global domains (Physical Functioning and Mental Health).

Substance Use

For substance use, brief screening measures that assess current alcohol and substance abuse have most often been used. The three-item Alcohol Use Disorders Identification Test—Consumption (Bush, Kivlahan, McDonell, Fihn, & Bradley, 1998) and the Two-Item Conjoint Screen (Brown, Leonard, Saunders, & Papasouliotis, 2001) have been used for these purposes in clinical research with patients with TMD. The Pain Medication Questionnaire (Adams et al., 2004; Buelow, Haggard, & Gatchel, 2009; Dowling, Gatchel, Adams, Stowell, & Bernstein, 2007; Holmes et al., 2006) has also been found to be clinically useful.

Psychiatric Symptoms

Multiple self-report measures have been used to screen for and assess the severity of psychiatric symptoms in TMD-related clinical research. The Patient Health Questionnaire is an 18-item self-report screening tool that assesses for symptoms of the most prevalent psychiatric diagnoses that present in health care settings (Spitzer, Williams, Kroenke, Hornyak, & McMurray, 2000). It specifically assesses symptoms of major depressive disorder, general anxiety and panic disorder, bulimia nervosa and binge-eating disorder, alcohol abuse or dependence, and somatoform disorder. The Beck Depression Inventory—II (Beck et al., 1996) and the Symptom Checklist—90 (Derogatis, Rickels, & Rock, 1976; Derogatis & Unger, 2010) are useful depression screening tools.

Coping Style

As reviewed earlier, the Multidimensional Pain Inventory is frequently used to identify potentially maladaptive styles of coping in clinical research with patients with TMD. This 52-item self-report measure contains 12 individual indices that are calibrated to yield a coping-related profile classification (e.g., Adaptive Coper, Interpersonally Distressed, Dysfunctional Coping; Kerns, Turk, & Rudy, 1985). The individual scales include Pain Severity, Pain-Related Life Interference, Perceived Support, Perceived Life Control, Affective Distress, Pain-Related Response Pattern of Significant Other (e.g., punishing responses, solicitous responses, and distracting responses), and activity-related indices (e.g., ability to engage in household chores, outdoor work, activities away from home, social activities, and overall activity level). The Somatization scale of the Symptom Checklist—90 is a 12-item screening tool included in the RDC–TMD. It assesses a respondent's tendency to report nonspecific physical symptoms as causing difficulties and categorizes patients as having normal, moderate, or severe symptom levels along this dimension (Derogatis & Unger, 2010).

CASE STUDY

Ms. D. is a 29-year-old Caucasian graduate student with a history of TMD symptoms for approximately the past 2 years.[1] She acknowledged that the onset of her symptoms coincided with stressful life changes in recent years. Ms. D. broke off her engagement to her fiancé after being accepted into a reputable graduate program in her field of interest; this program was located in a state several thousand miles from where Ms. D. grew up and where her family still resides. Although she initially experienced difficulty adjusting to the transition, Ms. D. reported that she has excelled in her studies and describes herself as a high-functioning, independent woman despite her ongoing TMD-related pain and disability.

About 5 months into her graduate studies, Ms. D. began waking up several mornings each week with soreness in her face and neck and began noticing that throughout the day she would intermittently clench her teeth. Her jaw would pop when she attempted to open her mouth completely.

---

[1]Details of this case have been altered to protect the patient's identity.

Eventually, she found chewing solid foods so painful that she often avoided them for softer foods. She decided to visit her dentist, who referred her to an orthodontist to adjust her bite with an occlusal splint. In the interim, Ms. D. was prescribed hydrocodone by her primary care physician to alleviate her jaw pain and eventually began running out of her prescription earlier each month, visiting different pharmacies in hopes of having her prescription refilled at an earlier date. After several months, she had not observed significant improvement from splint therapy alone, so her orthodontist recommended physical therapy, which Ms. D. promptly declined, stating that she did not have the time to commit to such a treatment and wanted to be referred for surgical intervention "so I can get this thing fixed and move on with my life."

At this time, Ms. D. visited an orofacial surgery clinic to be assessed for surgical candidacy. She presented well to the surgeon conducting the evaluation, and surgery was determined to be an appropriate biomedical intervention given the history and nature of her TMD symptoms. During the consultation, Ms. D. described her academic program as rigorous and demanding of her time, and she acknowledged that she would have little time to recover from the surgical procedure before returning to school. Additionally, when asked about scheduling the procedure, Ms. D. was hesitant to identify who would be responsible for her transportation to and from the appointment as well as for assistance in aftercare. At this point, the surgeon decided that further presurgical psychosocial screening (PPS) beyond the current consultation was appropriate in Ms. D.'s case.

Ms. D. was referred to a licensed psychologist affiliated with the clinic for a psychosocial screening. On reviewing the psychologist's report, the surgeon realized that Ms. D.'s psychosocial difficulties were beyond the expected anxiety and stress related to being a graduate student. Ms. D. indicated that she had also been experiencing multiple symptoms of depression and had felt socially isolated since moving away from her family and friends and terminating her romantic relationship. Her lack of local social support had prompted her to seek out an alternative means of coping with stress and alienation on her own time: substance use. When her surgeon followed up with her about her endorsement of consuming more drugs or alcohol on occasions other than she intended to in the past year, Ms. D disclosed that she had been combining her hydrocodone with other illicit substances to intensify the effects of the medication. She also shared that she drinks several glasses of wine alone in her apartment most nights to unwind from the stresses of the day. Ms. D. was observed to be tearful at certain points in this discussion.

Ms. D.'s treatment team (the surgeon, psychologist, and orthodontist) decided that surgery would not be scheduled at the time of this evaluation. Participation in individual psychotherapy on an outpatient basis was recommended to Ms. D., and her primary care physician was notified of her high-risk behavior involving her medication. Ms. D. was also referred to a psychiatrist for further assessment of her psychiatric symptoms. As for her TMD symptoms, Ms. D. agreed to continue seeing her orthodontist and stated that she would make time to participate in physical therapy. Ms. D. came to an agreement with her treatment team that she would be reassessed for surgical candidacy in 6 months if her symptoms persisted and were not adequately managed by the alternative treatments.

Discussion and Administration Considerations

This case demonstrates several practical considerations to address once the surgeon has decided to conduct a PPS. Specific questions include who will administer and interpret the measures, what type of training is required to perform such a screening, in what setting the screening should occur, and how and to whom a dental provider should refer a patient if a psychosocial screen is warranted. Multiple medicolegal and ethical factors emerge when a candidate for TMD-related surgery undergoes psychosocial screening before the proposed procedure. What follows is a discussion of these topics and related issues.

In our case example, a fairly easy presurgical assessment of the prospective surgical candidate was conducted, in that the dental provider and his staff were attuned to subtle clues and accessed a consulting psychologist who was trained in presurgical assessment and determination. Unfortunately, this is not often the case in most dental practices. Consequently, we discuss the administration and related medicolegal aspects of presurgical evaluation in two primary settings: (a) an ongoing clinician referral relationship exists and (b) no such referral relationship exists. With that said, however, in both situations the initial phase is the same and occurs between the surgeon and the patient. Once a surgeon determines that from a biomedical standpoint surgery is the preferred treatment route, the surgeon and the patient still need to have an important conversation. At this time, the surgeon needs to subtly inquire, as part of his or her evaluation, about possible yellow flags or indicators, including disability; symptoms of psychosocial disorders; and prolonged or excessive use of opiates, benzodiazepines, alcohol, or other drugs (Turner & Dworkin, 2004). This inquiry may occur as part of a conversation or begin on the basis of a history–intake form in the provider's office before the surgical consultation. When yellow flags are identified, the next steps are determined by the presence or absence of a clinician referral relationship.

Ongoing Clinician Referral Relationship Exists

Ideally, a dental provider has such a relationship, because clinicians who perform presurgical evaluations are specifically trained to elicit information that will help identify barriers to a successful surgical outcome. Once a surgeon identifies a yellow flag, a referral should occur. The physician should explain the rationale behind his or her recommendation that a psychosocial or behavioral evaluation will help determine the surgical candidate's readiness for surgery, ensuring correct timing of the surgical intervention, to achieve the most successful results. Additionally, patients are typically more comfortable being referred to a behavioral health specialist than to a psychologist. What seems mere semantics may actually mean a great deal to a surgical candidate because the former term carries less negative cultural weight.

Given clinicians' greater familiarity with legal and ethical standards as they pertain to a psychosocial interview and assessment, a clinician will be able to offset some of the medicolegal risk that a dental surgeon generally incurs when performing surgery. Before psychosocial evaluation, the clinician will also review the limits of confidentiality for the evaluation and obtain a necessary consent to release protected health information to the referring dental provider before proceeding with the referral. The clinician will then typically provide a brief report back to the referring surgeon with one of the following recommendations: (a) no psychosocial barriers, proceed with surgery; (b) defer surgery until completion of a specified number of behavioral health sessions or until a particular pending stressor has passed (e.g., final exams); or (c) surgical intervention not recommended at this time because of intervening psychosocial factors (e.g., ongoing prescription medication misuse [multisourcing], active suicidal ideation); consider for reevaluation in 6 months. Although the surgeon is not obligated to rely on such psychosocial evaluation feedback, it may prove immensely helpful in making a surgical determination, improving surgical outcomes, and reducing medicolegal risk.

No Clinician Referral Relationship Exists

If the physician does not have a referral relationship with a licensed clinician qualified to perform a more extensive psychosocial screen, an appropriate referral may be found by contacting a local psychological association or local psychology graduate school program. Dental surgeons who do not have a referral relationship may be tempted to administer some of the measures mentioned earlier in the chapter and score them in the office, without the consultation or oversight of a licensed clinician. Although this is not unheard of, and is now no longer unethical and illegal for many tests, providers need to be cautious about what information is obtained and by whom. For example, if a dental office decides to use the Beck Depression Inventory—II as a quick measure of depression, has the receptionist hand it out on the patient's first visit, and then scores it before the patient meets with the doctor, the medicolegal risk is huge. Although this measure was formerly only permitted to be scored and interpreted by a licensed mental health provider, that is no longer the case. In 2011, the publishers (Pearson; http://psychcorp.pearsonassessments.com) and authors of the test changed the administration qualifications for the Beck measures, including the Beck Depression Inventory, Beck Anxiety Inventory, and Beck Hopelessness Scale, among others (C. Ault, personal communication, April 3, 2012), to allow providers who have a "degree or license to practice in the healthcare or allied healthcare field" to administer, score, and interpret the measures to facilitate use in medical settings and aid in determining the need for more intensive psychological intervention. That said, precautions must still be taken, and in some ways the medicolegal risk for the medical provider actually increases. For example, if a patient endorses active suicidal thought and no one notices or inquires further and the patient leaves the office and commits suicide, the medical provider will likely be held liable or, at a minimum, have a lot of explaining to do to his or her board and surviving family members. For these reasons, it is important to consider how to introduce the screen and ensure that all those involved in the administration, scoring, and interpretation are closely following the procedures set forth in the test manual.

As a consequence of these changes in rules regarding screening measures, some testing companies are now actively marketing measures directly to medical providers, although no known direct marketing to dental providers has begun, and no measures directly written for dental providers have been identified. This marketing may indeed lead to increased screening and, consequently, improved outcomes; however, providers are strongly cautioned to closely monitor screening procedures and ideally establish a relationship with a mental health provider to regularly provide on-site training in the use of such measures and issues that may arise.

Additional Considerations

Because of the personal nature of questions asked during a psychosocial evaluation, approaching the evaluation process with sensitivity and understanding is important. A nonthreatening environment for the screening may be facilitated by validating the patient's pain experience because, regardless of its etiology, the pain perception is very real to the patient and has likely caused several difficulties that have resulted in disabling pain and compromised function. Patients may be fearful that if they disclose symptoms of psychiatric illness or reveal an inadequate support system, their opportunity for surgical treatment may be taken away, and they will be forced to live with the pain and functional difficulties indefinitely. For this reason, the rationale behind screening for psychosocial factors should be explained to the patient before the evaluation, with an emphasis on treatment outcome as it pertains to the patient and how best to time the surgery. If it becomes evident that psychosocial factors will negatively affect the outcome of surgery and the recovery process, alternative treatments should be explored. If alternative treatment options have been exhausted and surgery is strongly indicated for the patient, psychosocial screening still holds value because it draws attention to factors that influence the postsurgical recovery process.

When inquiring about difficulties related to psychiatric symptoms, the physician considering referring a patient for PPS must be prepared to address serious issues raised by the patient, such as current suicidal ideation, a history of previous suicide attempts or a current plan for suicide, or self-damaging behaviors involving drugs, and/or alcohol. Patients who acknowledge that they are imminently suicidal should be referred for further assessment. A patient's endorsement of current substance use or suicidality represents initial factors that may delay the patient's surgery and cause potential harm to the patient–doctor relationship. The overriding concern, if either is present, is the safety of the patient and the potential need for acute care.

Less salient psychosocial contributors to the patient's symptom experience and dysfunction may still warrant a referral to a clinician and should undoubtedly be considered when determining whether the patient is a good candidate for surgical intervention. When discussing this decision with the patient, the health care provider can explain that participation in mental health treatment may be helpful in reducing the negative impact of the patient's pain on his or her quality of life. More specifically, health care providers can explain that common difficulties (i.e., depression and acute stressors) are often associated with chronic pain and can worsen predicted surgical outcomes. One should also emphasize to the patient that the findings of the PPS will not permanently contraindicate surgery as a treatment option. One should explain that the patient could be reevaluated if indications for surgery persist after participation in recommended psychosocial treatment modalities.

In the event that a patient does not fully understand the process, the disclosure of results that could contraindicate surgery may create confusion and anger in the patient. In such a scenario, the patient could react in any number of undesirable ways to individuals associated with their care (e.g., verbal confrontation, termination of treatment with the provider, legal action). Attendance to these concerns and basic assessment of cognitive status is standard practice for mental health professionals who conduct PPS. However, diligence in explaining those issues and determining that the patient is informed during the consent process becomes more important for non–mental health providers, staff, or paraprofessionals who have limited experience with it. Individual consultation with a licensed clinician or legal practitioner is therefore advisable before implementing presurgical screening in a medical practice setting. In such consultation, additional medicolegal factors that pertain to particular states or professions should be identified and applied, as indicated.

IMPLICATIONS FOR THE FUTURE

As we have discussed, the use of evidence-based PPS for TMD affords the opportunity to identify factors for which intervention may improve outcomes. The assessment and administrative considerations described in this chapter provide the basic tools, rationale, and framework with which the PPS process can be carried out. However, future clinical research could expand on the utility of this process in several directions. Greater efficiency and usability could be achieved through the development of a quick screen that incorporates only the most predictive components of existing measures. Usability of such a quick screen would partly hinge on its ease of administration and interpretive demands. Optimally, the development of such a quick screen would be tailored so that dental staff could quickly, reliably, legally, and ethically administer and interpret it. Previous clinical research has developed brief self-report measures whose results translate into easily interpreted risk categories for opioid misuse (Adams et al., 2004; Dowling et al., 2007). Other such measures have been developed for elective implantable pain management devices (Heckler et al., 2007; Schocket et al., 2008). More detailed screening has been successfully developed for spine surgery candidates (Block, Gatchel, Deardorff, & Guyer, 2003). As with existing measures, a respondent's score on such a quick screen for candidates for TMD surgery could correspond with clear psychosocial risk categories. Categories related to TMDs warranting empirical investigation to develop such a quick screen should include, but not be limited to, psychiatric symptoms, psychosocial stressors, substance abuse or dependence, and disability and disability-related claims (see Table 7.2). As a potential model, the resultant psychosocial risk categories would correspond to specific recommendations that could be discussed with patients and initiated by staff and providers. These categories could include high-risk, moderate-risk, and low-risk categories that correspond to the likelihood of poor psychosocial outcomes from undergoing a surgical procedure. For example, a high-risk categorization would necessitate a referral for a separate psychosocial or behavioral evaluation, whereas moderate risk might correspond to the provision of resources for the patient to electively pursue psychosocial services or evaluation. Moreover, a low-risk categorization would reflect no contraindicating psychosocial factors. To be fully usable by staff and providers, specific guidelines for scoring, interpreting, and implementing recommendations would be necessary. The development and implementation of

TABLE 7.2

Summary of Factors to Consider for Inclusion in a Prospective
Temporomandibular Disorder Presurgical Psychosocial Screen
to be Administered in a Dental Setting, Based on Prior Research

Factor	Related research
Disproportionate pain rating based on presentation and Characteristic Pain Inventory score	Dworkin & LeResche (1992); Garofalo, Gatchel, Wesley, & Ellis (1998); Von Korff et al. (1992); Wright et al. (2004)
Anxiety	de Groot et al. (1997); Gatchel, Garofalo, Ellis, & Holt (1996); Gatchel et al. (2007); Wright et al. (2004)
Depression	Beck Depression Inventory—Beck, Steer, Ball, & Ranieri (1996); Gatchel (2005); Gatchel et al. (1996)
Prolonged or excessive use or misuse of opiates, benzodiazepines, alcohol, or other drugs, whether prescription or illicit	Edwards, Gatchel, Adams, & Stowell (2006); Turner & Dworkin (2004)
Dysfunctional coping style	Dahlström, Widmark, & Carlsson (1997); Epker (1999); Multidimensional Pain Inventory—Epker & Gatchel (2000); Rudy et al. (1989)
Ongoing pain-related litigation or disability claims	Gatchel et al. (2007); Turner & Dworkin (2004)
Numerous or significant stressors, such as moving, change in relationship status, job change	Auerbach, Laskin, Frantsve, & Orr (2001); Gatchel et al. (1996); Kinney, Gatchel, Ellis, & Holt (1992); Turner & Dworkin (2004); Wright et al. (2004)

a quick screen would be of benefit to both patients (through improvement of patient outcomes) and providers (through greater efficiency in the delivery of patient care).

REFERENCES

Adams, L. L., Gatchel, R. J., Robinson, R. C., Polatin, P., Gajraj, N., Deschner, M., & Noe, C. (2004). Development of a self-report screening instrument for assessing potential opioid medication misuse in chronic pain patients. *Journal of Pain and Symptom Management, 27,* 440–459. doi:10.1016/j.jpainsymman.2003.10.009

American Academy of Orofacial Pain. (2004). *TMD symptoms.* Mount Royal, NJ: Author.

American Psychiatric Association. (2000). *Diagnostic and statistical manual of mental disorders* (4th ed., text rev.). Washington, DC: Author.

Auerbach, S. M., Laskin, D. M., Frantsve, L. M., & Orr, T. (2001). Depression, pain, exposure to stressful life events, and long-term outcomes in temporomandibular disorder patients. *Journal of Oral and Maxillofacial Surgery, 59*, 628–633.

Beck, A. T., Steer, R. A., Ball, R., & Ranieri, W. F. (1996). Comparison of Beck Depression Inventories-IA and -II in psychiatric outpatients. *Journal of Personality Assessment, 67*, 588–597. doi:10.1207/s15327752jpa6703_13

Block, A. R., Gatchel, R. J., Deardorff, W. W., & Guyer, R. D. (2003). *The psychology of spine surgery*. Washington, DC: American Psychological Association. doi:10.1037/10613-000

Brown, R. L., Leonard, T., Saunders, L. A., & Papasouliotis, O. (2001). A two-item conjoint screen for alcohol and other drug problems. *Journal of the American Board of Family Practice, 14*, 95–106.

Buelow, A. K., Haggard, R., & Gatchel, R. J. (2009). Additional validation of the Pain Medication Questionnaire in a heterogeneous sample of chronic pain patients. *Pain Practice, 9*, 428–434. doi:10.1111/j.1533-2500.2009.00316.x

Bush, K., Kivlahan, D. R., McDonell, M. B., Fihn, S. D., & Bradley, K. A. (1998). The AUDIT Alcohol Consumption Questions (AUDIT-C): An effective brief screening test for problem drinking. *Archives of Internal Medicine, 158*, 1789–1795. doi:10.1001/archinte.158.16.1789

Dahlström, L., Widmark, G., & Carlsson, S. (1997). Cognitive-behavioral profiles among different categories of orofacial pain patients: Diagnostic and treatment implications. *European Journal of Oral Sciences, 105*(5, Pt. 1), 377–383.

de Groot, K. I., Boeke, S., van den Berge, H. J., Duivenvoorden, H. J., Bonke, B., & Passchier, J. (1997). Assessing short- and long-term recovery from lumbar surgery with pre-operative biographical, medical and psychological variables. *British Journal of Health Psychology, 2*, 229–243. doi:10.1111/j.2044-8287.1997.tb00538.x

Derogatis, L. R., Rickels, K., & Rock, A. F. (1976). The SCL-90 and the MMPI: A step in the validation of a new self-report scale. *British Journal of Psychiatry, 128*, 280–289. doi:10.1192/bjp.128.3.280

Derogatis, L. R., & Unger, R. (2010). *Symptom Checklist-90-Revised*. New York, NY: Wiley.

Dersh, J., Gatchel, R. J., Mayer, T., Polatin, P., & Temple, O. R. (2006). Prevalence of psychiatric disorders in patients with chronic disabling occupational spinal disorders. *Spine, 31*, 1156–1162. doi:10.1097/01.brs.0000216441.83135.6f

Dimitroulis, G. (2005). The role of surgery in the management of disorders of the temporomandibular joint: A critical review of the literature: Part 2. *International Journal of Oral and Maxillofacial Surgery, 34*, 231–237.

Dolwick, M. F. (2007). Temporomandibular joint surgery for internal derangement. *Dental Clinics of North America, 51*, 195–208. doi:10.1016/j.cden.2006.10.003

Dowling, L. S., Gatchel, R. J., Adams, L. L., Stowell, A. R., & Bernstein, D. (2007). An evaluation of the predictive validity of the Pain Medication Questionnaire with a heterogeneous group of patients with chronic pain. *Journal of Opioid Management, 3*, 257–266.

Drangsholt, M., & LeResche, L. (1999). Temporomandibular disorder pain. In I. K. Crombie, P. R. Croft, S. J. Linton, L. LeResche, & M. Von Korff (Eds.), *Epidemiology of pain* (pp. 203–233). Seattle, WA: IASP Press.

Dworkin, S. F., & LeResche, L. (1992). Research diagnostic criteria for temporomandibular disorders: Review, criteria, examinations and specifications, critique. *Journal of Craniomandibular Disorders: Facial & Oral Pain, 6*, 301–355.

Dworkin, S. F., LeResche, L., Fricton, J., Mohl, N., Sommers, E., & Truelove, E. (1992). Research diagnostic criteria, Part II, Axis I: Clinical TMD conditions [Review]. *Journal of Craniomandibular Disorders, 6*, 327–330.

Edwards, D., Gatchel, R., Adams, L., & Stowell, A. W. (2006). Emotional distress and medication use in two acute pain populations: Jaw and low back. *Pain Practice, 6*, 242–253. doi:10.1111/j.1533-2500.2006.00093.x

Epker, J., & Gatchel, R. J. (2000). Coping profile differences in the biopsychosocial functioning of patients with temporomandibular disorder. *Psychosomatic Medicine, 62*, 69–75.

Epker, J., Gatchel, R. J., & Ellis, E. (1999). A model for predicting chronic TMD: Practical application in clinical settings. *Journal of the American Dental Association, 130*, 1470–1475.

Fernandez, E., & Turk, D. C. (1992). Sensory and affective components of pain: Separation and synthesis. *Psychological Bulletin, 112*, 205–217. doi:10.1037/0033-2909.112.2.205

Garofalo, J. P., Gatchel, R. J., Wesley, A. L. V., & Ellis, E. (1998). Predicting chronicity in acute temporomandibular joint disorders using the research diagnostic criteria. *Journal of the American Dental Association, 129*, 438–447.

Gatchel, R. J. (2005). *Clinical essentials of pain management.* Washington, DC: American Psychological Association. doi:10.1037/10856-000

Gatchel, R. J., & Dersh, J. (2002). Psychological disorders and chronic pain: Are there cause-and-effect relationships? In D. C. Turk & R. J. Gatchel (Ed.), *Psychological approaches to pain management: A practitioner's handbook* (2nd ed., pp. 30–51). New York, NY: Guilford Press

Gatchel, R. J., Garofalo, J. P., Ellis, E., & Holt, C. (1996). Major psychological disorders in acute and chronic TMD: An initial examination. *Journal of the American Dental Association, 127*, 1365–1370, 1372, 1374.

Gatchel, R. J., Peng, Y. B., Peters, M. L., Fuchs, P. N., & Turk, D. C. (2007). The biopsychosocial approach to chronic pain: Scientific advances and future directions. *Psychological Bulletin, 133*, 581–624. doi:10.1037/0033-2909.133.4.581

Gatchel, R. J., Potter, S. M., Hinds, C. W., & Ingram, M. (2011). Early treatment of TMJ may prevent chronic pain and disability. *Practical Pain Management, 11*, 95–100.

Heckler, D. R., Gatchel, R. J., Lou, L., Whitworth, T., Bernstein, D., & Stowell, A. W. (2007). Presurgical Behavioral Medicine Evaluation (PBME) for implantable devices for pain management: A 1-year prospective study. *Pain Practice, 7,* 110–122. doi:10.1111/j.1533-2500.2007.00118.x

Holmes, C. P., Gatchel, R. J., Adams, L. L., Stowell, A. W., Hatten, A., Noe, C., & Lou, L. (2006). An opioid screening instrument: Long-term evaluation of the utility of the Pain Medication Questionnaire. *Pain Practice, 6,* 74–88. doi:10.1111/j.1533-2500.2006.00067.x

Kerns, R. D., Turk, D. C., & Rudy, T. E. (1985). The West Haven-Yale Multi-dimensional Pain Inventory (WHYMPI). *Pain, 23,* 345–356. doi:10.1016/0304-3959(85)90004-1

Kinney, R. K., Gatchel, R. J., Ellis, E., & Holt, C. (1992). Major psychological disorders in chronic TMD patients: Implications for successful management. *Journal of the American Dental Association, 123,* 49–54.

Klasser, G. D., & Greene, C. S. (2009). The changing field of temporomandibular disorders: What dentists need to know. *Journal of the Canadian Dental Association, 75,* 49–53.

LeResche, L. (1997). Epidemiology of temporomandibular disorders: Implications for the investigation of etiologic factors. *Critical Reviews in Oral Biology and Medicine, 8,* 291–305. doi:10.1177/10454411970080030401

Ohrbach, R., & Dworkin, S. F. (1998). Five-year outcomes in TMD: Relationship of changes in pain to changes in physical and psychological variables. *Pain, 74,* 315–326. doi:10.1016/S0304-3959(97)00194-2

Reston, J. T., & Turkelson, C. M. (2003). Meta-analysis of surgical treatments for temporomandibular articular disorders. *Journal of Oral and Maxillofacial Surgery, 61,* 3–10. doi:10.1053/joms.2003.50000

Rudy, T. E., Kerns, R. D., & Turk, D. C. (1988). Chronic pain and depression: Toward a cognitive-behavioral mediation model. *Pain, 35,* 129–140. doi:10.1016/0304-3959(88)90220-5

Rudy, T. E., Turk, D. C., Zaki, H. S., & Curtin, H. D. (1989). An empirical taxometric alternative to traditional classification of temporomandibular disorders. *Pain, 36,* 311–320. doi:10.1016/0304-3959(89)90090-0

Schocket, K. G., Gatchel, R. J., Stowell, A. W., Deschner, M., Robinson, R., Lou, L., . . . Bernstein, D. (2008). Presurgical behavioral medicine evaluation: Categorizing patients for potential treatment efficacy for spinal cord stimulation and intra-thecal drug therapy. *Neuromodulation, 11,* 237–248. doi:10.1111/j.1525-1403.2008.00171.x

Sessle, B. J., Bryant, P. S., & Dionne, R. (1995). *Temporomandibular disorders and related pain conditions.* Seattle, WA: IASP Press

Spitzer, R. L., Williams, J. B., Kroenke, K., Hornyak, R., & McMurray, J. (2000). Validity and utility of the PRIME-MD Patient Health Questionnaire in assess-ment of 3000 obstetric-gynecologic patients: The PRIME-MD Patient Health

Questionnaire Obstetrics-Gynecology Study. *American Journal of Obstetrics and Gynecology*, *183*, 759–769. doi:10.1067/mob.2000.106580

Stowell, A. W., Gatchel, R. J., & Wildenstein, L. (2007). Cost-effectiveness of treatments for temporomandibular disorders: Biopsychosocial intervention versus treatment as usual. *Journal of the American Dental Association*, *138*, 202–208.

Tan, G., Jensen, M. P., Robinson-Whelen, S., Thornby, J. I., & Monga, T. (2002). Measuring control appraisals in chronic pain. *Journal of Pain*, *3*, 385–393. doi:10.1054/jpai.2002.126609

Turk, D. C., & Monarch, E. S. (2002). Biopsychosocial perspective on chronic pain. In D. C. Turk & R. J. Gatchel (Eds.), *Psychological approaches to pain management: A practitioner's handbook* (2nd ed., pp. 3–29). New York, NY: Guilford Press.

Turk, D. C., Okifuji, A., & Scharff, L. (1995). Chronic pain and depression: Role of perceived impact and perceived control in different age cohorts. *Pain*, *61*, 93–101. doi:10.1016/0304-3959(94)00167-D

Turner, J. A., & Dworkin, S. F. (2004). Screening for psychosocial risk factors in patients with chronic orofacial pain: Recent advances. *Journal of the American Dental Association*, *135*, 1119–1125.

Von Korff, M., Dworkin, S. F., Fricton, J., & Ohrbach, R. (1992). Axis II: Pain-related disability and psychological status. *Journal of Craniomandibular Disorders: Facial and Oral Pain*, *6*, 330–334.

Von Korff, M., Dworkin, S., & LeResche, L. (1990). Graded chronic pain status: An epidemiologic evaluation. *Pain*, *40*, 279–291. doi:10.1016/0304-3959(90)91125-3

Ware, J. E., & Sherbourne, C. D. (1992). The MOS 36-Item Short-Form Health Survey (SF-36): I. Conceptual framework and item selection. *Medical Care*, *30*, 473–483. doi:10.1097/00005650-199206000-00002

Wright, A. R., Gatchel, R. J., Wildenstein, L., Riggs, R., Buschang, P., & Ellis, E. (2004). Biopsychosocial differences between high-risk and low-risk patients with acute TMD-related pain. *Journal of the American Dental Association*, *135*, 474–483.

8

RECONSTRUCTIVE PROCEDURES

CANICE E. CRERAND AND LEANNE MAGEE

In 2010, more than 5 million reconstructive surgical procedures were performed in the United States to address functional and aesthetic problems related to acquired injuries (e.g., lacerations), disease (e.g., tumor removal), congenital conditions (e.g., cleft lip and palate), and developmental abnormalities (e.g., breast reconstruction for asymmetry or macromastia; American Society of Plastic Surgeons [ASPS], 2011). A large literature on the psychological aspects of plastic surgery has developed over the past 50 years, owing largely to the interests of both surgeons and mental health professionals in understanding why individuals seek to surgically alter their appearance (e.g., Sarwer, 2006; Sarwer & Crerand, 2004; Sarwer, Wadden, Pertschuk, & Whitaker, 1998). Much of this research has focused on the psychological aspects of cosmetic procedures; psychosocial influences on reconstructive surgery have been far less researched. At the same time, a large body of social psychological research has suggested that physically attractive people are

DOI: 10.1037/14035-009
Presurgical Psychological Screening: Understanding Patients, Improving Outcomes, Andrew R. Block and David B. Sarwer (Editors)

rated more favorably and receive preferential treatment in a variety of situations across the life span (e.g., Sarwer & Magee, 2006). This beauty bias likely contributes to interest in pursuing cosmetic procedures, just as it may factor into the decision to undergo a reconstructive procedure to improve an "abnormal" or disfigured feature.

In this chapter, we review the psychological aspects of reconstructive surgical procedures as they pertain to adults, as well as to children and adolescents. We include a discussion of how a disfiguring injury or condition can affect social and psychological functioning and conclude with suggestions for conducting psychological assessments with patients who seek reconstructive procedures.

PSYCHOLOGICAL ASPECTS OF RECONSTRUCTIVE SURGERY

Reconstructive procedures are performed on physical defects caused by trauma, disease, and congenital or developmental anomalies with the purpose of restoring functional status and appearance. Although the literature is somewhat limited regarding the psychological aspects of reconstructive procedures, the growing body of research on psychological aspects of disfigurement can inform the evaluation of patients who present for reconstructive surgery, because disfigurement has been associated with body image concerns, anxiety, depression, and social difficulties.

Body Image and Disfigurement

People who experience a disfigurement are faced with the challenge of integrating various images of the self into a comprehensive and adaptive body image: the complete body before the traumatic injury, the healing body, and the body as it appears after the injury (Rybarczyk, Nyenhuis, Nicholas, Cash, & Kaiser, 1995). Adaptation to one's changed body image is considered a critical aspect of psychosocial adjustment to a disfiguring injury or illness (Pruzinsky, 2004). Body image disturbances are likely when an individual is unable to incorporate the disfiguring changes in appearance and function of the body into his or her reconceptualized body image. Experiencing a significant change in one's physical appearance has the potential to set up a series of emotional, perceptual, and psychological reactions that can lead to long-term body image disturbances, manifested as appearance-related distress and impairment in daily functioning (Cash, Phillips, Santos, & Hrabosky, 2004). Moreover, individuals who are overly invested in their physical appearance (e.g., appearance plays an important part of their self-concept and identity) may be at greater risk for psychosocial difficulties (Pruzinsky, 2002).

Factors such as social support, social skills, the importance of appearance to an individual's self-concept, and predisfigurement psychosocial functioning are thought to influence body image adaptation to disfigurement and psychosocial adjustment in general (Pruzinsky, 2002).

Although this result is perhaps counterintuitive, studies have typically demonstrated little to no correlation between severity of disfigurement and the individual's body image (e.g., Rumsey, Clarke, & White, 2003). Rather, subjective perceptions of severity and disfigurement appear to be the most critical predictors of distress and functional impairment. However, the visibility of the disfigurement may play a role in adjustment to it. Visible differences in appearance, those not routinely covered by clothing, are associated with low self-confidence and negative self-image across the life span, as well as with difficulties establishing and maintaining relationships and experiences of social stigmatization (e.g., staring, unsolicited comments or questions from others, appearance-based teasing; Rumsey & Harcourt, 2004). Facial disfigurements can be especially problematic. The face plays a key role in one's identity and serves the primary social functions of communicating and expressing emotion. Disfigurements that affect the communication triangle of the face—formed by the eyes and mouth—are thought to be particularly noticeable to others and can lead to shame and embarrassment for the affected individual (Partridge, 1993). Individuals affected by facial disfigurements are often vulnerable to difficulties with social interactions and may experience social anxiety and depression.

However, some evidence has suggested that adjustment may be easier for individuals with major, visible disfigurements than for those with minor or hidden changes in appearance. Facial or hand disfigurements that are more visible may force the affected individual to process and adapt to others' reactions (Pruzinsky, 2002; Rumsey, 2002). In contrast, people with concealable disfigurements may be not be confronted by the reality of their changed appearance on a regular basis, and so they may come to rely on concealment strategies and avoidance of situations in which their difference in appearance may be noticed.

Psychological Impact of Disfigurement

In addition to body image disturbances, individuals with disfigurement who present for reconstructive surgical procedures may be at risk for other types of psychological distress, including depression and social anxiety disorder, as well as acute stress disorder and posttraumatic stress disorder (PTSD). Identification of these disorders is critical because these conditions, if left untreated, can greatly affect adjustment and may present difficulties during the pre- and postoperative periods.

Individuals who experience disfigurement may be particularly vulnerable to depression and anxiety. A study of 458 patients presenting for treatment of a range of disfiguring conditions found that 25% reported clinically significant symptoms of depression and 48% reported clinically significant symptoms of anxiety, particularly in relation to social situations (Rumsey, Clarke, White, Wyn-Williams, & Garlick, 2004). Depression is not unexpected given the functional and aesthetic losses that can accompany disfigurement (e.g., role changes, inability to work) in addition to social stigmatization (scrutiny and negative evaluation). Such negative social experiences can in turn lead to worry and avoidance of social situations in an effort to reduce distress.

Particularly in cases in which patients have suffered an unexpected traumatic injury resulting in disfigurement, symptoms of PTSD may be present. Although most people experience symptoms of emotional and physiological distress immediately after a traumatic event, these symptoms often subside quickly and without treatment. In some cases, symptom onset may persist for a longer period, leading to a diagnosis of acute stress disorder, or may worsen and continue for prolonged periods, leading to a diagnosis of PTSD. Surprisingly, few studies to date have examined rates of acute or posttraumatic stress among people with disfigurement. The prevalence rate of PTSD among people who have survived accidents and nonsexual assault has been reported to be as high as 42% (O'Donnell, Creamer, Bryant, Schnyder, & Shalev, 2003). It has been hypothesized that disfigurement (e.g., scarring, missing body part) could serve as a stimulus for the development and maintenance of PTSD (van Loey, Maas, Faber, & Taal, 2003) because patients have a visible reminder of their trauma.

Social Impact of Disfigurement

People with disfigurement may experience difficulties in forming relationships, particularly romantic relationships. They may also receive negative social responses from strangers (e.g., stares) and experience stigmatization or outright discrimination in numerous settings (Rumsey & Harcourt, 2004). In general, people offer less help to and try to avoid or increase physical distance from those with appearance differences (Macgregor, 1990). Stigmatization can be overt (e.g., rude comments) or subtle (e.g., avoidance of eye contact), and it can contribute to poor body image, social isolation, and loss of anonymity among those with appearance differences (Bull & Rumsey, 1988; Rumsey & Harcourt, 2004). Comments from friends and family, both critical and positive, may draw unwanted attention to an appearance feature and contribute to the desire to pursue surgery. The media can also add to the stigmatization in its portrayal of individuals with burns and other disfigurements as evil. Stigmatization experiences may directly contribute to an individual's desire to undergo reconstructive surgery and may contribute to the development or maintenance of social anxiety, depression, and body image disturbances.

RECONSTRUCTIVE SURGERY IN ADULT POPULATIONS

In 2010, the five most common reconstructive procedures performed on adults were (a) tumor removal, (b) laceration repair, (c) scar revision, (d) hand surgery, and (e) breast reconstruction after breast cancer treatment (ASPS, 2011). The following sections highlight the significant psychosocial issues associated with the first four of these conditions; Chapter 9 provides a detailed discussion of the fifth. We also briefly discuss the emerging fields of hand and face transplantation. Psychologists and other mental health professionals who work with these patients typically do so on an as-needed basis; presurgical psychological screening is only included if the treating surgeon has identified some significant psychological issues and requests a consultation before surgery.

Tumor Removal

Tumor removal includes a variety of procedures to remove benign and malignant tissue throughout the body and optimize remaining structures and function. Surgical removal of internal tumors may result in little more than scars from incisions, but removal of tumors that involve surface tissue or bone may result in more significant disfigurement. A large body of literature has examined psychosocial functioning among postoperative cancer patients (e.g., Dropkin, 1999; White & Hood, 2011), which we summarize briefly here.

Research examining body image in cancer patients has largely focused on breast and head and neck cancers. Patients treated for these cancers have reported postoperative dissatisfaction with body image (i.e., Arora et al., 2001; Dropkin, 1999; White & Hood, 2011). A descriptive study of patients after head and neck cancer surgery found that successful body image reintegration after disfiguring surgery, or assimilation of surgical defects into one's self-concept, is characterized by effective use of self-care and socialization as coping strategies (Dropkin, 1999). As noted earlier, the severity of the disfigurement does not predict psychological distress; individuals with minor disfigurement may experience distress equal to or more than those with more severe appearance differences (e.g., Moss, 2005). In addition, postoperative changes in appearance and functioning among head and neck cancer patients may lead to disruptions in eating, swallowing, and speaking. Communication difficulties and related social distress have commonly been reported by patients with head and neck cancers, particularly those involving the mouth and tongue (Dropkin, 1999; Haman, 2008).

Laceration Repairs

Laceration repairs involve closing open wounds to the skin, tissue, and muscle. The exact method for wound closure depends on the location, size, and severity of the wound. Although most physicians are able to repair lacerations, plastic surgeons have received additional training in wound management and techniques to minimize scarring.

The psychosocial research on basic laceration repair is limited and often overlaps with research on scar management and revision, which is discussed next. In a retrospective study of adults with facial lacerations 3 centimeters (1.2 inches) or longer or fractured facial bones requiring surgical intervention (Levine, Degutis, Pruzinsky, Shin, & Persing, 2005), those with facial injuries (compared with nondisfigured controls) exhibited significantly lower satisfaction with life, more negative perception of body image, higher incidence of PTSD, higher incidence of alcoholism, and an increase in depression as well as higher incidence of marital problems, binge drinking, incarceration, posttrauma unemployment, and lower attractiveness ratings 2 years after their facial injury. In a subsequent study (Tebble, Adams, Thomas, & Price, 2006), patients with minor facial lacerations who completed an Appearance Scale and the State–Trait Anxiety Inventory at 1 week and 6 months after injury endorsed higher self-consciousness and anxiety scores than the general population, which continued at 6-month follow-up, despite some improvements. Thus, even minor lacerations to the face can have a significant and lasting impact on appearance and anxiety concerns.

Scar Revision

Scar revision is performed by plastic surgeons to improve the condition or appearance of a scar. No scar can be removed completely. A scar forms as skin heals after an injury or surgical incision and may vary on the basis of the size, depth, and location of the wound; age of the individual; hereditary factors; and skin characteristics, including pigmentation. Individuals may seek scar revision surgery because of concerns with discoloration or surface irregularities (e.g., acne scars or scars remaining from prior surgical incisions), scar hypertrophy (e.g., red, raised, and widened scar tissue), keloids (e.g., red, puckered scars with a different texture and color than surrounding skin, extending beyond the original scar margins), or scar contractures that restrict movement of muscles, joints, and tendons.

Patients seeking reconstructive surgery for revision of existing scars have characteristics similar to those seeking cosmetic procedures, particularly if scars are not associated with pain or restricted movement. Although scar revision may result in increased range of motion, or decreased stiffness and bulkiness at the scar site, patients are often attuned to the aesthetics of the scar. Patients' subjective perceptions of scar severity and visibility were associated with psychosocial distress, but objective scar severity ratings by a clinician were not (B. C. Brown, Moss, McGrouther, & Byat, 2010). Patients with nonvisible scars also reported greater appearance concerns, lower quality of life, and greater psychosocial distress than patients with visible scars.

In a clinical interview study of 97 patients with scarring after routine surgery, a majority expressed embarrassment about visible and hidden scars and indicated that they would value even small improvements in the appearance of scars through revision (Young & Hutchison, 2009). Ninety-two percent indicated that they wished the scar was less noticeable, 60% reported being unhappy with the scar, and 55% reported trying to hide the scar. Clinicians who perform surgical procedures were asked similar questions via telephone interview; all clinicians expressed intent to prevent or improve scarring, and 96% reported that their patients were significantly concerned about scarring. However, 71% of patients reported that they were more concerned with scarring than their surgeon seemed to be, and 60% of patients thought their surgeon could have been more sensitive to their feelings about scarring. Results suggested that patients were highly invested in and concerned with scarring after elective surgery and that clinicians and patients had room for improvement in their discussion of anticipated outcomes for scarring after elective procedures (Young & Hutchison, 2009).

Hand Surgery

In 2010, 105,711 reconstructive hand procedures were performed in the United States (ASPS, 2011). Such procedures are often performed as a result of traumatic injuries resulting from industrial accidents, self-inflicted injuries, traffic accidents, crush injuries, assaults, and sports-related injuries. In some instances, injuries may result in amputation of fingers or the hand itself. Hand injuries can have a significant physical and psychological impact on affected individuals because hands are critical to an individual's ability to perform a multitude of tasks (e.g., self-care, work, socializing, and communication; Grunert, 2006). Hand injuries are visible not only to the affected individual but also to others. As a result, hand disfigurements can result in appearance concerns for the affected individual and may also elicit negative responses from others.

Hand surgeries related to traumatic injuries are often performed on an emergent basis. Thus, often little time is available for assessment of psychological status (Grob, Papadopulos, Zimmerman, Biemer, & Kovacs, 2008). Nonetheless, the psychological aspects of hand trauma have been relatively well studied. PTSD is the most commonly reported psychological problem associated with hand injury (Grunert, 2006). Flashbacks have been noted to occur frequently in populations with hand injuries, and those who attribute injuries to external causes appear to have a greater likelihood of experiencing flashbacks and other PTSD symptoms, such as avoidance, than those who attribute their injury to internal causes (Grunert et al., 1992). Depression is also common and frequently co-occurs with PTSD (Williams, Newman, Ozer, Juarros, Morgan, & Smith, 2009). Hand injuries can also take a toll on interpersonal relationships. For example, in a study of 120 patients, 49% reported sexual dysfunction within the first 2 months after injury, and 19% continued to report sexual difficulties 6 months postinjury (Grunert, Devine, Matloub, Sanger, & Yousif, 1988). Taken together, these findings suggest that patients who experience hand injuries are at risk for a variety of intra- and interpersonal problems that could have an impact on postoperative outcomes for those who undergo reconstructive surgery.

Hand and Face Transplantation

With recent advances in microsurgery, as well as the use of composite tissue allographs, reconstructive surgeons have begun to refine hand and face transplantation surgeries. As of 2011, surgeons worldwide had completed 29 hand transplants and 12 face transplants. Given that this field is in its infancy, relatively little has been published about the psychological aspects of these procedures (see Clarke, 2012, for a review). Issues of emotional distress, body image and identity concerns, and ethical implications are critical areas of concern in both hand and face transplantation. In contrast to the reconstructive procedures discussed earlier, it is encouraging that presurgical psychological screening has already become an established part of these developing specialties.

In reviewing outcomes among recipients of hand and face transplants, psychological criteria have proven to be among the most crucial determinants of success and failure (Clarke, 2012; Soni et al., 2010). Psychological difficulties have been noted to contribute to nonadherence to immunosuppression medications, which can in turn lead to rejection of the transplant and, in some instances, even death (Soni et al., 2010). Thus, careful preoperative screening is critical for this patient population, with particular attention paid to motivations and expectations for transplantation, ability to adhere to lifelong immunosuppression therapy, current and past psychological history (e.g., history of trauma and PTSD; lack of psychosis, cognitive disabilities, homicidality, suicidality), social support system, and body image and degree of adjustment to disfigurement (Soni et al., 2010).

During the postoperative period and beyond, patients require psychosocial support to navigate challenges such as integration of the new hand or face into their body image and sense of identity and coping with the reactions of others to their altered appearance. A recent case report of a patient who underwent face transplantation described postoperative improvements in body image, depressive symptoms, and quality of life and reductions in social stigmatization (Coffman, Gordon, & Siemionow, 2010). Additional studies of postoperative outcomes and their relationship to preoperative psychological characteristics are needed.

PEDIATRIC RECONSTRUCTIVE PROCEDURES

The most commonly performed reconstructive surgical procedures among children and adolescents include craniofacial surgeries, such as cleft lip and palate repair, and reconstructive procedures to correct developmental breast and chest anomalies. In this section, we review the psychological aspects of these procedures. Craniofacial care often occurs at major medical centers and uses a multidisciplinary approach to treatment that typically involves assessment and treatment provided by mental health professionals. Thus, presurgical psychological screening is a relatively routine aspect of care with children and adolescents.

Birth Defect Reconstruction

In 2010, more than 34,000 surgeries were performed to repair birth defects (ASPS, 2011), most of which were performed on children born with cleft lip and palate or other birth defects of the head and face. These craniofacial conditions are among the most common birth defects, typically affecting one in every 750 babies born in the United States each year (National Birth Defects Prevention Network, 2006). Craniofacial conditions can result in speech, hearing, breathing, and dental problems as well as deformities of the bone and soft tissue and facial asymmetries.

Reconstructive procedures play a significant role in ameliorating the functional and aesthetic problems that are associated with congenital craniofacial conditions. Staged surgical procedures are typically performed over the course of childhood, adolescence, and potentially into adulthood to restore functional abilities such as eating, breathing, and speaking, as well as appearance (e.g., closure of a cleft lip, creation of a more normal skull shape).

As physical growth is completed, further procedures can be performed to improve the appearance of scars and other residual appearance differences (e.g., scar revision, tip rhinoplasty).

The psychosocial aspects of these craniofacial conditions have been well documented (e.g., Collett & Speltz, 2007). Internalizing disorders (e.g., anxiety, social inhibition) and externalizing behaviors (e.g., attention and behavior problems) appear to be more common among affected children than among their nondisfigured peers (see Collett & Speltz, 2007, for a review). These concerns can play a role in determining the timing of surgery. For example, a child who presents with significant self-consciousness may benefit from reconstructive surgery at an earlier age than a child who is well adjusted and not reporting concerns about appearance.

Despite the best efforts of reconstructive surgeons, most children with craniofacial conditions will have some degree of residual and permanent disfigurement. Speech difficulties, such as problems with intelligibility and articulation, are also common and can contribute to psychosocial difficulties. These aesthetic and functional concerns can leave affected individuals vulnerable to peer teasing and rejection. Additionally, youths with craniofacial conditions have the burden of coping with multiple surgical procedures. Often, there is frustration with the timing of procedures (e.g., having to wait until growth is completed for rhinoplasty or jaw surgery) as well as the stress of school absences and time away from extracurricular activities. Psychosocial factors, including developmental stage and psychological adjustment, are thought to be important factors in the timing of surgical procedures and satisfaction with treatment outcome. Because of these issues, regular psychosocial screenings are recommended for children and adolescents affected by craniofacial conditions (American Cleft Palate-Craniofacial Association, 2004). Most multidisciplinary clinics in major medical centers that provide this care routinely involve psychological screening of patients when they return for annual visits to monitor growth.

Gynecomastia Correction

Gynecomastia is a condition characterized by abnormal proliferation of breast tissue in boys and men, resulting in enlargement of one or both breasts as well as discomfort, nipple irritation, painful swelling, and skin redundancy. In 2010, more than 18,000 surgical procedures were performed in the United States for the correction of gynecomastia. Boys and men with this condition frequently experience significant distress because of the feminine appearance of their chest (Greydanus, Matytsina, & Gains, 2006; Ridha, Colville, & Vesely, 2009). Emotional distress and shame about appearance are considered to be indications for surgery (ASPS, 2002; Fisher & Fornari, 1990).

Clinically, adolescents with gynecomastia usually report embarrassment in social situations, low self-esteem, body image disturbances, teasing related to breast enlargement, and avoidance of situations and activities in which their chest may be exposed (e.g., locker room, athletic activities; Fisher & Fornari, 1990). Many report camouflaging the appearance of their chests by wearing loose or oversized shirts and binding their chests with tape or other restrictive materials. Case reports have described social isolation, eating pathology, depressive symptoms, and social anxiety among affected male adolescents (Storch et al., 2004). Although many of the psychosocial problems associated with gynecomastia are thought to resolve postoperatively, clinical experience has suggested that surgery does not improve psychosocial functioning for all. Although surgery removes excess breast tissue, it will typically result in some degree of scarring, which can be problematic for some patients. Furthermore, evidence has shown that some patients are dissatisfied with their postoperative outcome even after technically successful procedures (Fisher & Fornari, 1990; Ridha et al., 2009). Such reports have suggested that psychosocial factors such as body image, social skills, and social support may play an important role in predicting postoperative outcomes.

Female Breast Reduction Surgery

In 2010, 4,645 adolescent girls underwent breast reduction surgery (ASPS, 2011). Breast reduction is commonly performed on patients in their late teens because surgeons usually delay surgery until breast development is completed. Breast reduction is typically sought because of physical limitations (e.g., inability to participate in athletics) and pain associated with large breasts (Young & Watson, 2006). Most candidates present with a desire to have breasts of average size that are proportional to the rest of their body. Although physical complaints often motivate affected women to seek surgery, significant psychosocial concerns, including body image dissatisfaction, symptoms of anxiety and depression, low self-esteem, and social isolation may also influence their decision to reduce the size of their breasts, particularly among younger women (Saariniemi, Joukamma, Raitasalo, & Kuokkanen, 2009). Teasing and bullying from peers and unwanted attention, particularly from adolescent boys, can be significant concerns for those affected. Clinically, young women with large breasts may engage in behaviors to camouflage their breasts, such as wearing baggy clothing, adopting a hunched posture, or intentionally gaining or losing weight with the intention of making their breasts more proportional to their body frame. Others avoid activities and situations in which their breast size may be more noticeable, such as the gym or the beach.

Studies have suggested that breast reduction patients are highly satisfied with their postoperative outcomes, with more than 90% reporting that they would have surgery again or recommend it to others (A. P. Brown, Hill, & Khan, 2000; Dabbah, Lehman, Parker, Tantri, & Wagner, 1995). Post-operative improvements in self-esteem, body image, anxiety, depressive symptoms, and quality of life have also been reported (Behmand, Tang, & Smith, 2000; Rogliani, Gentile, Labardi, Donfrancesco, & Cervelli, 2009; Saariniemi et al., 2009; Shakespeare & Cole, 1997).

Two case series have examined the outcome of breast reduction in adolescent girls and young adult women with bulimia nervosa (Kreipe, Lewand, Dukarm, & Caldwell, 1997; Losee, Serletti, Kreipe, & Caldwell, 1997). In both reports, patients attributed their eating-disordered behaviors to a desire to reduce the size of their breasts and to achieve a more proportionate body. Most patients in both reports experienced post-operative improvements in their eating disorder symptoms (Kreipe et al., 1997; Losee et al., 1997) that were evident as much as 10 years post-operation (Losee et al., 2004). These findings suggest that large breast size may play a role in the etiology of eating disorders for some women, and breast reduction surgery may play a role in reducing eating pathology. However, given that these findings are based on case reports, concluding that breast reduction surgery is an effective treatment for eating pathology is clearly premature. Mental health professionals should be aware of the risk for eating disorders in this patient population.

PSYCHOLOGICAL ASSESSMENT OF RECONSTRUCTIVE SURGERY PATIENTS

As we have reviewed, patients who experience disfigurements resulting from congenital, developmental, or acquired conditions are at risk for psychosocial problems including depression, anxiety, PTSD, and body image disturbances, all of which can compromise daily functioning and quality of life. Recognizing such concerns, hospitals throughout the country are increasingly including psychological support services in their departments of plastic surgery. Among craniofacial teams at major medical centers that have been approved by the American Cleft Palate-Craniofacial Association, the standard of care requires access to psychological and social services as a part of the interdisciplinary team such that children with craniofacial anomalies and their families have the opportunity for periodic assessment, treatment, and psychological consultation.

Next, we outline a strategy for conducting presurgical psychological screening with prospective reconstructive surgery patients, based on a model that was developed for screening plastic surgery patients (e.g., Crerand & Sarwer, 2009; Sarwer, 2006; Sarwer, Crerand, & Magee, 2011). A thorough evaluation should include a clinical interview and use of psychometrically sound assessment instruments.

Clinical Interview

A presurgical psychological evaluation should begin with a clinical interview that assesses a patient's motivations and expectations for surgery, concerns about physical appearance and body image, current psychological status and history of psychological and psychiatric treatment, and social support network.

Motivations and Expectations

A semistructured interview is recommended and should begin with an assessment of the patient's motivations for surgery and expectations about any functional and appearance changes that may affect his or her daily life. It is important to gauge a patient's understanding of the procedure, its purpose, and its risks and benefits, including the potential impact on physical functioning and complications. An assessment of the timing of surgery (e.g., why is the patient pursuing surgery now?) can also help identify whether the desire for surgery is motivated by internal factors (e.g., a desire to have a more normal appearance, improvement in body image and confidence in social situations) as opposed to external factors (e.g., to eliminate teasing). Although reconstructive surgery may improve appearance and reduce the visibility of the disfigurement, individuals who pursue reconstructive surgery for purely external reasons, as with patients who seek cosmetic surgery, may be at risk for poor psychological outcomes (Honigman, Phillips, & Castle, 2004). Patients should be reminded that it is impossible to predict or control how others will respond to their altered appearance. Some individuals may find that few people notice the change in their appearance, and others may receive comments about their postoperative appearance. Although some patients may find this attention pleasurable, others may find it uncomfortable, particularly if others make comments about how much improved or "better" they appear compared with their preoperative appearance.

Particularly in the case of individuals with congenital disfigurements, expectations may run high that a long-awaited surgery will finally help them look "normal." Some patients may have put certain aspects of their life on hold in hopes that surgery will improve their chances of success (e.g., dating). Most patients who require reconstructive surgery, particularly those with congenital conditions, will have some degree of residual disfigurement, so it is important to ascertain whether the patient's expectations for surgical outcomes are realistic.

Body Image

A core component of the presurgical clinical interview entails the assessment of the patient's body image concerns. Patients should be asked what aspects of their appearance bother them. Providers can initiate a dialogue about appearance concerns by asking patients whether their appearance makes them feel self-conscious or isolated, whether they worry a lot about how they look, or whether they avoid places or situations in which other people might notice their appearance difference. Experiences of social stigmatization (e.g., unwanted attention, staring, rude comments, teasing) should also be evaluated. Such information can help providers to quickly gather information about body image disturbances, validate the patient's concerns, and determine those who will likely benefit from psychological or psychiatric support.

Although some degree of body image dissatisfaction and even disturbance is likely to be common among reconstructive surgery populations, some patients presenting for treatment of objectively mild or slight concerns (e.g., revision of a barely perceptible scar) may possibly have body dysmorphic disorder (BDD). BDD is a psychiatric condition characterized by preoccupation with an imagined or slight defect in appearance that results in significant distress or impairment in functioning. Individuals with BDD experience intrusive thoughts about their perceived defect and frequently spend inordinate amounts of time engaged in compulsive behaviors (e.g., mirror checking, camouflaging the perceived defect) in an attempt to reduce their distress (Phillips, Menard, Fay, & Weisberg, 2005). Although individuals with BDD frequently seek surgical interventions to address their appearance concerns, they rarely benefit from these procedures (e.g., Crerand, Menard, Phillips, 2010). Patients with suspected BDD should be referred for further psychological and psychiatric evaluation before surgery.

Psychological Status and History

As with any mental health assessment, patients should be asked about their past and current psychological functioning. Patients presenting for reconstructive surgery are at risk for depression and anxiety disorders (e.g., social anxiety, PTSD). Patients should also be assessed for substance use and abuse, particularly when drugs and alcohol may be used to self-medicate psychological symptoms stemming from difficulty coping with appearance differences. Physical pain can cause significant disruptions in daily functioning as well as sleep and can also have a negative impact on mood. Some patients may resort to inappropriate use of pain medications, illicit substances, or alcohol to manage pain. An assessment of current pain, coping strategies, substance use history, and current pain management regimen should be incorporated into the preoperative evaluation.

For patients who are prescribed pain medications for symptoms related to their appearance difference or to manage postoperative pain, the dosage, frequency, duration, and nature of medication use should be routinely evaluated at all medical visits.

Evaluation of the mood, affect, and overall presentation of a patient provides important clues to the presence of a mood disorder. Clinicians should inquire about disturbances in sleep, appetite, and concentration as well as crying spells, irritability, anhedonia, social isolation, feelings of hopelessness, and the presence of suicidal thoughts. To assess symptoms of anxiety, clinicians should ask patients whether they are avoiding social activities or leisure activities that they used to enjoy and about the impact of these concerns on their daily functioning and quality of life. Patients should also be screened for PTSD, acute stress disorder, or both. Refusal to talk about the injury or to view the injured body part may also be indicative of PTSD, and disturbances of mood, concentration, or sleep may indicate the presence of hyperarousal symptoms of PTSD. The mental health professional can also ask whether the patient's family has noticed any changes in behavior or demeanor since the traumatic injury. Finally, it is important to assess for the use of substances such as drugs and alcohol or excessive use of pain medication because they may also be indicators of PTSD or other psychological difficulties.

Among individuals who seek breast reduction or gynecomastia correction, eating disorders may occur with greater frequency. Patients with a body mass index less than 20 kilograms per meter squared (e.g., a 66-inch woman weighing less than 120 pounds) should be asked about recent weight fluctuations, ongoing dieting efforts, binge eating, purging, and other compensatory behaviors (e.g., excessive amounts of exercise, laxative use). Young women should be asked about amenorrhea.

For patients who already are engaged in psychiatric or psychological treatment, the consulting mental health professional should ask patients whether their treatment provider is aware of their decision to pursue reconstructive treatment. Their mental health providers should be contacted to verify that the timing of the surgery is appropriate. Requesting permission to review medical records, a treatment summary, or both from previous mental health professionals is also useful, particularly if a patient is a poor historian. Such information can also be helpful in ensuring that the consulting mental health professional has an accurate and unbiased accounting of previous mental health treatment.

Social Support

Given the potential for social stigmatization among people with disfigurement, assessing the patient's social support network is important.

Providers should ask about how a person's injury or illness has affected his or her relationships with family and peers, social and extracurricular activities, and the degree of support they receive from family and friends. Patients should also be asked to consider how they expect reconstructive surgery will affect their relationships. If patients report significant social isolation or difficulties coping with the social impact of their condition, therapy can be recommended to help improve social skills and increase support.

Particularly in the case of pediatric patients, it is important to determine how family and peer relationships have factored into the decision to seek surgery. Children and adolescents should be asked about when they first started thinking about surgery to determine whether the interest in surgery is internally derived or strongly influenced by parental or peer pressure. In some instances, parents may report concerns about the child's appearance difference and worries about how it will affect the child's social relationships and emotional well-being, when in fact the child may be functioning well at home and school and coping effectively with his or her appearance difference. In such cases, it may be recommended that surgery be postponed until the child expresses an independent desire to change his or her appearance.

Psychometric Assessment

Although a clinical interview yields important information about a patient's psychosocial functioning, a thorough evaluation will also include validated psychometric assessments. Table 8.1 lists recommended measures for the quantitative assessment of mood, anxiety, body image, and other psychosocial concerns among patients presenting for reconstructive surgery. Many mental health professionals use these as a matter of routine; others use the measures on an as-needed basis. Psychometric assessments can be used to supplement and quantify the information gathered in the clinical interview (e.g., scores on the Beck Depression Inventory—II can help a clinician rate the severity of a patient's depressive symptoms). They can also be used to measure changes between pre- and postoperative psychosocial functioning.

CONCLUSION

Each year, millions of patients undergo reconstructive surgical procedures to improve both physical functioning and appearance. Research has suggested that patients are at risk for psychological difficulties, including body image disturbances, social stigmatization, depression, and anxiety disorders. Mental health professionals can play a key role in maximizing outcomes for reconstructive surgery patients by identifying patients who are experiencing

TABLE 8.1

Self-Report Questionnaires for Use With Reconstructive
Surgery Populations

Name of measure	Reference	Description
Brief Symptom Inventory	Derogatis & Melisaratos (1983); Derogatis & Spencer (1982)	53-item measure of general psychological distress
Beck Depression Inventory—II	Beck, Steer, & Brown (1996)	21-item measure of the existence and severity of symptoms of clinical depression
Beck Anxiety Inventory	Beck, Epstein, Brown, & Steer (1988)	21-item measure of physiological and cognitive symptoms of anxiety
Children's Depression Inventory 2	Kovacs (1992, 2010)	27-item assessment of the presence and severity of depressive symptoms in children and adolescents; a parent version and teacher version are also available for multiple informant assessment. Ages 7–17
Hospital Anxiety and Depression Scale	Zigmond & Snaith (1983)	14-item measure of cognitive symptoms of depression and anxiety designed for use in outpatient medical settings
Derriford Appearance Scale	Carr, Moss, & Harris (2005); http://www.derriford.info	24-item measure of appearance concerns and distress
Body Image Disturbance Questionnaire	Cash, Phillips, Santos, & Hrabosky (2004)	7-item measure to assess concerns about physical appearance, including appearance-related dissatisfaction, appearance investment, and psychosocial impairment related to body image
Body Image Quality of Life Inventory	Cash & Fleming (2002)	19-item measure of the impact of body image on personal relationships, sex life, self-worth, moods, and other aspects of quality of life
Perceived Stigmatization Questionnaire	Lawrence, Fauerbach, Heinberg, Doctor, & Thombs (2006)	21-item measure used to assess perceptions of being stigmatized by others on the basis of appearance differences, including undue attention and staring, avoidance behavior, confused behavior, rude behavior and teasing, bullying, and external pressure to change one's appearance
Social Comfort Questionnaire	Lawrence et al. (2006)	8-item measure designed to assess two factors: a subjective sense of social isolation and the violation-of-privacy effect

difficulties and directing them to appropriate resources and interventions, or even recommending a delay in surgery until the patient becomes more motivated and emotional distress is better controlled.

REFERENCES

American Cleft Palate Craniofacial Association. (2004). *Parameters for evaluation and treatment of patients with cleft lip/palate or other craniofacial anomalies*. Chapel Hill, NC: Author.

American Society of Plastic Surgeons. (2002). *Position paper: Gynecomastia*. Arlington Heights, IL: Author.

American Society of Plastic Surgeons. (2011). *2011 report of the 2010 National Clearinghouse of Plastic Surgery Statistics*. Arlington Heights, IL: Author.

Arora, N. K., Gustafson, D. H., Hawkins, R. P., McTavish, F., Cella, D. F., Pingree, S., . . . Mahvi, D. M. (2001). Impact of surgery and chemotherapy on the quality of life of younger women with breast carcinoma: A prospective study. *Cancer, 92*, 1288–1298. doi:10.1002/1097-0142(20010901)92:5<1288::AID-CNCR1450>3.0.CO;2-E

Beck, A. T., Epstein, N., Brown, G., & Steer, R. A. (1988). An inventory for measuring clinical anxiety: Psychometric properties. *Journal of Consulting and Clinical Psychology, 56*, 893–897. doi:10.1037/0022-006X.56.6.893

Beck, A. T., Steer, R. A., & Brown, G. (1996). *Manual for Beck Depression Inventory II (BDI-II)*. San Antonio, TX: Psychological Corporation.

Behmand, R. R., Tang, D. H., & Smith, D. J., Jr. (2000). Outcomes in breast reduction surgery. *Annals of Plastic Surgery, 45*, 575–580.

Brown, A. P., Hill, C., & Khan, K. (2000). Outcome of reduction mammoplasty—A patient's perspective. *British Journal of Plastic Surgery, 53*, 584–587.

Brown, B. C., Moss, T. P., McGrouther, D. A., & Byat, A. (2010). Skin scar preconceptions must be challenged: Importance of self-perception in skin scarring. *Journal of Plastic, Reconstructive & Aesthetic Surgery, 63*, 1022–1029. doi:10.1016/j.bjps.2009.03.019

Bull, R. H. C., & Rumsey, N. (1988). *The social psychology of facial appearance*. New York, NY: Springer-Verlag.

Carr, T., Moss, T., & Harris, D. (2005). The DAS24: A short form of the Derriford Appearance Scale DAS59 to measure individual responses to living with problems of appearance. *British Journal of Health Psychology, 10*, 285–298. doi:10.1348/135910705X27613

Cash, T. F., & Fleming, E. C. (2002). The impact of body image experiences: Development of the Body Image Quality of Life Inventory. *International Journal of Eating Disorders, 31*, 455–460. doi:10.1002/eat.10033

Cash, T. F., Phillips, K. A., Santos, M. T., & Hrabosky, J. I. (2004). Measuring "negative body image": Validation of the Body Image Disturbance Questionnaire in a nonclinical population. *Body Image*, *1*, 363–372. doi:10.1016/j.bodyim.2004.10.001

Clarke, A. (2012). Facial transplants. In T. F. Cash (Ed.), *Encyclopedia of body image and human appearance* (pp. 431–443). London, England: Academic Press.

Coffman, K. L., Gordon, C., & Siemionow, M. (2010). Psychological outcomes with face transplantation: Overview and case report. *Current Opinion in Organ Transplantation*, *15*, 236–240.

Collett, B.R., & Speltz, M. L. (2007). A developmental approach to mental health for children and adolescents with orofacial clefts. *Orthodontics and Craniofacial Research*, *10*, 138–148.

Crerand, C. E., Menard, W., & Phillips, K. A. (2010). Surgical and minimally invasive cosmetic procedures among persons with body dysmorphic disorder. *Annals of Plastic Surgery*, *65*, 11–16. doi:10.1097/SAP.0b013e3181bba08f

Crerand, C. E., & Sarwer, D. B. (2009). Psychological evaluation of cosmetic surgery patients. In V. L. Young (Ed.), *Patient safety in plastic surgery* (pp. 259–278). St. Louis, MO: Quality Medical Publishing.

Dabbah, A., Lehman, J. A., Jr., Parker, M. G., Tantri, D., & Wagner, D. S. (1995). Reduction mammoplasty: An outcome analysis. *Annals of Plastic Surgery*, *35*, 337–341.

Derogatis, L. R., & Melisaratos, N. (1983). The Brief Symptom Inventory: An introductory report. *Psychological Medicine*, *13*, 595–605. doi:10.1017/S0033291700048017

Derogatis, L. R., & Spencer, M. S. (1982). *The Brief Symptom Inventory (BSI): Administration, scoring, and procedures manual—I.* Baltimore, MD: Johns Hopkins University School of Medicine, Clinical Psychometrics Research Unit.

Dropkin, M. J. (1999). Body image and quality of life after head and neck cancer surgery. *Cancer Practice*, *7*, 309–313. doi:10.1046/j.1523-5394.1999.76006.x

Fisher, M., & Fornari, V. (1990). Gynecomastia as a precipitant of eating disorders in adolescent males. *International Journal of Eating Disorders*, *9*, 115–119.

Greydanus, D. E., Matytsina, L., & Gains, M. (2006). Breast disorders in children and adolescents. *Primary Care: Clinics in Office Practice*, *33*, 455–502.

Grob, M., Papadopulos, N. A., Zimmermann, A., Biemer, E., & Kovacs, L. (2008). The psychological impact of severe hand injury. *Journal of Hand Surgery*, *33*, 358–362. doi:10.1177/1753193407087026

Grunert, B. K. (2006). Hand trauma. In D. B. Sarwer, T. Pruzinsky, T. F. Cash, R. M. Goldwyn, J. A. Persing, & L. A. Whitaker (Eds.), *Psychological aspects of reconstructive and cosmetic plastic surgery: Clinical, empirical, and ethical perspectives* (pp. 145–159). Philadelphia, PA: Lippincott Williams & Wilkins.

Grunert, B. K., Devine, C. A., Matloub, H. S., Sanger, J. R., & Yousif, N. J. (1988). Sexual dysfunction following traumatic hand injury. *Annals of Plastic Surgery*, *21*, 46–48. doi:10.1097/00000637-198807000-00009

Grunert, B. K., Hargarten, S. W., Matloub, H. S., Sanger, J. R., Hanel, D. P., & Yousif, N. J. (1992). Predictive value of psychological screening in acute hand injuries. *Journal of Hand Surgery, 17,* 196–199. doi:10.1016/0363-5023(92)90389-7

Haman, K. L. (2008). Psychologic distress and head and neck cancer: Part 1—Review of the literature. *Journal of Supportive Oncology, 6,* 155–163.

Honigman, R. J., Phillips, K. A., & Castle, D. J. (2004). A review of psychosocial outcomes for patients seeking cosmetic surgery. *Plastic and Reconstructive Surgery, 113,* 1229–1237. doi:10.1097/01.PRS.0000110214.88868.CA

Kovacs, M. (1992). *Children's Depression Inventory (CDI).* New York, NY: Multi-Health Systems.

Kovacs, M. (2010). *Children's Depression Inventory, Second Edition (CDI-2).* New York, NY: Multi-Health Systems.

Kreipe, R. E., Lewand, A. G., Dukarm, C. P., & Caldwell, E. H.(1997). Outcome for patients with bulimia and breast hypertrophy after reduction mammoplasty. *Archives of Pediatrics and Adolescent Medicine, 151,* 176–180.

Lawrence, J. W., Fauerbach, J. A., Heinberg, L. J., Doctor, M., & Thombs, B. D. (2006). The reliability and validity of the Perceived Stigmatization Questionnaire (PSQ) and the Social Comfort Questionnaire (SCQ) among an adult burn survivor sample. *Psychological Assessment, 18,* 106–111. doi:10.1037/1040-3590.18.1.106

Levine, E., Degutis, L., Pruzinsky, T., Shin, J., & Persing, J. A. (2005). Quality of life and facial trauma: Psychological and body image effects. *Annals of Plastic Surgery, 54,* 502–510. doi:10.1097/01.sap.0000155282.48465.94

Losee, J. E., Jiang, S., Long, D. E., Kreipe, R. E., Caldwell, E. H., & Serletti, J. M. (2004). Macromastia as an etiologic factor in bulimia nervosa: 10-year follow-up after treatment with reduction mammoplasty. *Annals of Plastic Surgery, 52,* 452–457.

Losee, J. E., Serletti, J. M., Kreipe, R. E., & Caldwell, E. H. (1997). Reduction mammoplasty in patients with bulimia nervosa. *Annals of Plastic Surgery, 39,* 443–446.

Macgregor, F. C. (1990). Facial disfigurement: Problems and management of social interaction and implication for mental health. *Aesthetic Plastic Surgery, 14,* 249–257. doi:10.1007/BF01578358

Moss, T. (2005). The relationships between objective and subjective ratings of disfigurement severity, and psychological adjustment. *Body Image, 2,* 151–159.

National Birth Defects Prevention Network. (2006). Birth defects surveillance data from selected states, 1999-2003. *Birth Defects Research Part A, 76,* 894–958.

O'Donnell, M. L., Creamer, M., Bryant, R. A., Schnyder, U., & Shalev, A. (2003). Post-traumatic disorders following injury: An empirical and methodological review. *Clinical Psychology Review, 23,* 587–603. doi:10.1016/S0272-7358(03)00036-9

Partridge, J. (1993). The psychological effects of facial disfigurement. *Journal of Wound Care, 2,* 168–171.

Phillips, K. A., Menard, W., Fay, C., & Weisberg, R. (2005). Demographic characteristics, phenomenology, comorbidity, and family history in 200 individuals with body dysmorphic disorder. *Psychosomatics, 46*, 317–325. doi:10.1176/appi.psy.46.4.317

Pruzinsky, T. (2002). Body image adaptation to reconstructive surgery. In T. F. Cash & T. Pruzinsky (Eds.), *Body image: A handbook of theory, research, and clinical practice* (pp. 440–449). New York, NY: Guilford Press.

Pruzinsky, T. (2004). Enhancing quality of life in medical populations: A vision for body image assessment and rehabilitation as standards of care. *Body Image, 1,* 71–81. doi:10.1016/S1740-1445(03)00010-X

Ridha, H., Colville, R. J. I., & Vesely, M. J. J. (2009). How happy are patients with their gynecomastia reduction surgery? *Journal of Plastic, Reconstructive, and Aesthetic Surgery, 62,* 1473–1478.

Rogliani, M., Gentile, P., Labardi, L., Donfrancesco, A., & Cervelli, V. (2009). Improvement of physical and psychological symptoms after breast reduction. *Journal of Plastic, Reconstructive, and Aesthetic Surgery, 62,* 1647–1649.

Rumsey, N. (2002). Optimizing body image in disfiguring congenital conditions. In T. F. Cash & T. Pruzinsky (Eds.), *Body image: A handbook of theory, research, and clinical practice* (pp. 431–439). New York, NY: Guilford Press.

Rumsey, N., Clarke, A., & White, P. (2003). Exploring the psychological concerns of outpatients with disfiguring conditions. *Journal of Wound Care, 12,* 247–252.

Rumsey, N., Clarke, A., White, P., Wyn-Williams, M., & Garlick, W. (2004). Altered body image: Appearance-related concerns of people with visible disfigurements. *Journal of Advanced Nursing, 48,* 443–453. doi:10.1111/j.1365-2648.2004.03227.x

Rumsey, N., & Harcourt, D. (2004). Body image and disfigurement: Issues and interventions. *Body Image, 1,* 83–97. doi:10.1016/S1740-1445(03)00005-6

Rybarczyk, C., Nyenhuis, D. L., Nicholas, J. J., Cash, S. M., & Kaiser, J. (1995). Body image, perceived social stigma, and the prediction of psychosocial adjustment to leg amputation. *Rehabilitation Psychology, 40,* 95–110. doi:10.1037/0090-5550.40.2.95

Saariniemi, K. M., Joukamma, M., Raitasalo, R., & Kuokkanen, H. O. (2009). Breast reduction alleviates depression and anxiety and restores self-esteem: A prospective randomized clinical trial. *Scandinavian Journal of Plastic and Reconstructive Surgery and Hand Surgery, 43,* 320–324.

Sarwer, D. B. (2006). Psychological assessment of cosmetic surgery patients. In D. B. Sarwer, T. Pruzinsky, T. F. Cash, R. M. Goldwyn, J. A. Persing, & L. A. Whitaker (Eds.), *Psychological aspects of reconstructive and cosmetic plastic surgery: Clinical, empirical, and ethical perspectives* (pp. 267–283). Philadelphia, PA: Lippincott Williams & Wilkins.

Sarwer, D. B., & Crerand, C. E. (2004). Body image and cosmetic medical treatments. *Body Image, 1,* 99–111. doi:10.1016/S1740-1445(03)00003-2

Sarwer, D. B., Crerand, C. E., & Magee, L. (2011). Cosmetic surgery and changes in body image. In T. F. Cash & L. Smolak (Eds.), *Body image: A handbook of science, practice, and prevention* (2nd ed., pp. 394–403). New York, NY: Guilford Press.

Sarwer, D. B., & Magee, L. (2006). Physical appearance and society. In D. B. Sarwer, T. Pruzinsky, T. F. Cash, R. M. Goldwyn, J. A. Persing, & L. A. Whitaker (Eds.), *Psychological aspects of reconstructive and cosmetic plastic surgery: Clinical, empirical and ethical perspectives* (pp. 23–36). Philadelphia, PA: Lippincott Williams & Wilkins.

Sarwer, D. B., Wadden, T. A., Pertschuk, M. J., & Whitaker, L. A. (1998). The psychology of cosmetic surgery: A review and reconceptualization. *Clinical Psychology Review, 18*, 1–22. doi:10.1016/S0272-7358(97)00047-0

Shakespeare, V., & Cole, R. P. (1997). Measuring patient-based outcomes in a plastic surgery service: Breast reduction surgical patients. *British Journal of Plastic Surgery, 50*, 242–248.

Soni, C. V., Barker, J. H., Pushpakumar, S. B., Furr, L. A., Cunningham, M., Banis, J. C., Jr., & Frank, J. (2010). Psychosocial considerations in facial transplantation. *Burns, 36*, 959–964. doi:10.1016/j.burns.2010.01.012

Storch, E., Lewin, A., Geffken, G., Heidgerken, A., Stawser, M., Baumeister, A., & Silverstein, J. (2004). Psychosocial adjustment of two boys with gynecomastia. *Journal of Pediatrics and Child Health, 40*, 331.

Tebble, N. J., Adams, R., Thomas, D. W., & Price, P. (2006). Anxiety and self-consciousness in patients with facial lacerations one week and six months later. *British Journal of Oral & Maxillofacial Surgery, 44*, 520–525. doi:10.1016/j.bjoms.2005.10.010

van Loey, N. E., Maas, C. J., Faber, A. W., & Taal, L. A. (2003). Predictors of chronic posttraumatic stress symptoms following burn injury: Results of a longitudinal study. *Journal of Traumatic Stress, 16*, 361–369. doi:10.1023/A:1024465902416

White, C. A., & Hood, C. (2011). Body image issues in oncology. In T. F. Cash & L. Smolak (Eds.), *Body image: A handbook of science, practice, and prevention* (2nd ed., pp. 333–341). New York, NY: Guilford Press.

Williams, A. E., Newman, J. T., Ozer, K., Juarros, A., Morgan, S. J., & Smith, W. R. (2009). Posttraumatic stress disorder and depression negatively impact general health status after hand injury. *Journal of Hand Surgery, 34*, 515–522. doi:10.1016/j.jhsa.2008.11.008

Young, V. L., & Hutchison, J. (2009). Insights into patient and clinician concerns about scar appearance: Semiquantitative structured surveys. *Plastic and Reconstructive Surgery, 124*, 256–265. doi:10.1097/PRS.0b013e3181a80747

Young, V. L., & Watson, M. E. (2006). Breast reduction. In D. B. Sarwer, T. Pruzinsky, T. F. Cash, R. M. Goldwyn, J. A. Persing, & L. A. Whitaker (Eds.), *Psychological aspects of reconstructive and cosmetic plastic surgery: Clinical, empirical and ethical perspectives* (pp. 189–206). Philadelphia, PA: Lippincott Williams & Wilkins.

Zigmond, A. S., & Snaith, R. P. (1983). The Hospital Anxiety and Depression Scale. *Acta Psychiatrica Scandinavica, 67*, 361–370. doi:10.1111/j.1600-0447.1983.tb09716.x

9

BREAST CANCER SURGERY

SARAH J. MILLER, JULIE B. SCHNUR, AND GUY H. MONTGOMERY

This year, more than 280,000 women will be diagnosed with breast cancer (American Cancer Society, 2012b). The vast majority of these women will undergo surgical treatment to remove the tumor and accurately stage the disease (American Cancer Society, 2011). Surgery is a critical component of the diagnostic and curative treatment of breast cancer; however, it is not without costs. Women undergoing breast cancer surgery often experience both psychological and physical side effects of the procedure (e.g., Dunn, Steginga, Occhipinti, Wilson, & McCaffrey, 1998; Jung, Ahrendt, Oaklander, & Dworkin, 2003).

Empirical research has found that a woman's preoperative thoughts, feelings, and coping strategies can have a negative impact on her postoperative psychological and physical recovery (e.g., Den Oudsten, Van Heck, Van der Steeg, Roukema, & De Vries, 2009a). There is great potential for health

DOI: 10.1037/14035-010
Presurgical Psychological Screening: Understanding Patients, Improving Outcomes, Andrew R. Block and David B. Sarwer (Editors)

care providers to identify and address such presurgical psychological factors to help reduce postsurgical suffering.

BREAST CANCER SURGERY OVERVIEW

The purposes of this chapter are to describe the experiences of patients with breast cancer from diagnosis to surgery, to review the literature on preoperative predictors of postoperative outcomes, to provide guidance on conducting an assessment in the breast cancer surgical context, to recommend an assessment battery to administer before breast cancer surgery, and to discuss practical implications of the suggested assessment battery. The goal of the suggested assessment is twofold: (a) to help identify women at risk for increased postsurgical side effects and (b) to guide interventions designed to reduce presurgical psychological risk factors and, in doing so, reduce postsurgical suffering.

This section provides an overview of the breast cancer surgical experience. In particular, the section discusses (a) detection of breast cancer, (b) surgeries used to diagnose and treat breast cancer, (c) physical and psychological side effects of such diagnostic and curative surgeries, (d) factors that place a woman at risk for experiencing such side effects, and (e) the role of mental health professionals in the breast cancer surgical setting.

Detection of Breast Cancer

Each woman with breast cancer has a personal story of how she detected an abnormality in her breast and subsequently was referred for diagnostic and curative surgery. Most often, breast cancer is first identified through breast self-exams, clinical breast exams, and mammograms. If a breast abnormality is detected, a woman is often referred for follow-up testing such as a breast ultrasound or MRI. When a suspicious mass is found, some women may undergo a nonsurgical breast biopsy to further examine the pathology.

The period of time leading up to a definitive diagnosis is often endured with emotional distress. During this waiting period, women are faced with the possibility of having a life-threatening disease, and thus it is not surprising that the diagnostic process can be frightening, distressing, and often chaotic (M. Montgomery, 2010; M. Montgomery & McCrone, 2010).

Breast Cancer Surgery

When the screening and diagnostic tests yield suspicious results, women are recommended to undergo one or more breast cancer surgical procedures. These procedures include surgical breast biopsy, sentinel node biopsy, mastectomy, breast-conserving surgery, and breast reconstruction (American Cancer Society, 2012a).

- *Surgical breast biopsy.* Some women undergo a surgical biopsy (rather than a needle biopsy) to help diagnose and stage the tumor. This procedure involves the partial–incisional or full–excisional removal of the tumor and the surrounding areas.
- *Sentinel node biopsy.* If breast cancer has metastasized, it will first spread to a lymph node, referred to as the *sentinel node*. A sentinel node biopsy involves the removal and examination of the sentinel lymph node to help determine whether the cancer has spread.
- *Mastectomy.* A mastectomy involves the removal of the entire breast. Depending on the type of mastectomy, the unaffected breast, muscle under the breast, and axillary lymph nodes may also be removed during the procedure.
- *Breast-conserving surgery.* Unlike a mastectomy, breast-conserving surgery (i.e., lumpectomy or quandrantectomy) preserves part of the breast tissue. A lumpectomy removes the tumor and the surrounding margins of normal tissues, whereas a quandrantectomy removes one quarter of the breast tissue. Lymph nodes may also be removed during the operative procedure.
- *Breast reconstruction surgery.* Although the focus of this chapter is diagnostic and curative surgeries for breast cancer, it is important to acknowledge that many patients may also elect to undergo reconstructive breast surgery. For example, many women choose to have an implant inserted during a mastectomy procedure. However, when the skin on the breast is too tight or flat, a breast expander may be inserted behind the breast muscle for 4 to 6 months to create space for an implant. As an alternative to receiving a breast implant, some women elect to have a tissue flap procedure (e.g., transverse rectus abdominis muscle flap) in which tissues from the abdomen, back, thighs, or buttocks are used to rebuild the breast. The extensive literature on the psychosocial aspects of breast reconstruction is beyond the focus of this chapter. For relatively recent reviews of this literature, the reader is referred to Reavey and McCarthy (2008) as well as Rosson et al. (2010).

Side Effects of Breast Cancer Surgery

Breast cancer surgery can cause both acute and chronic physical side effects, including pain, fatigue, numbness in the chest wall, difficulty sleeping, and nausea (e.g., Ewertz & Jensen, 2011; Jung et al., 2003; Shimozuma, Granz, Petersen, & Hirji, 1999; Tasmuth, von Smitten, & Kalso, 1996). Additionally, when operative procedures involve the removal of lymph nodes, patients may also develop lymphedema, a severe uncomfortable swelling of the arm (American Cancer Society, 2011). Not only are such side effects distressing, but they may also hinder recovery from the surgery, increase the necessity of pharmacological interventions, and delay discharge from the hospital (Hirsch, 1994; Marla & Stallard, 2009; Pavlin et al., 1998; Pavlin, Chen, Penaloza, Polissar, & Buckley, 2002).

Breast cancer surgery can also take a toll on a woman's psychological well-being and overall quality of life. Research has reported that after breast cancer surgery, women may suffer from disruptions in body image, decreased quality of life, depressive symptoms, fear of cancer recurrence, and general psychological distress (e.g., Dunn et al., 1998; Ewertz & Jensen, 2011; Fann et al., 2008; Shimozuma et al., 1999).

Presurgical Psychological Predictors of Postsurgical Morbidity

The literature has indicated that most surgical patients with breast cancer will experience some physical (e.g., pain, nausea and vomiting, fatigue) or psychological (e.g., emotional distress) sequelae (e.g., Bender, Ergun, Rosenzweig, Cohen, & Sereika, 2005; Gan, Ginsberg, Grant, & Glass, 2004; Gartner et al., 2009; Oddby-Muhrbeck, Jakobsson, Andersson, & Askergren, 1994). Understanding the predictive factors for such sequelae is of particular clinical importance.

The literature on modifiable presurgical factors that facilitate or hinder recovery after breast cancer surgery is summarized in Tables 9.1 and 9.2. The following presurgical psychological factors have been shown to place a woman at risk for psychological and physical morbidity after breast cancer surgery: emotional distress, expectations of poor surgical outcomes, concern about appearance, fatigue, lack of sleep, and avoidant coping.

Mental Health Professionals in Breast Cancer Surgical Settings

To our knowledge, few cancer surgical settings employ clinicians on staff to address patients' psychosocial needs before breast cancer surgery. These clinicians are most likely found in large comprehensive cancers centers housed in major medical centers. Indeed, these clinicians may be a luxury for a fortunate few. Their most common role is as a referral for difficult cases rather than as a member of the standing multidisciplinary surgical team involved in the care of all women. However, with a new focus on evidence-based medicine within the U.S. health care system and clear evidence emerging supporting

TABLE 9.1
Presurgical Predictors of Postsurgical Physical Side Effects

Predictor	Assessment	Sample	Physical outcome (time postsurgery)	Direction of effect	Citation
Anxiety symptoms	State–Trait Anxiety Inventory, State version	N = 114 Lumpectomy, or lumpectomy with nodes, or mastectomy	Pain (Day 2) Persistence of pain (Day 2 to Day 30)	+ +	Katz et al. (2005)
Pain expectancy	Pain expectancy VAS	N = 101 Excisional breast biopsy or lumpectomy	Pain severity (7 days) Pain intensity (hospital discharge) Pain unpleasantness (hospital discharge)	+ +	G. H. Montgomery, Schnur, Erblich, Diefenbach, & Bovbjerg (2010)
Nausea expectancy	Nausea expectancy VAS	N = 101 Excisional breast biopsy or lumpectomy	Nausea (7 days)	+	G. H. Montgomery, Schnur, et al. (2010)
Fatigue expectancy	Fatigue expectancy VAS	N = 101 Excisional breast biopsy or lumpectomy	Fatigue (7 days) Fatigue (hospital discharge)	+ +	G. H. Montgomery, Schnur, et al. (2010)
Distress	Tension–Anxiety subscale of the Short Version of the Profile of Mood States	N = 101 Excisional breast biopsy or lumpectomy	Pain severity (7 days) Fatigue Severity (7 days)	+ +	G. H. Montgomery, Schnur, et al. (2010)
Distress	Distress VAS	N = 63 Excisional breast biopsy or lumpectomy	Nausea (hospital discharge) Fatigue (hospital discharge) Discomfort (hospital discharge)	+ + +	G. H. Montgomery & Bovbjerg (2004)

Note. VAS = visual analogue scale.

TABLE 9.2
Presurgical Predictors of Postsurgical Psychological Side Effects

Predictor	Assessment	Sample	Psychological outcomes (time postsurgery)	Direction of effect	Citation
Concern about appearance	Concern about appearance scale	N = 66 Lumpectomy or mastectomy	Emotional distress (3 months) Emotional distress (6 months)	+ +	Carver et al. (1998)
Depressive symptoms	Center for Epidemiological Studies Depression Scale	N = 144 Lumpectomy or mastectomy	Depression (12 months)	+	Den Oudsten, Van Heck, Van der Steeg, Roukema, & De Vries (2009a)
Mood symptoms	Hospital Anxiety and Depression Scale	N = 91 Modified radical mastectomy or breast conservation therapy	Mood disorder (within 1 year)	+	Ramirez, Richards, Jarrett, & Fentiman (1995)
Acceptance coping	Acceptance subscale of the COPE Inventory	N = 70 Breast conservation surgery or mastectomy	Distress (1 year) Positive mood (1 year)	− +	Stanton, Danoff-Burg, & Huggins (2002)
Avoidant coping	Avoidance subscale of the COPE Inventory	N = 70 Breast conservation surgery or mastectomy	Distress (3 months) Fear of recurrence (1 year)	− +	Stanton, Danoff-Burg, & Huggins (2002)
Cognitive avoidant coping	Cognitive–Escape Avoidance factor of the Ways of Coping Questionnaire—Cancer Version	N = 36 Breast conservation surgery or mastectomy	Negative affect (3 weeks) Vigor (3 weeks)	+ −	Stanton & Snider (1993)
Fatigue	Fatigue Assessment Scale	N = 144 Lumpectomy or mastectomy	Depression (12 months)	+	Den Oudsten et al. (2009a)
Rest and sleep difficulties	Sleep and Rest facet of the World Health Organization Quality of Life instrument	N = 144 Lumpectomy or mastectomy	Depression (12 months)	+	Den Oudsten et al. (2009a)

the clinical and cost-effectiveness of psychological interventions with cancer surgical patients (e.g., Jacobsen & Jim, 2008; G. H. Montgomery et al., 2007), we hope that more widespread inclusion of clinicians in breast cancer surgical settings is on the horizon.

PSYCHOLOGICAL ASSESSMENT BEFORE BREAST CANCER SURGERY

On the basis of the empirical literature, clinicians are advised to assess patients' psychological well-being before breast cancer surgery. Components of a psychological assessment, in and of itself, can have therapeutic benefits (Burton et al., 1995). A presurgery psychological assessment can be used to (a) help identify women at risk for poor postsurgical side effects; (b) guide clinical and psychopharmacological interventions designed to reduce presurgical psychological risk factors; and (c) limit postoperative distress. Brief presurgical interventions can significantly improve psychological and physical recovery from surgery. For example, our research group found that a 15-minute presurgical hypnosis intervention significantly improves postsurgical pain, fatigue, and nausea by addressing women's response expectancies (e.g., surgery-related pain expectancy) and reducing their anticipatory distress (G. H. Montgomery, Hallquist, et al., 2010). Research in other cancer surgical contexts has also found that preoperative psychosocial interventions (e.g., psychoeducation, stress management) can significantly improve postoperative psychological and physical recovery (e.g., Ali & Khalil, 1989; Parker et al., 2009).

Setting the Stage for the Assessment

Next, we outline suggestions for and information about conducting a presurgical psychological assessment in a breast cancer surgical setting.

Considerations

As previously discussed, women may experience notable psychological distress and elevated feelings of uncertainty before breast cancer surgery (M. Montgomery, 2010; M. Montgomery & McCrone, 2010). Thus, when conducting a preoperative assessment, it is imperative that the mental health professional be sensitive to and mindful of the psychological burden of the breast cancer diagnostic process, as well as the distress related to the impending breast surgery.

Timing

Optimally, the assessment should occur several weeks before the scheduled surgery to allow time for preventive interventions. At the same time, we have found that 1 week, although often too brief for promoting personality change or treating chronic psychiatric disorders (e.g., major depression), is sufficient time to address acute psychological issues. Randomized trials have demonstrated that brief behavioral medicine interventions administered within 1 week of surgery can reduce presurgical emotional distress and prevent aversive postsurgical outcomes (e.g., G. H. Montgomery et al., 2007).

Setting

We have found that candidates for breast cancer surgery are often extremely busy with appointments and follow-up procedures. Therefore, assessments should be administered in whatever setting is most convenient and least burdensome for the patient. For example, an assessment may be administered in an exam room before or after a scheduled medical appointment. Although conducting a clinical interview in person is ideal (see the next section), if the patient has minimal time to meet with a clinician, she can complete the self-report questionnaires at her convenience (e.g., at home) and perhaps complete the interview via telephone. Research in other contexts has found that telephone assessments are comparable to in-person assessments (e.g., Smith, Illiq, Friedler, Hamilton, & Ottenbacher, 1996); however, telephone assessments limit the ability to have a well-controlled testing environment and the opportunity to consider nonverbal communication cues (Soet & Basch, 1997).

Role of the Clinician

Patients may not be accustomed to meeting with a mental health professional in a medical setting (or in general) and may not expect to discuss their psychological health during breast cancer surgical appointments. Therefore, clinicians should clarify the rationale for the assessment and the role of the clinician in the surgical setting to set appropriate expectations and ease any discomfort or ambivalence.

The assessment can be introduced in the following manner:

> Sometimes the way you think or feel emotionally may affect how you feel physically. For example, have you ever gotten a headache or stomachache when you were stressed? We are checking in on your thoughts and feelings before surgery so that we can help you feel better after surgery.

Presurgical Psychological Battery

We recommend a brief psychological battery to administer before breast cancer surgery. The suggested battery consists of a clinical interview, a mental status exam, and a series of self-report measures.

Clinical Interview

As with all psychological assessments, a face-to-face interview can provide rich, clinically relevant data. In the breast cancer surgical context (i.e., a busy medical practice), clinicians may have as little as 25 to 30 minutes to complete a clinical interview. As such, establishing rapport quickly and asking directive, specific questions is critical. Although patients frequently meet with their medical treatment team, medical providers may not ask patients about their psychological well-being and emotional needs. We have found utility in beginning an interview by stating, "Tell me about your thoughts and feelings leading up to surgery."

After assessing current symptoms and distress, clinicians should also assess psychiatric history. Drawing from the empirical literature, a trauma history, particularly of sexual abuse, can place a woman at risk for worsened psychological distress after breast cancer surgery (Wyatt, Loeb, Desmond, & Ganz, 2005). We have found that women who have a history of sexual abuse often have heightened distress before surgery because aspects of breast cancer surgery (e.g., exposure of the breast, lack of power and control, physical pain and discomfort) can parallel aspects of sexual trauma (Schnur & Goldsmith, 2011).

In addition, brief needs assessment can help determine whether the patient would benefit from additional referrals (e.g., social work, support groups, psychiatry). For example, the clinician may assess the patient's needs for psychosocial support, financial and insurance planning, psychosexual concerns, and so forth. Richardson, Medina, Brown, and Sitzia (2007) summarized 15 measures to assess cancer patients' clinical, health, and support needs.

Mental Status Exam

Given the brevity of the clinical interview, behavioral observations can contribute to the assessment in fundamental ways. In particular, the patient's overall appearance, affect, behaviors, and mood can provide valuable data regarding well-being and psychological needs. An assessment of patients' cognitive functioning can help determine whether they are capable of providing informed consent for treatment and for treatment decisions, such as (a) surgical treatment options (e.g., mastectomy vs. breast-conserving therapy), (b) personal and familial genetic testing, and (c) participation in a clinical trial (Takasugi et al., 2005). Assessment tools, such as the Mini-Mental State Examination, could be used to obtain information about the patient's cognitive functioning (e.g., Sorger, Rosenfeld, Pessin, Timm, & Cimino, 2007). More extensive neuropsychological testing may be warranted if cognitive dysfunction or decline is suspected.

Self-Report Assessment Measures

To obtain quantifiable data regarding presurgical psychological status, patients can be asked to complete a series of self-report questionnaires designed to assess mood, thoughts, response expectancies, coping strategies, fatigue, and sleep. Drawing from the empirical literature, we have generated an evidence-informed pre–breast cancer surgery assessment battery that we use with most patients. When creating the battery, we considered stable variables (e.g., trait characteristics) that may place a woman at risk for poor surgical side effects. For example, empirical studies have found that demographic variables (e.g., age; Katz et al., 2005) and personality characteristics (e.g., pessimism; Schou, Ekeberg, Ruland, Sandvik, & Karesen, 2004) predict the occurrence of postoperative side effects. However, to minimize patient burden and maximize the utility of assessment results, we aimed to create a battery that is efficient and can directly inform clinical presurgical interventions. Therefore, we decided to exclusively assess presurgical psychological constructs that are amenable to brief psychological or pharmacological intervention.

Anxiety Symptoms. The State–Trait Anxiety Inventory, State version (Spielberger, Gorsuch, Lushene, Vagg, & Jacobs, 1983), is a 20-item self-report measure that assesses context-dependent feelings of tension, apprehension, and nervousness. The State version of STAI has shown excellent internal consistency (Cronbach's α = .92) and validity.

The Tension–Anxiety subscale of the Short Version of the Profile of Mood States is a six-item scale that assesses current level of anxiety and tension. The scale has shown excellent internal consistency in a sample with breast cancer (Cronbach's α = .86). Validation studies conducted with patients with breast cancer have shown that the Tension–Anxiety subscale of the Short Version of the Profile of Mood States can differentiate between a sample of patients with breast cancer and a healthy sample (DiLorenzo, Bovbjerg, Montgomery, Valdimarsdottir, & Jacobsen, 1999).

Depressive Symptoms. The Center for Epidemiologic Studies Depression Scale (Radloff, 1977) is a widely used, 20-item self-report measure that assesses the presence and frequency of depressive symptoms over the past week. When used with a breast cancer population, the internal consistency is good (Cronbach's α = .89; Hann, Winter, & Jacobsen, 1999). Validation studies have shown that the Center for Epidemiologic Studies Depression Scale can effectively differentiate between clinically depressed and healthy populations, and the scale has been found to correlate with other validated measures of depressive symptoms (Radloff, 1977).

Mixed Depression and Anxiety Symptoms. The Hospital Anxiety and Depression Scale is a 14-item self-report questionnaire that assesses anxiety and depression symptoms in individuals with mood and somatic complaints.

The scale has two subscales: Anxiety (Cronbach's α = .80) and Depression (Cronbach's α = .76; Mykletun, Stordal, & Dahl, 2001). Validation studies have found that the Hospital Anxiety and Depression Scale correlates with other measures of anxiety and depression (Bjelland, Dahl, Haug, & Neckelmann, 2002).

Distress. The distress visual analogue scale (VAS) is a single item that assesses current emotional distress. Patients are asked to indicate the intensity of their level of distress by drawing a slash through a 100-millimeter line with anchors (i.e., *not upset at all, as upset as I could be*). The distress VAS has been both efficient and valid in breast cancer treatment clinics and experimental settings (Cella & Perry, 1986; DiLorenzo et al., 1995; G. H. Montgomery & Bovbjerg, 1997; Schnur et al., 2007). See Figure 9.1 for an example of a distress VAS.

Response Expectancies. A response expectancy VAS is a single item that assesses presurgical expectations of the intensity of a postsurgery side effect such as pain, nausea, or fatigue. Patients are asked to indicate the intensity of response expectancy by drawing a slash through a 100-millimeter line with anchors (e.g., *no pain at all, as much pain as there could be*). For example, a patient may be asked,

Distress Visual Analog Scale

1. Right now, how <u>emotionally upset</u> do you feel?

Not upset at all	As Upset as I Could Be

Response Expectancy Visual Analog Scales

1. After surgery, how <u>fatigued</u> do you expect to be?

Not Fatigued at All	As Fatigued as I Could Be

2. After surgery, how <u>nauseated</u> do you think you will feel?

Not at All Nauseated	As Nauseated as I Could Be

3. After surgery, how much <u>pain</u> do you think you will feel?

No Pain at all	As Much Pain as There Could Be

Figure 9.1. Distress and Response Expectancy Visual Analogue Scales.

"After surgery, how much pain do you think you will feel?" The response expectancy VAS has been both efficient and valid in breast cancer treatment clinics and experimental settings (e.g., G. H. Montgomery & Bovbjerg, 2004; Schnur et al., 2007). See Figure 9.1 for an example of a response expectancy VAS.

Body Image. The Concerns About Appearance Scale was developed by Carver et al. (1998) to assess concern about physical appearance. More specifically, the four-item scale assesses the extent to which a woman's positive feelings about herself are dependent on her physical appearance. The scale demonstrated adequate internal consistency (Cronbach's $\alpha = .78$) in a breast cancer surgical setting (Carver et al., 1998).

Fatigue and Sleep. The Fatigue Assessment Scale is a 10-item self-report measure that assesses the presence and frequency of cognitive and physiological fatigue. Previous research has found the measure to have excellent internal consistency (Cronbach's $\alpha = .91$). Validation studies have shown that the Fatigue Assessment Scale can differentiate between a fatigued medical population, such as individuals diagnosed with sarcoidosis, and a healthy population (Michielsen, De Vries, Drent, & Peros-Golubicic, 2005). In addition, the Fatigue Assessment Scale has been found to significantly correlate with other empirically validated fatigue scales (Michielsen, De Vries, & Van Heck, 2003).

The Sleep and Rest facet of the World Health Organization Quality of Life Instrument (*WHOQOL–100*) is a four-item self-report measure that assesses the presence and severity of sleep problems. For example, one item reads, "Do you have any difficulties with sleeping?" (WHOQOL Group, 1998). Previous research with a breast cancer sample has found that the Rest and Sleep facet of the WHOQOL–100 has excellent internal consistency (Cronbach's $\alpha = .92$). In validation studies, the Sleep and Rest facet has been significantly correlated with related constructs such as general health, mental health, fatigue, and energy (Den Oudsten, Van Heck, Van der Steeg, Roukema, & De Vries, 2009b).

Coping Strategies. The Avoidance subscales of the COPE Inventory consist of Mental Disengagement (four items), Behavioral Disengagement (four items), and Denial (four items). These subscales assess avoidant coping strategies (Carver, Scheier, & Weintraub, 1989). In a breast cancer surgical setting, the total avoidance subscales demonstrated adequate internal reliability (Cronbach's $\alpha = .67$; Stanton, Danoff-Burg, & Huggins, 2002).

The Acceptance subscale of the COPE Inventory (four items) assesses a tendency to accept difficult situations (Carver et al., 1989). In a breast cancer setting, the Acceptance subscale demonstrated adequate internal consistency (Cronbach's $\alpha = .69$; Stanton et al., 2002).

The Cognitive–Escape Avoidance factor of the Ways of Coping Questionnaire—Cancer Version is a nine-item self-report measure that assesses mental avoidance. In a cancer setting, the Cognitive–Escape Avoidance factor demonstrated adequate internal consistency (Cronbach's $\alpha = .78$; Dunkel-Schetter, Feinstein, Taylor, & Falke, 1992; Stanton & Snider, 1993).

Ideal Versus Real-World Assessment Battery

An evidence-informed presurgical battery such as the one we describe consists of 12 scales, would have a total of 107 items, and would likely take approximately 30 minutes to complete. Ideally, item response theory would be used to reduce the full battery, yielding a final, concise, psychometrically sound scale that maximizes information gained while minimizing patient burden. However, such analyses have not yet been conducted. We recognize that to further minimize patient burden, clinicians may be interested in a briefer assessment battery, in which case we recommend the following: the Short Version of the Profile of Mood States, response expectancies (fatigue, pain, nausea), the Concerns About Body Image scale, the Center for Epidemiologic Studies Depression Scale, the Sleep and Rest Facet of the WHOQOL-100, and the Avoidance and Acceptance subscales of the COPE Inventory. The shortened battery would consist of 53 items and would take approximately 10 to 15 minutes to complete.

Interpreting the Assessment Results

Empirical research has reported incremental predictive relationships between the outlined assessment tools and postsurgical side effects. In other words, as presurgical psychological functioning declines, the risk of postsurgical side effects increases. This is not to say, however, that someone with higher levels of presurgical functioning is entirely protected from postoperative distress. To date, no cutoffs have been established to determine the threshold at which treatment is necessary or most beneficial. As such, the results of this assessment battery should be viewed more as a means to identify patients at risk and psychotherapeutic targets than as a threshold for treatment. This view is further supported by the high degree of benefit patients can receive from participating in brief behavioral medicine interventions (e.g., a brief relaxation exercise) and the extremely low incidence of side effects of such interventions. Drawing on information obtained through psychometric testing can help the clinician and patient collaborate to determine the most critical psychological targets for intervention.

Applying the Assessment Results

The proposed assessment battery should not be used to determine patients' eligibility or appropriateness for surgical treatment. Rather, it should be used to inform brief presurgical interventions designed to (a) improve psychological functioning and (b) improve postsurgical recovery (e.g., decrease pain, distress, fatigue, nausea). Although a large menu of psychotherapeutic treatment options are available to address psychosocial difficulties, when selecting a psychological treatment approach clinicians should consider (a) what treatment options have been supported by empirical research (preferably in the breast cancer surgical setting), (b) what resources are available at the breast cancer surgical setting (e.g., psychiatrists, psychologists, social workers, nurses), and (c) whether the intervention can produce the desired results in the time between assessment and surgery.

Case Study

J. M. entered her surgical consultation appointment with both her mind and heart racing, feeling what she described as pure "shock and terror."[1] Only 7 days earlier, her primary care physician had found an abnormal lump in her breast. Now, at age 55, J. M. was scheduled to have a bilateral mastectomy, followed by reconstruction. Her diagnosis was Stage III breast carcinoma. Immediately after J. M.'s consultation with the treating breast surgeon, a clinician conducted a brief interview and administered a series of self-report measures to assess her current psychological functioning. During the interview, J. M. spoke of her sweaty palms and frayed nerves. Her scores on the Anxiety subscale of the Hospital Anxiety and Depression Scale and distress VAS further confirmed elevated anxiety and distress. In addition, J. M. indicated that she expected to feel severe pain, nausea, and fatigue after surgery. The results suggested that she was at an elevated risk for increased postsurgical side effects: Pain, fatigue, nausea, and emotional distress were likely. In an effort to prevent or reduce such outcomes, the treating clinician led J. M. through a brief hypnosis intervention, gave her audio materials to practice with at home, and discussed cognitive–behavioral techniques to reduce her symptoms of anxiety and set more positive expectancies for breast cancer surgery. With these new skills, J. M. was able to reduce her level of presurgical distress, improve expectancies, and in turn improve her postsurgical recovery. After surgery, she reported minimal to no physical and psychological side effects.

FUTURE DIRECTIONS

Although we believe that the preoperative assessment approach described in this chapter has a great deal of clinical utility, we also recognize that it has some limitations. One limitation is that no research to

---

[1]Details of this case have been altered to protect the patient's identity.

date has applied item response theory to this set of assessment items as a whole. In the future, item response theory should be used to reduce the number of items and to refine the assessment battery (Lipscomb, Gotay, & Snyder, 2005).

A second limitation is that the current literature has focused almost entirely on women undergoing breast cancer surgery. Therefore, it is unclear whether this battery has similar predictive power for male breast cancer patients. An estimated 2,190 men will be newly diagnosed with breast cancer this year (American Cancer Society, 2012b), but no research to date has focused on how their thoughts, feelings, and coping strategies before breast cancer surgery affect their postsurgical recovery.

Finally, research to date has focused exclusively on paper-and-pencil assessment measures. Presently, approximately 60% of adults living with chronic disease report going online (Fox & Purcell, 2010). Therefore, to keep up with patient preferences, we recommend that this battery be tested in an online format, which can provide a greater sense of privacy and a decreased sense of interpersonal risk for patients who are reluctant to disclose emotional distress because of perceived stigma.

Although this chapter's focus was on breast cancer surgery assessments, it is important to note that the assessment process should be ongoing throughout the course of breast cancer treatment and survivorship. The psychological factors (e.g., thoughts, feelings) identified as predictors of postsurgical side effects have also been shown to be predictive of clinical outcomes in the chemotherapy and radiation oncology settings (e.g., Vearncombe et al., 2009). As such, throughout the course of treatment, understanding patients' pretreatment acute psychological status is a step toward improving their quality of life during and after treatment.

CONCLUSION

Breast cancer affects hundreds of thousands of U.S. women each year. Surgery is often an essential component of the diagnostic and curative treatment of breast cancer; however, it can cause grueling physical and psychological side effects. Empirical research has drawn a clear connection between a woman's presurgical thoughts, feelings, and coping strategies and her physical well-being and health-related quality of life after surgery. In this chapter, we provided guidance on the tools needed to identify critical components of presurgical psychological functioning. It is our hope that the proposed assessment battery can directly inform presurgical interventions designed to reduce postsurgical suffering in women with breast cancer.

REFERENCES

Ali, N. S., & Khalil, H. Z. (1989). Effect of psychoeducational intervention on anxiety among Egyptian bladder cancer patients. *Cancer Nursing, 12,* 236–242. doi:10.1097/00002820-198908000-00006

American Cancer Society. (2011). *Breast cancer facts and figures 2011-2012.* Atlanta, GA: Author.

American Cancer Society. (2012a). *Breast cancer overview.* Atlanta, GA: Author.

American Cancer Society. (2012b). *Cancer facts and figures 2012.* Atlanta, GA: Author.

Bender, C. M., Ergun, F. S., Rosenzweig, M. Q., Cohen, S. M., & Sereika, S. M. (2005). Symptom clusters in breast cancer across 3 phases of the disease. *Cancer Nursing, 28,* 219–225. doi:10.1097/00002820-200505000-00011

Bjelland, I., Dahl, A. A., Haug, T. T., & Neckelmann, D. (2002). The validity of the Hospital Anxiety and Depression Scale: An updated literature review. *Journal of Psychosomatic Research, 52,* 69–77. doi:10.1016/S0022-3999(01)00296-3

Burton, M. V., Parker, R. W., Farrell, A., Bailey, D., Conneely, J., Booth, S., & Elcombe, S. (1995). A randomized controlled trial of preoperative psychological preparation for mastectomy. *Psycho-Oncology, 4,* 1–19. doi:10.1002/pon.2960040102

Carver, C. S., Pozo-Kaderman, C., Price, A. A., Noriega, V., Harris, S. D., Derhagopian, R. P., . . . Moffat, F. L., Jr. (1998). Concern about aspects of body image and adjustment to early stage breast cancer. *Psychosomatic Medicine, 60,* 168–174.

Carver, C. S., Scheier, M. F., & Weintraub, J. K. (1989). Assessing coping strategies: A theoretically based approach. *Journal of Personality and Social Psychology, 56,* 267–283. doi:10.1037/0022-3514.56.2.267

Cella, D. F., & Perry, S. W. (1986). Reliability and concurrent validity of three visual-analogue mood scales. *Psychological Reports, 59,* 827–833. doi:10.2466/pr0.1986.59.2.827

Den Oudsten, B. L., Van Heck, G. L., Van der Steeg, A. F., Roukema, J. A., & De Vries, J. (2009a). Predictors of depressive symptoms 12 months after surgical treatment of early-stage breast cancer. *Psycho-Oncology, 18,* 1230–1237. doi:10.1002/pon.1518

Den Oudsten, B. L., Van Heck, G. L., Van der Steeg, A. F., Roukema, J. A., & De Vries, J. (2009b). The WHOQOL-100 has good psychometric properties in breast cancer patients. *Journal of Clinical Epidemiology, 62,* 195–205. doi:10.1016/j.jclinepi.2008.03.006

DiLorenzo, T. A., Bovbjerg, D. H., Montgomery, G. H., Valdimarsdottir, H., & Jacobsen, P. B. (1999). The application of a shortened version of the Profile of Mood States in a sample of breast cancer chemotherapy patients. *British Journal of Health Psychology, 4,* 315–325. doi:10.1348/135910799168669

DiLorenzo, T. A., Jacobsen, P. B., Bovbjerg, D. H., Chang, H., Hudis, C. A., Sklarin, N. T., & Norton, L. (1995). Sources of anticipatory emotional distress in women receiving chemotherapy for breast cancer. *Annals of Oncology, 6,* 705–711.

Dunkel-Schetter, C., Feinstein, L. G., Taylor, S. E., & Falke, R. L. (1992). Patterns of coping with cancer. *Health Psychology, 11,* 79–87. doi:10.1037/0278-6133.11.2.79

Dunn, J., Steginga, S. K., Occhipinti, S., Wilson, K., & McCaffrey, J. (1998). Profiles of distress in women following treatment for primary cancer. *The Breast, 7,* 251–254. doi:10.1016/S0960-9776(98)90090-X

Ewertz, M., & Jensen, A. B. (2011). Late effects of breast cancer treatment and potentials for rehabilitation. *Acta Oncologica, 50,* 187–193. doi:10.3109/0284 186X.2010.533190

Fann, J. R., Thomas-Rich, A. M., Katon, W. J., Cowley, D., Pepping, M., McGregor, B. A., & Gralow, J. (2008). Major depression after breast cancer: A review of epidemiology and treatment. *General Hospital Psychiatry, 30,* 112–126. doi:10.1016/j.genhosppsych.2007.10.008

Fox, S., & Purcell, K. (2010). *Chronic disease and the internet.* Washington, DC: Pew Internet & American Life Project.

Gan, T. J., Ginsberg, B., Grant, A. P., & Glass, P. S. A. (2004). Double-blind, randomized comparison of ondansetron and intraoperative propofol to prevent postoperative nausea and vomiting. *Anesthesiology, 85,* 1036–1042.

Gärtner, R., Jensen, M., Nielsen, J., Ewertz, M., Niels, K., & Kehlet, H. (2009). Prevalence of and factors associated with persistent pain following breast cancer surgery. *JAMA, 302,* 1985–1992. doi:10.1001/jama.2009.1568

Hann, D., Winter, K., & Jacobsen, P. (1999). Measurement of depressive symptoms in cancer patients: Evaluation of the Center for Epidemiological Studies Depression Scale (CES-D). *Journal of Psychosomatic Research, 46,* 437–443. doi: 10.1016/S0022-3999(99)00004-5

Hirsch, J. (1994). Impact of postoperative nausea and vomiting in the surgical setting. *Anaesthesia, 49*(Suppl.), 30–33. doi:10.1111/j.1365-2044.1994.tb03580.x

Jacobsen, P. B., & Jim, H. S. (2008). Psychosocial interventions for anxiety and depression in adult cancer patients: Achievement and challenges. *CA: A Cancer Journal for Clinicians, 58,* 214–230. doi:10.3322/CA.2008.0003

Jung, B. F., Ahrendt, G. M., Oaklander, A. L., & Dworkin, R. H. (2003). Neuropathic pain following breast cancer surgery: Proposed classification and research update. *Pain, 104,* 1–13. doi:10.1016/S0304-3959(03)00241-0

Katz, J., Poleshuck, E. L., Andrus, C. H., Hogan, L. A., Jung, B. F., Kulick, D. I., & Dworkin, R. H. (2005). Risk factors for acute pain and its persistence following breast cancer surgery. *Pain, 119,* 16–25. doi:10.1016/j.pain.2005.09.008

Lipscomb, J., Gotay, C. C., & Snyder, C. (Eds.). (2005). *Outcome assessments in cancer: Measures, methods, and applications.* New York, NY: Cambridge University Press.

Marla, S., & Stallard, S. (2009). Systematic review of day surgery for breast cancer. *International Journal of Surgery, 7,* 318–323. doi:10.1016/j.ijsu.2009.04.015

Michielsen, H. J., De Vries, J., Drent, M., & Peros-Golubicic, T. (2005). Psychometric qualities of the Fatigue Assessment Scale in Croatian sarcoidosis patients.

Sarcoidosis, Vasculitis, and Diffuse Lung Diseases, 22, 133–138. doi:10.1016/
S0022-3999(02)00392-6

Michielsen, H. J., De Vries, J., & Van Heck, G. L. (2003). Psychometric qualities
of a brief self-rated fatigue measure: The Fatigue Assessment Scale. *Journal of
Psychosomatic Research, 54,* 345–352. doi:10.1016/S0022-3999(02)00392-6

Montgomery, G. H., & Bovbjerg, D. H. (1997). The development of anticipatory
nausea in patients receiving adjuvant chemotherapy for breast cancer. *Physiology & Behavior, 61,* 737–741. doi:10.1016/S0031-9384(96)00528-8

Montgomery, G. H., & Bovbjerg, D. H. (2004). Pre-surgery distress and specific response
expectancies predict post-surgery outcomes in surgery patients confronting breast
cancer. *Health Psychology, 23,* 381–387. doi:10.1037/0278-6133.23.4.381

Montgomery, G. H., Bovbjerg, D. H., Schnur, J. B., David, D., Goldfarb, A., Weltz,
C. R., . . . Silverstein, J. H. (2007). A randomized clinical trial of a brief hyp-
nosis intervention to control side effects in breast surgery patients. *Journal of the
National Cancer Institute, 99,* 1304–1312. doi:10.1093/jnci/djm106

Montgomery, G. H., Hallquist, M. N., Schnur, J. B., David, D., Silverstein, J. H., &
Bovbjerg, D. H. (2010). Mediators of a brief hypnosis intervention to control side
effects in breast surgery patients: Response expectancies and emotional distress.
Journal of Consulting and Clinical Psychology, 78, 80–88. doi:10.1037/a0017392

Montgomery, G. H., Schnur, J. B., Erblich, J., Diefenbach, M. A., & Bovbjerg, D. H.
(2010). Pre-surgery psychological factors predict pain, nausea, and fatigue one
week after breast cancer surgery. *Journal of Pain and Symptom Management, 39,*
1043–1052. doi:10.1016/j.jpainsymman.2009.11.318

Montgomery, M. (2010). Uncertainty during breast diagnostic evaluation: State of
the science. *Oncology Nursing Forum, 37,* 77–83. doi:10.1188/10.ONF.77-83

Montgomery, M., & McCrone, S. H. (2010). Psychological distress associated with
the diagnostic phase for suspected breast cancer: Systematic review. *Journal of
Advanced Nursing, 66,* 2372–2390. doi:10.1111/j.1365-2648.2010.05439.x

Mykletun, A., Stordal, E., & Dahl, A. A. (2001). Hospital Anxiety and Depression (HAD) Scale: Factor structure, item analyses and internal consistency in
a large population. *The British Journal of Psychiatry, 179,* 540–544. doi:10.1192/
bjp.179.6.540

Oddby-Muhrbeck, E., Jakobsson, J., Andersson, L., & Askergren, J. (1994). Postoperative nausea and vomiting: A comparison between intravenous and inhala-
tion anesthesia in breast surgery. *Acta Anaesthesiologica Scandinavica, 38,* 52–56.
doi:10.1111/j.1399-6576.1994.tb03837.x

Parker, P. A., Pettaway, C. A., Babaian, R. J., Pisters, L. L., Miles, B., Fortier,
A., . . . Cohen, L. (2009). The effects of a pre-surgical stress management intervention for men with prostate cancer undergoing radical prostatectomy. *Journal
of Clinical Oncology, 27,* 3169–3176. doi:10.1200/JCO.2007.16.0036

Pavlin, D. J., Chen, C., Penaloza, D. A., Polissar, N. L., & Buckley, F. P. (2002). Pain
as a factor complicating recovery and discharge after ambulatory surgery. *Anesthesia and Analgesia, 95,* 627–634. doi:10.1213/01.ANE.0000025706.69612.1D

Pavlin, D. J., Rapp, S. E., Polissar, N. L., Malmgren, J. A., Koerschgen, M., & Keyes, H. (1998). Factors affecting discharge time in adult outpatients. *Anesthesia and Analgesia, 87,* 816–826.

Radloff, L. S. (1977). The CES-D Scale: A self-report depression scale for research in the general population. *Applied Psychological Measurement, 1,* 385–401. doi:10.1177/014662167700100306

Ramirez, A. J., Richards, M. A., Jarrett, S. R., & Fentiman, I. S. (1995). Can mood disorder in women with breast cancer be identified preoperatively? *British Journal of Cancer, 72,* 1509–1512. doi:10.1038/bjc.1995.538

Reavey, P., & McCarthy, C. M. (2008). Update on breast reconstruction in breast cancer. *Current Opinion in Obstetrics & Gynecology, 20,* 61–67. doi:10.1097/GCO.0b013e3282f2329b

Richardson, A., Medina, J., Brown, V., & Sitzia, J. (2007). Patients' needs assessment in cancer care: A review of assessment tools. *Supportive Care in Cancer, 15,* 1125–1144. doi:10.1007/s00520-006-0205-8

Rosson, G. D., Magarakis, M., Shridharani, S. M., Stapleton, S. M., Jacobs, L. K., Manahan, M. A., & Flores, J. I. (2010). A review of the surgical management of breast cancer: Plastic reconstructive techniques and timing implications. *Annals of Surgical Oncology, 17,* 1890–1900. doi:10.1245/s10434-010-0913-7

Schnur, J. B., & Goldsmith, R. E. (2011). Through her eyes. *Journal of Clinical Oncology, 29,* 4054–4056. doi:10.1200/JCO.2011.37.2409

Schnur, J. B., Hallquist, M. N., Bovbjerg, D. H., Silverstein, J. H., Stojceska, A., & Montgomery, G. H. (2007). Predictors of expectancies for post-surgical pain and fatigue in breast cancer surgical patients. *Personality and Individual Differences, 42,* 419–429. doi:10.1016/j.paid.2006.07.009

Schou, I., Ekeberg, O., Ruland, C. M., Sandvik, L., & Karesen, R. (2004). Pessimism as a predictor of emotional morbidity one year following breast cancer surgery. *Psycho-Oncology, 13,* 309–320. doi:10.1002/pon.747

Shimozuma, K., Granz, P. A., Petersen, L., & Hirji, K. (1999). Quality of life in the first year after breast cancer surgery: Rehabilitation needs and patterns of recovery. *Breast Cancer Research and Treatment, 56,* 45–57. doi:10.1023/A:1006214830854

Smith, P. M., Illiq, S. B., Fiedler, R. C., Hamilton, B. B., & Ottenbacher, K. J. (1996). Intermodal agreement of follow-up telephone functional assessment using the Functional Independence Measure in patients with stroke. *Archives of Physical Medicine and Rehabilitation, 77,* 431–435. doi:10.1016/S0003-9993(96)90029-5

Soet, J. E., & Basch, C. E. (1997). The telephone as a communication medium for health education. *Health Education & Behavior, 24,* 759–772. doi:10.1177/109019819702400610

Sorger, B. M., Rosenfeld, B., Pessin, H., Timm, A. K., & Cimino, J. (2007). Decision-making capacity in elderly, terminally ill patients with cancer. *Behavioral Sciences & the Law, 25,* 393–404. doi:10.1002/bsl.764

Spielberger, C. D., Gorsuch, R. L., Lushene, R., Vagg, P. R., & Jacobs, G. A. (1983). *State–Trait Anxiety Inventory (Form Y).* Redwood City, CA: Mind Garden.

Stanton, A. L., Danoff-Burg, S., & Huggins, M. E. (2002). The first year after breast cancer diagnosis: Hope and coping strategies as predictors of adjustment. *Psycho-Oncology, 11*, 93–102. doi: DOI: 10.1002/pon.574

Stanton, A. L., & Snider, P. R. (1993). Coping with a breast cancer diagnosis: A prospective study. *Health Psychology, 12*, 16–23. doi:10.1037/0278-6133.12.1.16

Takasugi, M., Iwamoto, E., Akashi-Tanaka, S., Kinoshita, T., Fukutomi, T., & Kubouchi, K. (2005). General aspects and specific issues of informed consent on breast cancer treatments. *Breast Cancer, 12*, 39–44. doi:10.2325/jbcs.12.39

Tasmuth, T., von Smitten, K., & Kalso, E. (1996). Pain and other symptoms during the first year after radical and conservative surgery for breast cancer. *British Journal of Cancer, 74*, 2024–2031. doi:10.1038/bjc.1996.671

Vearncombe, K. J., Rolfe, M., Wright, M., Pachana, N. A., Andrew, B., & Beadle, G. (2009). Predictors of cognitive decline after chemotherapy in breast cancer patients. *Journal of the International Neuropsychological Society, 15*, 951–962. doi:10.1017/S1355617709990567

WHOQOL Group. (1998). The World Health Organization Quality of Life Assessment (WHOQOL): Development and general psychometric properties. *Social Science & Medicine, 46*, 1569–1585. doi:10.1016/S0277-9536(98)00009-4

Wyatt, G. E., Loeb, T. B., Desmond, K. A., & Ganz, P. A. (2005). Does a history of childhood sexual abuse affect sexual outcomes in breast cancer survivors? *Journal of Clinical Oncology, 23*, 1261–1269. doi:10.1200/JCO.2005.01.150

10

GYNECOLOGIC SURGERY

ANDREA BRADFORD

Despite the advent of pharmacologic and hormonal management of many gynecologic conditions, surgery remains a mainstay in the treatment of both benign and malignant diseases of the female reproductive system. Although surgery for gynecologic disorders may provide relief of pain and other symptoms, it may also entail short- or long-term changes in sexual and reproductive function. Negative psychosocial outcomes are present in a small proportion of patients who undergo elective procedures for benign disease. Nevertheless, this minority represents a large number of women.

Hysterectomy, the surgical removal of the uterus, is the most common nonobstetric major surgical procedure among women of childbearing age in the United States. More than half a million U.S. women undergo hysterectomy each year, although rates have gradually declined during the past decade (Jacobson, Shaber, Armstrong, & Hung, 2007; Whiteman et al., 2008). Common indications for hysterectomy are benign leiomyoma (fibroid tumors),

DOI: 10.1037/14035-011
Presurgical Psychological Screening: Understanding Patients, Improving Outcomes, Andrew R. Block and David B. Sarwer (Editors)

abnormal uterine bleeding, uterine prolapse (descent of the uterus into the vaginal canal), endometriosis, and pelvic pain. *Radical hysterectomy*, performed to treat cancers of the cervix, uterus, and upper vagina, is a more extensive procedure that involves removal of additional pelvic tissues surrounding the uterus and sometimes the upper portion of the vagina. *Oophorectomy* (surgical removal of the ovaries) and *salpingo-oophorectomy* (surgical removal of the ovaries and fallopian tubes) account for more than 300,000 procedures per year (Centers for Disease Control and Prevention, 2011). These procedures are performed to treat both benign and malignant diseases of the ovaries and fallopian tubes and to reduce the risk of future ovarian cancer. Bilateral oophorectomy (removal of both ovaries) or salpingo-oophorectomy are performed concurrently with about 50% of hysterectomies (Novetsky, Boyd, & Curtin, 2011; Whiteman et al., 2008). More radical pelvic surgeries for gynecologic malignancies, although less common, are associated with greater functional impairment and psychosocial morbidity.

No current guidelines exist for presurgical psychological screening for routine gynecologic procedures. Thus, clinicians who perform presurgical screening in this population are most likely to be consulted on an as-needed basis. In this chapter, I review the prevalence of psychological problems encountered after common gynecologic surgeries, risk factors for these problems, and practical suggestions for psychological assessment in this heterogeneous patient population. I focus primarily on hysterectomy, bilateral salpingo-oophorectomy (BSO), and radical surgeries for gynecologic cancers. Obstetric and reproductive procedures, including cesarean section, pregnancy termination, and assisted reproduction interventions, are beyond the scope of this chapter. Readers are referred to existing resources for guidance on psychological assessment of candidates for surgical procedures for disorders of sex development (Consortium on the Management of Disorders of Sex Development, 2006; P. A. Lee, Houk, Ahmed, & Hughes, 2006) and gender dysphoria (Bockting, Knudson, & Goldberg, 2006; World Professional Association for Transgender Health, 2011).

PSYCHOLOGICAL ASPECTS OF GYNECOLOGIC SURGERY

As with any invasive procedure, gynecologic surgery is a stressor that has the potential to affect physical and emotional functioning, particularly among women with inadequate coping resources or other vulnerabilities. In addition to the potential physical, social, emotional, and financial toll of invasive surgery in general, gynecologic procedures are unique in that they specifically target reproductive organs. To the extent that a woman's identity is related to her reproductive functions, the removal of these organs may be

216   ANDREA BRADFORD

associated with feelings of loss. However, such reactions are not universal, nor are they necessarily typical. Concerns about sustaining a sexual relationship, managing pain, and maintaining one's health are also important factors to consider in psychosocial adjustment after gynecologic surgery. The most common aspects of psychosocial function associated with gynecologic surgery in the literature are described next.

Depression

Early retrospective studies showed an alarming prevalence of mood disturbance among women who had undergone hysterectomy (e.g., Richards, 1974). However, more recent research has reflected greater methodological sophistication and perhaps also changes in gynecologic practice over time. Women with benign gynecologic disorders such as pelvic pain and reproductive tract infections endorse elevated levels of depressive symptoms (e.g., Leithner et al., 2009), and hysterectomy appears to reduce the burden of depressive symptoms among this population (Farquhar, Harvey, Sadler, & Stewart, 2006; Ferroni & Deeble, 1996; Persson, Brynhildsen, & Kjølhede, 2010). The reasons for this are somewhat unclear, but one likely explanation is relief of symptoms and associated improvement in functioning. Factors related to depressive symptoms after hysterectomy include preoperative depression, preoperative pain, preoperative anxiety, and prior history of psychiatric problems (Vandyk, Brenner, Tranmer, & Van Der Kerkhof, 2011; Yen et al., 2008). New onset of depression is relatively uncommon, occurring in 6% to 8% of women within 6 months of hysterectomy (Vandyk et al., 2011; Yen et al., 2008).

Several studies have aimed to determine the effect of BSO on symptoms of depression among women undergoing hysterectomy. Rohl, Kjerulff, Langenberg, and Steege (2008) found that BSO did not confer greater risk of clinically significant self-reported depression symptoms 12 months after hysterectomy among a large sample of more than 1,000 premenopausal women. In this sample, BSO was actually associated with a reduced risk of depression among women who were not depressed at the time of surgery. This and other prospective studies have suggested that changes in mood symptoms do not distinguish women with and without a history of BSO, provided that the latter group of women receive estrogen replacement (Aziz, Bergquist, Nordholm, Möller, & Silfverstolpe, 2005; Everson, Matthews, Guzick, Wing, & Kuller, 1995).

Pain

Pain frequently accompanies uterine fibroids, ovarian cysts, pelvic inflammatory disease, and endometriosis and is a common symptom among women who are candidates for hysterectomy. Chronic pelvic pain results from numerous etiologies and is often present without an identifiable underlying pathology. Psychosocial risk factors for chronic pelvic pain include a prior history of childhood sexual abuse, lifetime sexual assault, psychiatric comorbidity, and sexual dysfunction (for review, see Latthe, Mignini, Gray, Hills, & Khan, 2006). The etiology of chronic pelvic pain among women with a history of traumatic stress or depression has been linked to chronic alteration in hypothalamic–pituitary–adrenal axis function (Heim, Ehlert, Hanker, & Hellhammer, 1998; Wingenfeld et al., 2009). Similar neuroendocrine mechanisms may contribute to the development of other medically unexplained conditions such as fibromyalgia and chronic fatigue syndrome that may be comorbid in this population (Riva, Mork, Westgaard, & Lundberg, 2012; Tanriverdi, Karaca, Unluhizarci, & Kelestimur, 2007).

Prospective studies have indicated that hysterectomy improves pelvic pain symptoms in most women, including many women with no identifiable pathology (Tay & Bromwich, 1998). However, hysterectomy does not consistently resolve pelvic pain, and 26% to 36% of women with preoperative pain report some degree of residual pain as many as 3 years after hysterectomy (Farquhar et al., 2006; Hillis, Marchbanks, & Peterson, 1995; Tay & Bromwich, 1998). Women at elevated risk for persistent pelvic pain after hysterectomy include those with no identifiable pelvic pathology, those with coexisting pain conditions elsewhere, and those for whom pain is the primary indication for surgery (Brandsborg, Dueholm, Nikolajsen, Kehlet, & Jensen, 2009; Brandsborg, Nikolajsen, Hansen, Kehlet, & Jensen, 2007; Hillis et al., 1995). Learman et al. (2011) reported that preoperative depression does not influence the effectiveness of hysterectomy for pelvic pain. In a 3-year prospective study of women undergoing hysterectomy for benign conditions, new-onset pelvic pain occurred in only 5% of patients (Farquhar et al., 2006). Unfortunately, few data exist on predictors of long-term pain outcomes associated with radical hysterectomy.

Sexual Function

Concerns about sexual function after gynecologic surgery are common, particularly among those who are younger and sexually active. A preponderance of evidence has indicated that sexual function is either unchanged or improves for most women after hysterectomy (Flory, Bissonnette, Amsel, & Binik, 2006; Kuppermann et al., 2005; Rhodes, Kjerulff, Langenberg, & Guzinski, 1999; Roovers, van der Bom, van der Vaart, & Heintz, 2003). However, a small proportion of women have poorer sexual function after hysterectomy. Risk factors for poorer sexual adjustment include the existence of sexual problems and depression before hysterectomy (Rhodes et al., 1999). The quality of the partner relationship may also be an important factor in predicting some aspects of sexual adjustment (Helström, Sörbom, & Bäckström, 1995; Rhodes et al., 1999; Zobbe et al., 2004).

The influence of BSO on sexual function is somewhat controversial. BSO results in an immediate onset of menopause (surgical menopause), and the resulting symptoms may be more severe and distressing than in natural menopause given their abrupt and premature nature. Prospective studies have not necessarily revealed an effect of BSO (vs. ovarian preservation) on sexual outcomes in the short term (Farquhar et al., 2006; Teplin, Vittinghoff, Lin, Learman, Richter, & Kuppermann, 2007). However, large, cross-sectional, population-based studies have identified surgical menopause as an independent risk factor for hypoactive sexual desire disorder (Dennerstein, Koochaki, Barton, & Graziottin, 2006; West, D'Aloisio, Agans, Kalsbeek, Borisov, & Thorp, 2008). Differences among these findings may reflect cohort differences in symptom duration or treatment. In addition to reduced sexual desire, vaginal dryness and vulvovaginal atrophy resulting from the loss of ovarian estradiol are clear deterrents to sexual activity and are prevalent in both surgically and naturally menopausal women.

The effects of radical hysterectomy and other invasive procedures for gynecologic cancer are difficult to separate from the impact of cancer itself and from the effects of adjuvant treatments such as chemotherapy, radiation, and endocrine therapy. Because radical hysterectomy may involve removal of a portion of the upper vagina, reduced vaginal dimension is a symptom reported by some women after radical hysterectomy (Bergmark, Åvall-Lundqvist, Dickman, Henningsohn, & Steineck, 1999). Hypothetically, radical hysterectomy also has greater potential to cause damage to nerves and blood vessels that regulate sexual response. However, studies of sexual adjustment have suggested that a large proportion of women eventually return to near-baseline levels of sexual function after undergoing radical hysterectomy (Frumovitz et al., 2005; Jongpipan & Charoenkwan, 2007). In a recent prospective study, radical hysterectomy was associated with more severe vaginal symptoms than simple hysterectomy; however, this comparison was confounded by receipt of adjuvant chemotherapy by the women who underwent radical hysterectomy (Plotti et al., 2011). Even so, frequency and enjoyment of sexual activity after radical hysterectomy did not differ substantially between the two groups (Plotti et al., 2011). Alternative treatment options, such as primary radiotherapy, have been associated with comparatively more long-term problems with sexual dysfunction (Frumovitz et al., 2005; Greimel, Winter, Kapp, & Haas, 2009; P. T. Jensen, Groenvold, Klee, Thranov, Petersen, & Machin, 2003). Despite the physical toll of these treatments, psychological interventions appear to improve sexual outcomes among survivors of gynecologic cancer (for a review, see Brotto, Yule, & Breckon, 2010).

Fertility-Related Distress

Treatment-related infertility appears to have a long-term impact on emotional well-being and quality of life among women treated for gynecologic diseases. One of the largest studies to date included more than 1,000 premenopausal women who underwent hysterectomy for benign conditions. In this sample, 14% of women indicated that they might have or definitely wanted to have a child or another child at the time of their treatment. This subgroup of women tended to be younger and nulliparous at the time of hysterectomy (Leppert, Legro, & Kjerulff, 2007). At a 2-year follow-up, women who had expressed an interest in childbearing at the time of hysterectomy reported more symptoms of depression and greater bother from pelvic pain than women who were not interested in further childbearing (Leppert et al., 2007).

Women who undergo elective hysterectomy may postpone treatment because of concerns about fertility. Delayed treatment is less often a viable option for women with malignant disease. Studies of cancer survivors with treatment-related infertility have suggested that distress over interrupted childbearing may persist for years after treatment and is associated with lower overall quality of life (Canada & Schover, 2012; Wenzel et al., 2005). Women who have had at least one child but wanted another are less distressed over time than those who are childless, but remain more distressed than those who completed their childbearing. Although fertility preservation options are available to many women with cancer (for a review, see S. J. Lee, Schover, et al., 2006), oncology providers do not necessarily raise the subject of fertility during treatment planning (Quinn, Vadaparampil, Bell-Ellison, Gwede, & Albrecht, 2008). Thus, potential roles for clinicians in the oncology setting include enhancing providers' awareness of the impact of infertility on patients' quality of life, helping patients cope with actual or potential loss of fertility, and assisting patients in decision making about assisted reproduction and other alternatives for family building.

SPECIAL POPULATIONS IN GYNECOLOGIC SURGERY

Several groups of patients experience unique psychosocial stressors by virtue of their medical condition or treatment. These groups, and considerations for their assessment, are summarized in this section.

Risk-Reducing Bilateral Salpingo-Oophorectomy

Healthy women who are genetically susceptible to breast and ovarian cancers owing to a mutation of the *BRCA1* or *BRCA2* genes may elect to undergo

BSO to reduce their risk of future malignancy (Haber, 2002). As use of genetic screening and testing increases, concerns about the outcomes of BSO are likely to become more common in women's health care settings. Several studies have demonstrated that recipients of risk-reducing oophorectomy are similar to the general population in terms of their emotional well-being and quality-of-life outcomes (Elit, Esplen, Butler, & Narod, 2001; Finch et al., 2011; Madalinska et al., 2005). Women with a high risk of ovarian cancer who undergo BSO report less cancer-related worry than those who opt for gynecologic screening as a preventive measure (Madalinska et al., 2005). However, they experience more difficulties with vasomotor symptoms and sexual dysfunction in addition to permanent infertility. Younger and nulliparous women are more likely to delay BSO after genetic counseling (Bradbury et al., 2008), and these women may benefit from psychological intervention to manage uncertainty, cope with cancer-related worry, and address concerns about fertility and family planning.

Vulvar Excision and Radical Vulvectomy

Vulvar cancers are rare, accounting for less than 1% of all cancers in women, but the incidence of vulvar preinvasive lesions associated with the human papillomavirus is increasing among younger women (Judson, Habermann, Baxter, Durham & Virnig, 2006). Treatment of vulvar cancer usually involves surgical excision of the malignant lesion or, in more advanced disease, removal of all or a portion of the vulva (vulvectomy). Treatment of vulvar cancer is associated with reduced quality of life and negative changes in sexual function, although not necessarily because of onset of depressive symptoms or anxiety (Janda, Obermair, Cella, Crandon, & Trimmel, 2004; Likes, Stegbauer, Tillmanns, & Pruett, 2007; McFadden, Sharp, & Cruickshank, 2009). Predictors of sexual dysfunction after vulvar surgery include patient age (older patients report greater sexual dysfunction) and the extensiveness of surgery (Likes et al., 2007). Unfortunately, empirical literature on psychosocial outcomes in this population is limited.

Pelvic Exenteration

Pelvic exenteration is a radical procedure involving the removal of all pelvic organs, usually including the bladder and rectum (total pelvic exenteration). It is a potentially curative treatment option, and possibly the only such option, for a subset of patients with locally advanced and recurrent cervical and endometrial cancers. However, the morbidity associated with pelvic exenteration is extensive, and the recovery period is lengthy. Moreover, the 5-year survival rate for women with locally recurrent cancers is roughly 50% or less after exenteration. The surgery also necessitates creation of a urostomy, colostomy, or both. Not surprisingly, women who have undergone pelvic exenteration have lasting decrements in quality of life, mood, body image, and sexual function (Andersen & Hacker, 1983; Carter et al., 2004; Hawighorst-Knapstein, Schönefuss, Hoffmann, & Knapstein, 1997; Ratliff et al., 1996). Vaginal reconstruction is an option that can help preserve sexual function, although in one study only about half of patients who received a vaginal reconstruction resumed sexual activity after surgery (Ratliff et al., 1996). People with both a urostomy and a colostomy may be at especially high risk for body image disturbance and poorer quality-of-life outcomes (Hawighorst-Knapstein et al., 2004). This patient population is likely to benefit from proactive psychological assessment given the extremely stressful and possibly traumatic nature of the surgery.

RECOMMENDATIONS FOR PRESURGICAL ASSESSMENT OF GYNECOLOGIC SURGERY CANDIDATES

At present, the most compelling indication for presurgical psychological assessment is to identify patients who might benefit from pre- or postoperative psychological intervention. In the nursing literature, studies have supported the efficacy of brief presurgical intervention for promoting self-care behaviors and reducing anxiety during recovery after simple hysterectomy (Oetker-Black et al., 2003). Cognitive–behavioral and other psychological interventions might likewise improve other psychosocial outcomes among patients with clinically significant distress before surgery. For example, the American College of Gynecology and Obstetrics (2004) has recommended psychotherapy as an adjunct to medical management of chronic pelvic pain. Cancer survivors, whose surgeries are often more extensive, may especially benefit from proactive identification of psychosocial needs.

Unmet psychoeducational needs, which are not consistently addressed during preoperative clinic visits, can also be more readily identified and addressed with psychological assessment. For instance, women who reported that a health care provider explained possible sexual side effects before hysterectomy also reported greater overall satisfaction with their surgery (Bradford & Meston, 2007). The assessment may, in some cases, help inform treatment selection (e.g., if concerns about loss of fertility emerge during the assessment), but at present there are no specific guidelines for use of psychological assessment data in treatment planning.

Assessment Format

Because most patients who undergo common gynecologic procedures will adjust well without intervention, routine psychological assessment of all gynecologic surgery candidates is not recommended. However, a screening approach may be useful for efficiently detecting those at increased risk for psychological distress after surgery and who may benefit from further evaluation. Implementing some form of psychological assessment for all patients who are planning to undergo radical vulvectomy, pelvic exenteration, or other procedures that are associated with high morbidity may also be helpful. Brief screening measures such as the Patient Health Questionnaire—9 (Kroenke, Spitzer, & Williams, 2001), Brief Symptom Inventory (Zabora et al., 2001), and Hospital Anxiety and Depression Scale (Zigmond & Snaith, 1983) can be used to identify women with elevated levels of psychiatric symptoms and other risk factors. Ideally, these measures should be administered during the diagnostic workup, rather than at the preoperative visit, to allow time for further assessment or intervention if indicated.

If further psychological assessment is warranted, a clinical interview is necessary to contextualize the patient's current symptoms and distress. The interviewer should take care to inform the patient of the nature and purpose of the interview and to provide reassurance that responses will not be used to withhold medical treatment. Patients may fear that their physical symptoms will be interpreted as psychogenic, and these concerns should be addressed sensitively. Clear evidence of collaboration with the referring provider may reduce the patient's discomfort with the assessment process (see Robinson & Reiter, 2007, for examples of scripts for medical providers referring to a mental health professional for consultation). Finally, questions about sexuality and other sensitive topics should be presented in a manner that normalizes these concerns and invites frank discussion. An example of such an interview question is "Many women who have this surgery wonder how it will affect their sex lives; what questions or concerns do you have?"

Table 10.1 lists several self-report measures that can be used as adjuncts to a clinical interview. The use of lengthier personality assessment instruments such as the Minnesota Multiphasic Personality Inventory—2 in populations with gynecologic disease has seldom been discussed in the recent literature, and at present no clear advantage of using these tools in routine assessment has been found.

Use of Assessment Data

The empirical literature has been slow to answer the question of how best to use psychological assessment data in the gynecologic care setting. Unfortunately, research on psychosocial outcomes of gynecologic surgery has chiefly remained focused on clarifying overall population-level outcomes, with relatively little emphasis on the identification and management of patients at risk for negative outcomes. In the absence of empirical evidence

TABLE 10.1
Assessment Domains for Candidates for Gynecologic Surgery

Domain	Key concepts for clinical interview	Validated self-report measures
Psychiatric symptoms	Depressed mood, anxiety, somatization	Beck Depression Inventory—II (Beck, Steer, & Brown, 1996); Patient Health Questionnaire—9 (Kroenke, Spitzer, & Williams, 2001); Hospital Anxiety and Depression Scale (Zigmond & Snaith, 1983); Beck Anxiety Inventory (Beck, Epstein, Brown, & Steer, 1988); Brief Symptom Inventory (Zabora et al., 2001)
Pain	Quality and severity of pelvic and nonpelvic pain, pain coping	McGill Pain Questionnaire (Melzack, 1975); Brief Pain Inventory (Cleeland & Ryan, 1994); Chronic Pain Coping Inventory (M. P. Jensen, Turner, Romano, & Strom, 1995); Coping Strategies Questionnaire (Rosenstiel & Keefe, 1983); Pain Catastrophizing Scale (Sullivan, Bishop, & Pivik, 1995)
Sexual function	Sexual desire, vaginal dryness, orgasm, dyspareunia, sexual pleasure and satisfaction	Female Sexual Function Index (Rosen et al., 2000); Changes in Sexual Functioning Questionnaire (Clayton, McGarvey, & Clavet, 1997); Female Sexual Distress Scale (Derogatis, Rosen, Leiblum, Burnett, & Heiman, 2002)
Infertility-related distress	Desire for parenthood, expectations of family and social group, impact of infertility on personal identity and relationship	Reproductive Concerns Scale (Wenzel et al., 2005); Fertility Problem Inventory (Newton, Sherrard, & Glavac, 1999)
Psychosocial risk and protective factors	Relationship adjustment, history of interpersonal violence or abuse, coping style	Dyadic Adjustment Scale (Spanier, 1976); Childhood Trauma Questionnaire (Bernstein et al., 1994); Trauma History Questionnaire (B. L. Green, 1996); COPE Inventory (Carver, Scheier, & Weintraub, 1989)

to support screening guidelines, the following indicators have been associated with poorer psychological adjustment after gynecologic surgery and may be screened for as triggers for further evaluation:

- clinically significant psychiatric symptoms (e.g., mood disturbance and anxiety);
- chronic pelvic pain in the absence of identifiable pathology or in conjunction with chronic pain conditions affecting other parts of the body;
- concern about sexual function (especially if other than dyspareunia);
- desire for future childbearing; and
- prior history of sexual or physical abuse.

Selection of appropriate interventions, referrals, or changes in the treatment plan should be based on collaborative discussions among the mental health clinician, medical provider, and patient. No evidence has suggested that routine gynecologic surgery should be delayed on the basis of psychological risk factors (a high risk of harm to self or others is a clear exception). However, it may be appropriate to request a priority follow-up visit or referral to a mental health provider if intervention before surgery is desirable.

The success of collaboration with the gynecologic care team depends on effective communication. The clinician's role and scope of practice should be made clear as early as possible to all parties directly involved in the consultation or referral process. Because many presurgical assessments will involve patients with complex psychosocial histories, clinicians may find themselves torn between advocating for a difficult patient and facilitating the work of the medical team. Ensuring role clarity and expectations can help prevent or mitigate these conflicts. Finally, timely feedback to the referring provider, whether formal or informal, is necessary to effectively close the communication loop and is an essential skill for collaborative practice. Feedback can also present an opportunity to orient providers to potentially appropriate interventions and refine misconceptions about psychogenesis.

FUTURE DIRECTIONS

The literature on psychosocial outcomes of gynecologic surgery has clarified that individual psychosocial factors are often more influential than specific clinical factors (e.g., route of surgery, use of hormone replacement) in predicting psychological adjustment. However, very little literature is available to inform best practices for psychological screening and assessment of women undergoing gynecologic procedures. Several areas require further clarification before guidelines for assessment can be developed.

Effectiveness of Presurgical Screening and Assessment

The recommendations provided in this chapter reflect what is known about risk factors for poorer psychosocial adjustment after gynecologic surgery. However, the effects of screening for these risk factors on health outcomes, well-being, and patient satisfaction are unknown. Controlled trials of screening programs are needed to determine whether routine identification of psychologically vulnerable patients results in better health and quality-of-life outcomes.

Cultural Differences in Risk Factors for Poorer Adjustment After Surgery

The literature concerning sociocultural disparities in the incidence and treatment of gynecologic diseases is sizable. However, far less is known about ethnic and cultural differences in the risk for negative psychological outcomes. Women of color and nonheterosexual women are underrepresented in studies of psychosocial outcomes of gynecologic surgery. Interactions with the health care system are an important avenue for future study. For instance, ineffective provider communication and distrust of health providers' motives, particularly among African Americans (Galavotti & Richter, 2000; Gamble, 1997), may influence satisfaction with treatment decisions or outcomes. Also, evidence that ethnicity and culture influence reproductive health outcomes, such as experiences of menopausal symptoms (Avis et al., 2001; R. Green & Santoro, 2009), has implications for understanding quality-of-life outcomes after gynecologic surgery.

Role of Intimate Partners and Family Members

Partners and family members are potentially pivotal figures in women's adjustment to gynecologic surgery. Concerns about sexuality and reproductive function, in particular, are the result not only of the woman's perception of her disease and treatment but also of her intimate partner's perception of it and their relationship. Although a few studies of sexual outcomes have explicitly addressed relationship adjustment, they have done so largely from the woman's point of view. Greater involvement of partners in the assessment process may yield greater opportunities to correct misconceptions, address maladaptive relational patterns, and better understand the causes and course of distressing psychological outcomes.

CONCLUSION

Gynecologic diseases and mental disorders have been associated for centuries in a variety of cultural and historical contexts. Because gynecologic conditions are associated with some degree of psychiatric morbidity that is not entirely relieved by treatment, mental health professionals have a potentially meaningful role to play in the gynecologic care setting. However, unlike psychological services in other areas of surgical practice, to date very little precedent exists for early screening and assessment of gynecologic surgery patients with the greatest psychosocial needs. Better integration of these services will be a promising step forward in improving the health outcomes of this population.

REFERENCES

American College of Obstetricians and Gynecologists. (2004). *Chronic pelvic pain* (ACOG Practice Bulletin No. 51). Washington, DC: Author.

Andersen, B. L., & Hacker, N. F. (1983). Psychosexual adjustment following pelvic exenteration. *Obstetrics and Gynecology, 61,* 331–338.

Avis, N. E., Stellato, R., Crawford, S., Bromberger, J., Ganz, P., Cain, V., & Kagawa-Singer, M. (2001). Is there a menopausal syndrome? Menopausal status and symptoms across racial/ethnic groups. *Social Science & Medicine, 52,* 345–356. doi:10.1016/S0277-9536(00)00147-7

Aziz, A., Bergquist, C., Nordholm, L., Möller, A., & Silfverstolpe, G. (2005). Prophylactic oophorectomy at elective hysterectomy: Effects on psychological well-being at 1-year follow-up and its correlations to sexuality. *Maturitas, 51,* 349–357. doi:10.1016/j.maturitas.2004.08.018

Beck, A. T., Epstein, N., Brown, G., & Steer, R. A. (1988). An inventory for measuring clinical anxiety: Psychometric properties. *Journal of Consulting and Clinical Psychology, 56,* 893–897. doi:10.1037/0022-006X.56.6.893

Beck, A. T., Steer, R. A., & Brown, G. K. (1996). *Beck Depression Inventory–II (BDI–II).* San Antonio, TX: Pearson.

Bergmark, K., Åvall-Lundqvist, E., Dickman, P. W., Henningsohn, L., & Steineck, G. (1999). Vaginal changes and sexuality in women with a history of cervical cancer. *The New England Journal of Medicine, 340,* 1383–1389. doi:10.1056/NEJM199905063401802

Bernstein, D. P., Fink, L., Handelsman, L., Foote, J., Lovejoy, M., Wenzel, K., . . . Ruggiero, J. (1994). Initial reliability and validity of a new retrospective measure of child abuse and neglect. *American Journal of Psychiatry, 151,* 1132–1136.

Bockting, W., Knudson, G., & Goldberg, J. M. (2006). *Counselling and mental health care of transgender adults and loved ones.* Retrieved from http://trans health.vch.ca/resources/library/tcpdocs/guidelines-mentalhealth.pdf

Bradbury, A. R., Ibe, C. N., Dignam, J. J., Cummings, S. A., Verp, M., White, M. A., . . . Olopade, O. I. (2008). Uptake and timing of bilateral prophylactic salpingo-oophorectomy among BRCA1 and BRCA2 mutation carriers. *Genetics in Medicine, 10,* 161–166. doi:10.1097/GIM.0b013e318163487d

Bradford, A., & Meston, C. M. (2007). Sexual outcomes and satisfaction with hysterectomy: Influence of patient education. *Journal of Sexual Medicine, 4,* 106–114. doi:10.1111/j.1743-6109.2006.00384.x

Brandsborg, B., Dueholm, M., Nikolajsen, L., Kehlet, H., & Jensen, T. S. (2009). A prospective study of risk factors for pain persisting 4 months after hysterectomy. *Clinical Journal of Pain, 25,* 263–268. doi:10.1097/AJP.0b013e31819655ca

Brandsborg, B., Nikolajsen, L., Hansen, C. T., Kehlet, H., & Jensen, T. S. (2007). Risk factors for chronic pain after hysterectomy: A nationwide questionnaire and database study. *Anesthesiology, 106,* 1003–1012. doi:10.1097/01.anes.0000265161.39932.e8

Brotto, L. A., Yule, M., & Breckon, E. (2010). Psychological interventions for the sexual sequelae of cancer: A review of the literature. *Journal of Cancer Survivorship, 4,* 346–360. doi:10.1007/s11764-010-0132-z

Canada, A. L., & Schover, L. R. (2012). The psychosocial impact of interrupted childbearing in long-term female cancer survivors. *Psycho-Oncology, 21,* 134–143.

Carter, J., Chi, D. S., Abu-Rustum, N., Brown, C. L., McCreath, W., & Barakat, R. R. (2004). Brief report: Total pelvic exenteration—A retrospective clinical needs assessment. *Psycho-Oncology, 13,* 125–131. doi:10.1002/pon.766

Carver, C. S., Scheier, M. F., & Weintraub, J. K. (1989). Assessing coping strategies: A theoretically based approach. *Journal of Personality and Social Psychology, 56,* 267–283. doi:10.1037/0022-3514.56.2.267

Centers for Disease Control and Prevention. (2011). *Number, rate, and standard error of all-listed surgical and nonsurgical procedures for discharges from short-stay hospitals, by selected procedure categories: United States, 2009.* Retrieved from http://www.cdc.gov/nchs/nhds/nhds_products.htm

Clayton, A. H., McGarvey, E. L., & Clavet, G. J. (1997). The Changes in Sexual Functioning Questionnaire (CSFQ): Development, reliability, and validity. *Psychopharmacology Bulletin, 33,* 731–745.

Cleeland, C. S., & Ryan, K. M. (1994). Pain assessment: Global use of the Brief Pain Inventory. *Annals of the Academy of Medicine, Singapore, 23,* 129–138.

Consortium on the Management of Disorders of Sex Development. (2006). *Clinical guidelines for the management of disorders of sex development in childhood.* Retrieved from http://www.accordalliance.org/dsd-guidelines.html

Dennerstein, L., Koochaki, P., Barton, I., & Graziottin, A. (2006). Hypoactive sexual desire disorder in menopausal women: A survey of Western European women. *Journal of Sexual Medicine, 3,* 212–222. doi:10.1111/j.1743-6109.2006.00215.x

Derogatis, L. R., Rosen, R., Leiblum, S., Burnett, A., & Heiman, J. (2002). The Female Sexual Distress Scale (FSDS): Initial validation of a standardized scale for assessment of sexually related personal distress in women. *Journal of Sex & Marital Therapy, 28*, 317–330. doi:10.1080/00926230290001448

Elit, L., Esplen, M. J., Butler, K., & Narod, S. (2001). Quality of life and psychosexual adjustment after prophylactic oophorectomy for a family history of ovarian cancer. *Familial Cancer, 1*, 149–156. doi:10.1023/A:1021119405814

Everson, S. A., Matthews, K. A., Guzick, D. S., Wing, R. R., & Kuller, L. H. (1995). Effects of surgical menopause on psychological characteristics and lipid levels: The Healthy Woman Study. *Health Psychology, 14*, 435–443. doi:10.1037/0278-6133.14.5.435

Farquhar, C. M., Harvey, S. A., Sadler, L., & Stewart, A. W. (2006). A prospective study of 3 years of outcomes after hysterectomy with and without oophorectomy. *American Journal of Obstetrics and Gynecology, 194*, 711–717. doi:10.1016/j.ajog.2005.08.066

Ferroni, P., & Deeble, J. (1996). Women's subjective experience of hysterectomy. *Australian Health Review, 19*, 40–55. doi:10.1071/AH960040a

Finch, A., Metcalfe, K. A., Chiang, J., Elit, L., McLaughlin, J., Springate, S., . . . Narod, S. A. (2011). The impact of prophylactic salpingo-oophorectomy on quality of life and psychological distress in women with a BRCA mutation. *Psycho-Oncology.* Advance online publication.

Flory, N., Bissonnette, F., Amsel, R. T., & Binik, Y. M. (2006). The psychosocial outcomes of total and subtotal hysterectomy: A randomized controlled trial. *Journal of Sexual Medicine, 3*, 482–491.

Frumovitz, M., Sun, C. C., Schover, L. R., Munsell, M. F., Jhingran, A., Wharton, J. T., . . . Bodurka, D. C. (2005). Quality of life and sexual functioning in cervical cancer survivors. *Journal of Clinical Oncology, 23*, 7428–7436. doi:10.1200/JCO.2004.00.3996

Galavotti, C., & Richter, D. L. (2000). Talking about hysterectomy: The experiences of women from four cultural groups. *Journal of Women's Health & Gender-Based Medicine, 9*(Suppl.), S63–S67. doi:10.1089/152460900318777

Gamble, V. N. (1997). Under the shadow of Tuskegee: African Americans and health care. *American Journal of Public Health, 87*, 1773–1778. doi:10.2105/AJPH.87.11.1773

Green, B. L. (1996). Psychometric review of Trauma History Questionnaire (self-report). In B. H. Stamm & E. M. Varra (Eds.), *Measurement of stress, trauma, and adaptation* (pp. 366–388). Lutherville, MD: Sidran.

Green, R., & Santoro, N. (2009). Menopausal symptoms and ethnicity: The Study of Women's Health Across the Nation. *Women's Health, 5*, 127–133. doi:10.2217/17455057.5.2.127

Greimel, E. R., Winter, R., Kapp, K. S., & Haas, J. (2009). Quality of life and sexual functioning after cervical cancer treatment: A long-term follow-up study. *Psycho-Oncology, 18*, 476–482. doi:10.1002/pon.1426

Haber, D. (2002). Prophylactic oophorectomy to reduce the risk of ovarian and breast cancer in carriers of BRCA mutations. *New England Journal of Medicine*, *346*, 1660–1662. doi:10.1056/NEJMed020044

Hawighorst-Knapstein, S., Fusshoeller, C., Franz, C., Trautmann, K., Schmidt, M., Pilch, H., . . . Koelbl, H. (2004). The impact of treatment for genital cancer on quality of life and body image—Results of a prospective longitudinal 10-year study. *Gynecologic Oncology*, *94*, 398–403. doi:10.1016/j.ygyno.2004.04.025

Hawighorst-Knapstein, S., Schönefuss, G., Hoffman, S. O., & Knapstein, P. G. (1997). Pelvic exenteration: Effects of surgery on quality of life and body image—A prospective longitudinal study. *Gynecologic Oncology*, *66*, 495–500.

Heim, C., Ehlert, U., Hanker, J. P., & Hellhammer, D. H. (1998). Abuse-related post-traumatic stress disorder and alterations of the hypothalamic-pituitary-adrenal axis in women with chronic pelvic pain. *Psychosomatic Medicine*, *60*, 309–318.

Helström, L., Sörbom, D., & Bäckström, T. (1995). Influence of partner relationship on sexuality after subtotal hysterectomy. *Acta Obstetricia et Gynecologica Scandinavica*, *74*, 142–146. doi:10.3109/00016349509008924

Hillis, S. D., Marchbanks, P. A., & Peterson, H. B. (1995). The effectiveness of hysterectomy for chronic pelvic pain. *Obstetrics and Gynecology*, *86*, 941–945. doi:10.1016/0029-7844(95)00304-A

Jacobson, G. F., Shaber, R. E., Armstrong, M. A., & Hung, Y.-Y. (2007). Changes in rates of hysterectomy and uterine conserving procedures for treatment of uterine leiomyoma. *American Journal of Obstetrics and Gynecology*, *196*, 601.e1–601.e6. doi: 10.1016/j.ajog.2007.03.009

Janda, M., Obermair, A., Cella, D., Crandon, A. J., & Trimmel, M. (2004). Vulvar cancer patients' quality of life: A qualitative assessment. *International Journal of Gynecological Cancer*, *14*, 875–881. doi:10.1111/j.1048-891X.2004.14524.x

Jensen, P. T., Groenvold, M., Klee, M. C., Thranov, I., Petersen, M. A., & Machin, D. (2003). Longitudinal study of sexual function and vaginal changes after radiotherapy for cervical cancer. *International Journal of Radiation Oncology, Biology, Physics*, *56*, 937–949. doi:10.1016/S0360-3016(03)00362-6

Jongpipan, J., & Charoenkwan, K. (2007). Sexual function after radical hysterectomy for early-stage cervical cancer. *Journal of Sexual Medicine*, *4*, 1659–1665. doi:10.1111/j.1743-6109.2007.00454.x

Judson, P. L., Habermann, E. B., Baxter, N. N., Durham, S. B., & Virnig, B. A. (2006). Trends in the incidence of invasive and in situ vulvar carcinoma. *Obstetrics and Gynecology*, *107*, 1018–1022. doi:10.1097/01.AOG.0000210268.57527.a1

Kroenke, K., Spitzer, R. L., & Williams, J. B. W. (2001). The PHQ-9: Validity of a brief depression severity measure. *Journal of General Internal Medicine*, *16*, 606–613. doi:10.1046/j.1525-1497.2001.016009606.x

Kuppermann, M., Summitt, R. L., Jr., Varner, R. E., McNeeley, S. G., Goodman-Gruen, D., Learman, L. A., . . . Washington, A. E. (2005). Sexual functioning after total compared with supracervical hysterectomy: A randomized trial. *Obstetrics and Gynecology*, *105*, 1309–1318. doi:10.1097/01.AOG.0000160428.81371.be

Latthe, P., Mignini, L., Gray, R., Hills, R., & Khan, K. (2006). Factors predisposing women to chronic pelvic pain: Systematic review. *BMJ, 332*, 749. doi:10.1136/bmj.38748.697465.55

Learman, L. A., Gregorich, S. E., Schembri, M., Jacoby, A., Jackson, R. A., & Kuppermann, M. (2011). Symptom resolution after hysterectomy and alternative treatments for chronic pelvic pain: Does depression make a difference? *American Journal of Obstetrics and Gynecology, 204*, 269.e1–269.e9

Lee, P. A., Houk, C. P., Ahmed, S. F., & Hughes, I. A. (2006). Consensus statement on management of intersex disorders. *Pediatrics, 118*, e488–e500. doi:10.1542/peds.2006-0738

Lee, S. J., Schover, L. R., Partridge, A. H., Patrizio, P., Wallace, W. H., Hagerty, K., . . . Oktay, K. (2006). American Society of Clinical Oncology recommendations on fertility preservation in cancer patients. *Journal of Clinical Oncology, 24*, 2917–2931. doi:10.1200/JCO.2006.06.5888

Leithner, K., Assem-Hilger, E., Fischer-Kern, M., Loeffler-Stastka, H., Sam, C., & Ponocny-Sellger, E. (2009). Psychiatric morbidity in gynecological and otorhinolaryngological outpatients: A comparative study. *General Hospital Psychiatry, 31*, 233–239. doi:10.1016/j.genhosppsych.2008.12.007

Leppert, P. C., Legro, R. S., & Kjerulff, K. H. (2007). Hysterectomy and loss of fertility: Implications for women's mental health. *Journal of Psychosomatic Research, 63*, 269–274. doi:10.1016/j.jpsychores.2007.03.018

Likes, W. M., Stegbauer, C., Tillmanns, T., & Pruett, J. (2007). Correlates of sexual function following vulvar excision. *Gynecologic Oncology, 105*, 600–603. doi:10.1016/j.ygyno.2007.01.027

Madalinska, J. B., Hollenstein, J., Bleiker, E., van Beurden, M., Valdimarsdottir, H. B., Massuger, L. F., . . . Aaronson, N. K. (2005). Quality-of-life effects of prophylactic salpingo-oophorectomy versus gynecologic screening among women at increased risk of hereditary ovarian cancer. *Journal of Clinical Oncology, 23*, 6890–6898. doi:10.1200/JCO.2005.02.626

McFadden, K. M., Sharp, L., & Cruickshank, M. E. (2009). The prospective management of women with newly diagnosed vulval intraepithelial neoplasia: Clinical outcome and quality of life. *Journal of Obstetrics & Gynaecology, 29*, 749–753. doi:10.3109/01443610903191285

Melzack, R. (1975). The McGill Pain Questionnaire: Major properties and scoring methods. *Pain, 1*, 277–299. doi:10.1016/0304-3959(75)90044-5

Newton, C. R., Sherrard, W., & Glavac, I. (1999). The Fertility Problem Inventory: Measuring perceived infertility-related stress. *Fertility and Sterility, 72*, 54–62. doi:10.1016/S0015-0282(99)00164-8

Novetsky, A. P., Boyd, L. R., & Curtin, J. P. (2011). Trends in bilateral oophorectomy at the time of hysterectomy for benign disease. *Obstetrics and Gynecology, 118*, 1280–1286.

Oetker-Black, S. L., Jones, S., Estok, P., Ryan, M., Gale, N., & Parker, C. (2003). Preoperative teaching and hysterectomy outcomes. *AORN, 77*, 1215–1231. doi:10.1016/S0001-2092(06)60983-6

Persson, P., Brynhildsen, J., & Kjølhede, P.; Hysterectomy Multicentre Study Group in South-East Sweden. (2010). A 1-year follow up of psychological wellbeing after subtotal and total hysterectomy—A randomized study. *BJOG: An International Journal of Obstetrics & Gynaecology, 117*, 479–487. doi:10.1111/j.1471-0528.2009.02467.x

Plotti, F., Sansone, M., Di Donato, V., Antonelli, E., Altavilla, T., Angioli, R., & Panici, P. B. (2011). Quality of life and sexual function after Type C2/Type III radical hysterectomy for locally advanced cervical cancer: A prospective study. *Journal of Sexual Medicine, 8*, 894–904. doi:10.1111/j.1743-6109.2010.02133.x

Quinn, G. P., Vadaparampil, S. T., Bell-Ellison, B. A., Gwede, C. K., & Albrecht, T. L. (2008). Patient-physician communication barriers regarding fertility preservation among newly diagnosed cancer patients. *Social Science & Medicine, 66*, 784–789. doi:10.1016/j.socscimed.2007.09.013

Ratliff, C. R., Gershenson, D. M., Morris, M., Burke, T. W., Levenback, C., Schover, L. R., . . . Wharton, J. T. (1996). Sexual adjustment of patients undergoing gracilis myocutaneous flap vaginal reconstruction in conjunction with pelvic exenteration. *Cancer, 78*, 2229–2235. doi:10.1002/(SICI)1097-0142(19961115)78:10<2229::AID-CNCR27>3.0.CO;2-#

Rhodes, J. C., Kjerulff, K. H., Langenberg, P. W., & Guzinski, G. M. (1999). Hysterectomy and sexual functioning. *JAMA, 282*, 1934–1941. doi:10.1001/jama.282.20.1934

Richards, D. H. (1974). A post-hysterectomy syndrome. *The Lancet, 304*, 983–985. doi:10.1016/S0140-6736(74)92074-1

Riva, R., Mork, P. J., Westgaard, R. H., & Lundberg, U. (2012). Comparison of the cortisol awakening response in women with shoulder and neck pain and women with fibromyalgia. *Psychoneuroendocrinology, 37*, 299–306.

Robinson, P. J., & Reiter, J. T. (2007). *Behavioral consultation and primary care: A guide to integrating services*. New York, NY: Springer. doi:10.1007/978-0-387-32973-4

Rohl, J., Kjerulff, K., Langenberg, P., & Steege, J. (2008). Bilateral oophorectomy and depressive symptoms 12 months after hysterectomy. *American Journal of Obstetrics & Gynecology, 199*, 22.e1–22.e5.

Roovers, J.-P. W. R., van der Bom, J. G., van der Vaart, C. H., & Heintz, A. P. M. (2003). Hysterectomy and sexual wellbeing: Prospective observational study of vaginal hysterectomy, subtotal abdominal hysterectomy, and total abdominal hysterectomy. *BMJ, 327*, 774. doi:10.1136/bmj.327.7418.774

Rosen, R., Brown, C., Heiman, J., Leiblum, S., Meston, C. M., Shabsigh, R., . . . D'Agostino, R., Jr. (2000). The Female Sexual Function Index (FSFI): A multidimensional self-report instrument for the assessment of female sexual function. *Journal of Sex & Marital Therapy, 26*, 191–208. doi:10.1080/009262300278597

Rosenstiel, A. K., & Keefe, F. J. (1983). The use of coping strategies in chronic low back pain patients: Relationship to patient characteristics and current adjustment. *Pain, 17,* 33–44. doi:10.1016/0304-3959(83)90125-2

Spanier, G. B. (1976). Measuring dyadic adjustment: New scales for assessing the quality of marriage and similar dyads. *Journal of Marriage and the Family, 38,* 15–28. doi:10.2307/350547

Sullivan, M. J. L., Bishop, S. R., & Pivik, J. (1995). The Pain Catastrophizing Scale: Development and validation. *Psychological Assessment, 7,* 524–532. doi:10.1037/1040-3590.7.4.524

Tanriverdi, F., Karaca, Z., Unluhizarci, K., & Kelestimur, F. (2007). The hypothalamo-pituitary-adrenal axis in chronic fatigue syndrome and fibromyalgia. *Stress, 10,* 13–25. doi:10.1080/10253890601130823

Tay, S.-K., & Bromwich, N. (1998). Outcome of hysterectomy for pelvic pain in premenopausal women. *Australian and New Zealand Journal of Obstetrics and Gynaecology, 38,* 72–76.

Teplin, V., Vittinghoff, E., Lin, F., Learman, L. A., Richter, H. E., & Kuppermann, M. (2007). Oophorectomy in premenopausal women: Health-related quality of life and sexual functioning. *Obstetrics and Gynecology, 109,* 347–354. doi:10.1097/01.AOG.0000252700.03133.8b

Vandyk, A. D., Brenner, I., Tranmer, J., & Van Der Kerkhof, E. (2011). Depressive symptoms before and after elective hysterectomy. *Journal of Obstetric, Gynecologic, and Neonatal Nursing, 40,* 566–576. doi:10.1111/j.1552-6909.2011.01278.x

Wenzel, L., Dogan-Ates, A., Habbal, R., Berkowitz, R., Goldstein, D. P., Bernstein, M., . . . Cella, D. (2005). Defining and measuring reproductive concerns of female cancer survivors. *JNCI Monographs, 2005,* 94–98. doi:10.1093/jncimonographs/lgi017

West, S. L., D'Aloisio, A. A., Agans, R. P., Kalsbeek, W. D., Borisov, N. N., & Thorp, J. M. (2008). Prevalence of low sexual desire and hypoactive sexual desire disorder in a nationally representative sample of US women. *Archives of Internal Medicine, 168,* 1441–1449. doi:10.1001/archinte.168.13.1441

Whiteman, M. K., Hillis, S. D., Jamieson, D. J., Morrow, B., Podgornik, M. N., Brett, K. M., & Marchbanks, P. A. (2008). Inpatient hysterectomy surveillance in the United States, 2000-2004. *American Journal of Obstetrics and Gynecology, 198,* 34.e1–34.e7. doi: 10.1016/j.ajog.2007.05.039

Wingenfeld, K., Hellhammer, D. H., Schmidt, I., Wagner, D., Meinlschmidt, G., & Heim, C. (2009). HPA axis reactivity in chronic pelvic pain: Association with depression. *Journal of Psychosomatic Obstetrics and Gynecology, 30,* 282–286. doi:10.3109/01674820903254732

World Professional Association for Transgender Health. (2011). *Standards of care for the health of transsexual, transgender, and gender nonconforming people* (7th ed.). Minneapolis, MN: Author. Retrieved from http://www.wpath.org/publications_standards.cfm

Yen, J.-Y., Chen, Y.-H., Long, C.-Y., Chang, Y., Yen, C.-F., Chen, C.-C., & Ko, C.-H. (2008). Risk factors for major depressive disorder and the psychological impact of hysterectomy: A prospective investigation. *Psychosomatics, 49,* 137–142. doi:10.1176/appi.psy.49.2.137

Zabora, J., Brintzenhofeszoc, K., Jacobsen, P., Curbow, B., Piantadosi, S., Hooker, C., . . . Derogatis, L. (2001). A new psychosocial screening instrument for use with cancer patients. *Psychosomatics, 42,* 241–246. doi:10.1176/appi. psy.42.3.241

Zigmond, A. S., & Snaith, R. P. (1983). The Hospital Anxiety and Depression Scale. *Acta Psychiatrica Scandinavica, 67,* 361–370. doi:10.1111/j.1600-0447.1983. tb09716.x

Zobbe, V., Gimbel, H., Andersen, B. M., Filtenborg, T., Jakobsen, K., Sørensen, H. C., . . . Tabor, A. (2004). Sexuality after total vs. subtotal hysterectomy. *Acta Obstetricia et Gynecologica Scandinavica, 83,* 191–196.

11

CARPAL TUNNEL SURGERY

M. SCOTT DeBERARD AND JASON T. GOODSON

The typical clinical picture of carpal tunnel syndrome (CTS) involves pain and paresthesia of the hand in the median nerve–innervated digits (thumb, index finger, middle finger, and half of the ring finger; Cantatore, Dell'Accio, & Lapadula, 1997; Rosenbaum & Ochoa, 2002; Szabo, 1998). Patients also commonly complain of pain that radiates into the forearm, upper arm, and even shoulder (Jarvik & Yuen, 2001). Pain and paresthesias are typically worse at night, and patients with CTS often report nighttime pain episodes that awaken them from sleep (Jarvik & Yuen, 2001; Padua, Padua, LoMonaco, Rommanini, & Tonali, 1998). Patients with CTS may obtain relief from pain and numbness by shaking their hand, which is referred to as the *flick test* and is itself a valid and reliable clinical sign of CTS (Pryse-Phillips, 1984). CTS-related paresthesias are frequently accompanied by sensory deficits in the median nerve–innervated regions of the hand

DOI: 10.1037/14035-012
Presurgical Psychological Screening: Understanding Patients, Improving Outcomes, Andrew R. Block and David B. Sarwer (Editors)

(e.g., reduced two-point discrimination, reduced perception of pin prick; Rosenbaum & Ochoa, 2002). Additional symptoms reported by patients include weakness or clumsiness of the hand, history of dropping objects from the hand, weak grip, dry skin, and swelling or color changes in the hand (American Academy of Neurology, American Association of Electrodiagnostic Medicine, and American Academy of Physical Medicine and Rehabilitation, 1993). Finally, in severe CTS, weakness and even wasting of the thumb muscles is common (Cantatore et al., 1997).

CTS is a common condition estimated to annually affect 5% to 7% of the working population and 1% to 3% of the general population (Silverstein et al., 2010; Wolf, Mountcastle, & Owens, 2009) The lifetime risk of developing CTS is estimated to be as high as 11%, although rates vary by the diagnostic definition used (Descatha, Dale, Franzblau, Coomes, & Evanoff, 2011). According to Leigh and Miller (1998), CTS is among the four most frequent causes of workers' compensation disability coverage (both permanent and temporary partial). In a study conducted by the National Institute for Occupational Safety and Health (Tanaka et al., 1994), the estimated prevalence of CTS was 1.5% (2.65 million) of the U.S. population. In addition to high prevalence rates, several investigators have reported an increasing incidence of CTS. Franklin, Haug, Heyer, Checkoway, and Peck (1991) found an increased trend in CTS workers' compensation claims in Washington State between 1984 and 1988. In their study, the incidence rate of these claims increased from 1.78 per 1,000 full-time employees in 1984 to 2.00 per 1,000 full-time employees in 1988. Bell and Crumpton (1997) stated that CTS was the "largest problem facing ergonomists and the medical community" and was "developing in epidemic proportions" (p. 790). Ergonomic factors that have been most consistently associated with CTS onset include hand tasks requiring frequent repetition (e.g., computer use), combined repetition and force, and vibration (Goodson, 2005). Examples of occupations that frequently involve combined repetition and force include assembly line and fish processing jobs.

In addition to its high occurrence rates, CTS is associated with considerable medical costs. Szabo (1998) noted that the nonmedical costs of CTS workers' compensation coverage settlement cases averaged $10,000 per hand, with the total cost (i.e., workers' compensation and medical costs) ranging from $20,000 to $100,000 per case. Likewise, Palazzo (1994) reported that a surgical workers' compensation case may cost between $25,000 and $100,000 per hand. Independent of workers' compensation costs, CTS results in medical costs that exceed $2 billion per year (Palmer, Paulson, Lane-Larsen, Peulen, & Olson, 1993). Carpal tunnel release is the most commonly performed hand operation, with more than 500,000 procedures carried out each year ("Who Gets Carpal Tunnel Syndrome," 2009).

The purposes of this chapter are to provide an overview of CTS and its surgical treatment and to provide an evidence-based rationale for conducting presurgical psychological screening (PPS) with patients with CTS. We provide recommendations regarding selection and measurement of specific PPS variables. Finally, we offer an illustrative case study using PPS assessment and associated interventions.

PATHOPHYSIOLOGY AND SURGICAL TREATMENT OF CARPAL TUNNEL SYNDROME

The carpal canal is an open-ended, fibro-osseus canal in the wrist through which pass the median nerve and the nine flexor tendons of the fingers and their sheaths (Viikari-Juntura & Silverstein 1999). The floor (dorsal and lateral sides) of the tunnel is formed by the eight carpal bones and the transverse carpal ligament, which forms the roof (volar side) of the canal to complete the oval-shaped tunnel (Cantatore et al., 1997; Rosenbaum & Ochoa, 2002). Although the carpal canal is an anatomically open-ended compartment, pressure does not freely transfer in and out of the canal, causing it to function as a closed structure (Cantatore et al., 1997; Viikari-Juntura & Silverstein, 1999). This leaves the carpal canal susceptible to high levels of pressure, which can result in damage to the median nerve induced by ischemia (low oxygen, usually resulting from obstruction of arterial blood flow) and subsequent CTS symptoms (Cantatore et al., 1997). In addition, high levels of canal pressure may result in irritation and swelling of the flexor tendons, palmar bowing of the transverse carpal ligament, or both, which may cause compression of the median nerve and symptoms of CTS (Jarvik & Yuen, 2001; Jeng, Radwin, & Rodriquez, 1994). Pressure-induced damage may lead to demyelination (loss of myelin with preservation of the axons or fiber tracts; Rosenbaum & Ochoa, 2002), and complete axonal loss may eventually occur (Jarvik & Yuen, 2001).

The first-line approach to managing CTS is typically nonoperative and involves immobilization via splinting, activity limitation, nonsteroidal anti-inflammatory drugs, and steroid injections designed to minimize inflammation. Approximately 20% of patients will not respond to initial nonoperative treatments or will have a recurrence of symptoms and progress to surgery. Surgery may be performed either in an open fashion or endoscopically. The primary purpose of the procedure is to decompress the carpal tunnel via complete division of the transverse carpal ligament (Brooks, Schiller, Allen, & Akelman, 2003). This procedure typically allows pressure in the carpal tunnel to decrease and a subsequent reduction in pain, sensory disturbances, and functional impairment.

PATIENT OUTCOMES AFTER CARPAL TUNNEL SURGERY

Between 70% and 90% of patients have good to excellent outcomes after carpal tunnel decompression (A. Turner, Kimble, Gulyás, & Ball, 2010). In general, outcome measures relative to clinical function (e.g., grip strength, nerve conduction velocities) reflect greater improvement than do outcomes for patient-oriented measures (e.g., activity, quality of life, satisfaction). Atroshi, Johnsson, and Ornstein (1998) found that 85% of CTS surgery patients were satisfied with their results 6 months after surgery. Katz et al. (2005) found 6- and 12-month work absence rates of 19% and 22%, respectively; return-to-work intervals ranged from 0 to 60 days with a mean of 19 days. Rosenbaum and Ochoa (2002) demonstrated substantially longer return-to-work intervals (typically more than 1 month work loss) for workers' compensation patients after CTS surgery.

RATIONALE FOR PERFORMING PRESURGICAL EVALUATIONS FOR PATIENTS WITH CARPAL TUNNEL SYNDROME

With many medical disorders, onset, severity, chronicity, and response to surgical intervention can be influenced by wide array of factors. Identification of such negative prognostic indicators before surgery can lead to avoidance of surgery or a delay in surgery while the patient receives appropriate psychological interventions designed to change mutable psychosocial factors (e.g., reduce depression and anxiety) for the positive. PPS also provides the patient with an opportunity to gain knowledge about the procedure and form appropriate expectations. Unfortunately, identification of prognostic factors for CTS surgery outcomes is in its early stages, and PPS procedures for CTS surgery are still in their infancy. However, in the next section we provide a comprehensive and current assessment of the relevant CTS outcome studies that form the basis for initial PPS recommendations among such patients.

PSYCHOLOGICAL FACTORS AND CARPAL TUNNEL SYNDROME SURGERY OUTCOMES

General Mental Health

Several studies have demonstrated that lower preoperative scores on measures of general mental health are associated with poorer CTS surgery outcomes (Gimeno, Amick, Habeck, Ossman, & Katz, 2005; Katz et al., 2001;

Lozano Calderón, Piava, & Ring, 2008). These measures typically involve assessment of symptoms of both depression and anxiety. For example, Katz et al. (1997) determined that worse mental health as assessed by the Short Form–36 Mental Health subscale was associated with lower return-to-work rates after CTS surgery. Katz et al. (2001) found that lower Mental Health Inventory—5 scores were associated with greater 18-month CTS surgery postoperative symptom severity, functional limitations, and dissatisfaction with surgery. Amick et al. (2004) found that lower scores on the Mental Health Inventory—5 at baseline were predictive of failure to return to work at 6 months after CTS surgery. Likewise, Lozano Calderón et al. (2008) found the presence of depression to be associated with lowered patient satisfaction after CTS surgery. However, Hobby, Venkatesh, and Motkur (2005) found that overall psychological distress as measured by the Hospital Anxiety and Depression Scale showed no association with CTS surgery outcomes at follow-up. Given the available studies, it appears prudent to consider general mental health indices (e.g., Short Form–36 Mental Health subscale; Ware & Sherbourne, 1992) as well as specific psychological symptoms (e.g., depression, anxiety) as likely prognostic indicators of CTS surgery outcomes.

Somatization

Somatization has been frequently correlated with patient outcomes across many surgical areas. Somatization has been less studied in CTS surgery studies; however, available studies have suggested that it may have some import in terms of predicting CTS surgery outcomes. Hamlin, Hitchcock, Hofmeister, and Owens (1996) determined that higher levels of somatization (as assessed via the Minnesota Multiphasic Personality Inventory—2 [MMPI–2]) were associated with low probabilities of pain relief and return to work after CTS surgery.

Personality Constructs

Although the MMPI has been consistently used in presurgical assessment for spine and other surgeries (e.g., Block, Gatchel, Deardorff, & Guyer, 2003), very few studies have used this measure in CTS surgery outcome studies. Hamlin et al. (1996) used scores on the original MMPI to create the Paindex, which afforded fairly good prediction of pain relief and return to work in a sample of 70 CTS surgery patients. Although the Paindex algorithm is proprietary, an earlier version known as the Pain Assessment Index used an algorithm based on the MMPI–2's Hypochondriasis, Hysteria, and Depression subscales (Smith & Duerksen, 1979). In an attempt to validate the Pain Assessment Index for lumbar surgery patients, J. A. Turner, Herron, and Weiner (1986) found that presurgical MMPI–2 Hypochondriasis scores predicted more than 83% of outcome variation, whereas the Pain Assessment Index accounted for 79% of variation. J. A. Turner et al. concluded that the Hypochondriasis scale alone might be a better predictor of surgical outcomes than the Pain Assessment Index but urged further research before making strong conclusions. Given the results of these prior studies, further investigation of the utility of the MMPI–2 with CTS surgery outcomes is clearly warranted. Particular elevations (more than 1.5 standard deviations above the mean) on the Depression, Hysteria, and Hypochondriasis scales should be considered.

Alcohol Use

Katz et al. (2001) found that drinking more than two alcoholic drinks per day before surgery was associated with more severe symptoms and less overall satisfaction after CTS surgery. Alcohol use is likely a marker for other lifestyle factors that contribute to decreases in general health. For instance, increased alcohol consumption may be associated with a decreased level of vigorous physical exercise, which has been associated with CTS onset. Alternatively, the presence of alcohol misuse before surgery may contribute to less adherence to postoperative recovery programs, thereby diminishing the surgery's effectiveness.

OCCUPATIONAL FACTORS AND WORKERS' COMPENSATION

Workers' Compensation

As is common with other medical conditions, workers' compensation patients who undergo CTS surgery appear to have generally worse outcomes than other CTS surgery patients. Agee et al. (1992) and Palmer et al. (1993) determined that workers' compensation patients took a greater average number of days to return to work after CTS surgery than their noncompensation counterparts. Katz et al. (1997) found that workers' compensation was associated with a greater likelihood of work absence at 6 months after CTS surgery (adjusted odds ratio = 5.7). Katz et al. (2005) found that compensation patients had significantly lower return-to-work rates than noncompensation patients at both 6 and 12 months after CTS surgery. Workers' compensation has long been associated with poorer outcomes across several surgery types (Harris, Mulford, Soloman, van Gelder, & Young, 2005), particularly spine surgery (DeBerard, LaCaille, Spielmans, & Parlin, 2009; DeBerard, Masters, Colledge, Schleusener, & Schlegel, 2001). Some have argued that the workers' compensation system may promote an adversarial system in which workers are forced to continually prove they have symptoms to ensure ongoing medical treatment and compensation (DeBerard et al., 2001).

Legal Representation

Katz et al. (2001) found that workers' compensation patients who hired a lawyer to represent their compensation claim were significantly less satisfied and reported more functional impairment and more severe symptoms after CTS surgery than did noncompensation patients and workers' compensation patients who did not hire a lawyer. Several other studies have also found lawyer representation to be a risk factor for poor CTS surgery outcomes (Butterfield, Spencer, Redmond, Rosenbaum, & Zirkle, 1997; Katz et al., 1997). In contrast, Braun, Doehr, Mosqueda, and Garcia (1999) found that representation by a lawyer was not associated with functional CTS surgical outcomes, nor was it associated with the medical decision-making process. The association of litigation with poor CTS surgical outcomes is consistent with low back surgery outcome studies, which have consistently found presurgical litigation to be a predictor of poor patient outcomes (DeBerard et al., 2001, 2009). DeBerard et al. (2001) have previously suggested that the presence of a lawyer may serve as an incentive to the patient to portray more severe symptoms to ensure ongoing disability and an increased likelihood of a larger legal settlement.

Employment Factors

Several studies have examined the influence of patient presurgery job status with outcomes after CTS surgery. Katz et al. (2005) found that high psychological job demands, lower control, lower job security, and low coworker social support were associated with higher work absence rates at 6 months after CTS surgery. Gimeno et al. (2005) found that "job strain," defined as high psychological job demands and low job control, was predictive of lower return-to-work rates at both 2 and 6 months after CTS surgery. Amick et al. (2004) found that self-efficacy and a supportive employer were each related to successful work-role functioning after CTS surgery. Thus, negative employment prognostic indicators deserve consideration in the context of PPS for CTS surgery patients.

Length of Work Absence

Katz et al. (1997) found that the length of preoperative work absence was positively correlated with less complete symptom relief at 6 months after CTS surgery. Hansen, Dalsgaard, Meldgaard, and Larsen (2009) found that

4 or more weeks of preoperative sick leave was associated with greater post-operative sick leave.

Other Variables Related to Outcomes

Several studies have determined that lower premorbid overall health status is related to more negative CTS surgical outcomes. Katz et al. (1998) determined that baseline Physical Component summary scores on the Short Form—12 were predictive of failure to return to work at 6 months after CTS surgery. Other studies have determined that older age (Porter, Venkateswaran, Stephenson, & Wray, 2002) and fewer years of education (Butterfield et al., 1997) are additional possible risk factors for poor outcomes after CTS surgery.

PHYSICIAN REFERRAL FOR PRESURGICAL PSYCHOLOGICAL SCREENING

As we have illustrated, several presurgical occupational, psychosocial, and psychological factors have been associated with worse CTS surgical outcomes. In our practice, patients typically present for surgical consultation with at least one and often multiple negative prognostic variables. Although no empirical evidence exists to support a cumulative risk effect, the more negative prognostic factors that are identified, the more strongly providers should consider PPS.

Table 11.1 summarizes the possible factors a physician might consider in referring a CTS patient for PPS. Rather than set a quantitative threshold for making a referral, we would suggest that the physician consider at least all of the red flag variables listed in the table and make a referral if any of them are positive. We also recommend the physician make use of a screening measure for assessing general mental health symptoms, such as the Brief Symptom Index—18 (Derogatis, 2000), which is a useful measure for assessing depression, anxiety, and somatization among patients with CTS (Goodson, 2005), as well as the CAGE questionnaire (Mayfield, McLeod, & Hall, 1974) for detecting potential problems with alcohol abuse or addiction. Patients whose scores exceed clinical cutoffs should be referred for PPS.

TENTATIVE STRUCTURE AND METHODS FOR CONDUCTING PRESURGICAL SCREENING WITH PATIENTS HAVING CARPAL TUNNEL SYNDROME

Table 11.2 outlines the structure and methods for conducting PPS for patients with CTS. Throughout the process, it is of considerable importance for the mental health clinician to maintain an empathic yet objective stance

TABLE 11.1
Possible Physician Referral Criteria for Presurgical Psychological Screening for Carpal Tunnel Surgery Candidates

Red flags[a]	Yellow flags[b]
Physical symptoms inconsistent with pathology	Older age
Failed prior carpal tunnel syndrome surgery	Limited education
Workers' compensation involvement	Poorer overall health status
Attorney representation	Cigarette smoking
Extended work absence before surgery	More than two alcoholic drinks per day
Poorer overall mental health status[c]	Job dissatisfaction
Presence or history of anxiety or depression	Lack of employer support
Presence or history of alcohol or drug use[d]	
Multiple comorbid health conditions	

[a]Red flags are those variables that are likely most strongly associated with the potential for poor carpal tunnel syndrome surgical outcomes. [b]Yellow flags are those variables for which the empirical support is somewhat less than red flag variables. [c]Brief mental health screening assessments include the Short Form–36 Version 2 Mental Health Composite (Ware & Sherbourne, 1992) and the Brief Symptom Index—18 (Derogatis, 2000). [d]Brief alcohol abuse screening assessment includes the CAGE (Mayfield, McLeod, & Hall, 1974).

and communicate nothing suggesting that the patient is mentally ill or that symptoms are fictitious. This process is more easily afforded in a multidisciplinary clinic but is also possible in a sole practice setting.

As in other areas of health psychology, conducting a medical chart review as an initial starting point for the PPS evaluation is wise. The first entry in the left column of Table 11.2 contains information relevant to such a chart review. The first entry in the right column lists the relevant variables that are likely available via this review. If the variable cannot be ascertained via the medical chart or the medical chart is unavailable, then the information should be obtained in the patient interview. The patient interview includes obtaining a comprehensive history and also assessing current psychological signs and symptoms. As with the chart review, the relevant variables to be assessed during the clinical interview are listed in the right column. Conducting a brief mental status examination is also recommended. Ascertaining patients' degree of satisfaction with their employer and their overall level of perceived job control would also be important. Some objective assessment of patients' pain experience is also critical, and we recommend specific procedures outlined by Turk and Robinson (2011). For example, pain intensity, pain quality, and pain modifiers would be important targets of such an assessment. Our experience has been that such clinical interviews take approximately 1 to 1.5 hours. Finally, the patient should be asked to complete a battery of objective paper-and-pencil measures, including the MMPI–2 Revised Form (Ben-Porath & Tellegen, 2008) and some measures of current psychological symptoms. Including a measure

TABLE 11.2
Factors to Consider in Presurgical Psychological Screening for Carpal Tunnel Surgery Candidates

Method of information collection	Relevant presurgical psychological screening variables
Medical chart review	Current carpal tunnel syndrome symptoms and treatment history
	Mental health history
	Prior alcohol or substance abuse
	Workers' compensation status
	Litigation
	Prior failed surgeries
	Comorbid health problems
Patient interview	Relevant developmental, educational, psychosocial, and mental health history
	Current psychological symptoms
	Satisfaction with work and employer
	Level of job control
	Pain behaviors
	Expectations for outcomes after surgery
Psychological assessments	Minnesota Multiphasic Personality Inventory—2 (Beck, Ward, Mendelson, Mock, & Erbaugh, 1961) or Minnesota Multiphasic Personality Inventory—2 Revised Form (Ben-Porath & Tellegen, 2008)
	Brief Symptom Inventory—18 (Derogatis, 2000)
	Beck Depression Inventory—II (Beck & Steer, 1993)
	State–Trait Anxiety Inventory (Spielberger, Gorsuch, Lushene, Vagg, & Jacobs, 1983)
	Adult Substance Abuse Subtle Screening Inventory—3 (Miller & Lazowski, 1999)
	Pain Coping Assessments (e.g., Coping Strategies Questionnaire [Rosenstiel & Keefe, 1983] or Pain Catastrophizing Scale [Sullivan, Bishop, & Privik, 1995])

of substance abuse such as the Adult Substance Abuse Subtle Screening Inventory—Version 3 (Miller & Lazowski, 1999) may also be appropriate. We have also found it useful to include some relevant measures of pain coping, such as the Coping Strategies Questionnaire (Rosenstiel & Keefe, 1983) or the Pain Catastrophizing Scale (Sullivan, Bishop, & Privik, 1995). In evaluating these questionnaires, it is useful to examine the range of pain coping responses available to a person (Coping Flexibility) and whether these coping mechanisms are predominantly adaptive (e.g., Pain Control and Rational Thinking subscales of the Coping Strategies Questionnaire) or maladaptive (e.g., Rumination, Magnification, and Helplessness subscales of the Pain Catastrophizing Scale). Presurgical interventions designed to enhance adaptive coping mechanisms may be warranted for some PPS patients.

COMMUNICATION OF PRESURGICAL PSYCHOLOGICAL
SCREENING RESULTS TO PHYSICIAN AND PATIENT

For purposes of PPS in the context of CTS, we believe recommending specific decision rules on the basis of any singular negative prognostic factor being present is somewhat premature. We suggest that clinicians look at all the data across all three domains of information (chart review, interview, and objective measures) and use sound clinical judgment along with assessment of the relevant prognostic variables in assessing risk for poor outcome.

It is also critical that the mental health clinician have a clear plan for coordinating, or in some cases providing, presurgical or postsurgical psychological services. We have found it useful to provide a brief report to the surgeon shortly after the evaluation with an overall judgment of risk for poor outcomes (high, medium, low) along with specific options for how to proceed (e.g., proceed, delay surgery, avoid surgery altogether).

Clearly, significant actuarial error occurs in predicting potential outcomes after any surgery, and CTS is certainly not an exception to this observation. Predicting with certainty the patient who will struggle after CTS surgery or the patient who might do well is impossible. Thus, clinicians making predictions for CTS patients on the basis of PPS should deliver conclusions and recommendations in a careful and prudent way to avoid any adverse medical or legal challenges. However, we have identified some fairly robust presurgical prognostic indicators of poor CTS outcomes. We believe that if PPS findings are brought to the attention of a hand surgeon in an appropriate and respectful manner, it would likely lead to an appropriate presurgical intervention designed to lessen or ameliorate such identified issues before surgery. This process will ultimately lead to better outcomes for CTS surgery patients.

We believe that results of the PPS evaluation are advisory and not prescriptive. Indeed, the surgeon may elect to operate despite the identification of negative risk factors, in which case it would be appropriate for the clinician to advocate for pre- and postsurgical psychosocial interventions that might be helpful to the patient in recovery.

POSSIBLE PRESURGICAL AND POSTSURGICAL INTERVENTIONS
FOR HIGH-RISK PATIENTS

In the case of severe depression, anxiety, or substance abuse, we almost universally recommend some brief psychotherapy before the surgery so that the patient can begin the process of addressing such symptoms and recognizing how they could adversely affect outcomes after surgery. Referral for psychiatric medication evaluation is also common. Although ameliorating all mental health issues before surgery is not realistic, with the increase in brief, time-limited evidence-based therapies, meaningful clinical improvement can be achieved. It is especially important to address addiction to substances (particularly pain medications) before surgery. As we have noted, a surgeon may elect to proceed with surgery despite adverse psychosocial indications, such as when the patient evidences high levels of pain and physical dysfunction and electrodiagnostic testing is consistent with median nerve compromise (Higgs, Edwards, Martin, & Weeks, 1997). Carefully following up with the patient after surgery and providing mental health services and appropriate referrals can be quite important for the patient. We often work quite closely with the multidisciplinary treatment team to ensure such surgical patients are at least provided the option for receiving these services.

POTENTIAL PROBLEMS WITH CONDUCTING PRESURGICAL PSYCHOLOGICAL SCREENING AMONG CARPAL TUNNEL SYNDROME SURGERY PATIENTS

Given the high success rate of CTS surgery, many surgeons may overlook the need for, or be wary of, the PPS process related to CTS. Therefore, explaining the rationale and empirical basis for PPS to both physician and patient is critical. We recommend providing the physician with a copy of Table 11.1 and briefly explaining the relative prognostic factors as well as the potential to improve patient outcomes by screening and providing appropriate interventions. We would urge the physician to refer patients for PPS as appropriate. The timeliness of providing PPS information to the provider and patient is critical. The results of and recommendations from a PPS must be communicated in a timely and clear manner to both the physician and the patient, and time must be allowed for the physician and patient to ask and receive answers to any questions they have.

CASE STUDY

Ms. M is a 40-year-old factory worker.[1] She is a single mother of three children and has worked on the production floor for a military contractor for the past 20 years, helping to assemble rocket booster engines. Her job requires frequent use of handheld tools. She has been off work for the past 3 months, is receiving workers' compensation benefits, and recently hired a lawyer to represent her because workers' compensation has been reluctant

---

[1]Details of this case have been altered to protect the patient's identity.

to pay for her treatment. She has severe signs and symptoms of CTS in her dominant right hand. Her symptoms have been present and gradually worsening for the past 5 years, and she has failed multiple courses of nonoperative therapy (e.g., physical therapy, splinting). Her symptoms were corroborated by both a physical examination by a physiatrist and nerve conduction tests. She was referred to a hand surgeon, who felt surgery was necessary. The surgeon screened Ms. M. using the Brief Symptom Index—18, and she exceeded the clinical cutoffs for somatization, depression, and anxiety. She was also administered the CAGE, and some symptoms of potential alcohol abuse were noted. As a result, Ms. M. was referred to a clinician for a presurgical psychological evaluation to determine psychosocial factors that could potentially place her at risk for poor surgical outcomes.

Ms. M. completed a comprehensive clinical interview as well as the MMPI–2 Revised Form, the Beck Depression Inventory—II (Beck & Steer, 1993), and the State–Trait Anxiety Inventory (Spielberger, Gorsuch, Lushene, Vagg, & Jacobs, 1983). During the clinical interview, Ms. M. indicated that she is distraught over her inability to work and fearful that she may never be able to return to work. She expressed significant concern that she will not be allowed to return to work because the company might hire a younger, stronger, and more highly skilled worker to replace her. She noted that her employer has not been understanding regarding her injury and time off work and has been pressuring her to return. She noted that some of her coworkers believe she is faking her symptoms. She expressed concerns about whether hand surgery will be successful because nothing she has tried (physical therapy, splints) has provided any relief. Ms. M. reported a long history of depressed mood and had for the past year noted increasing fatigue, lethargy, and anhedonia. She feels guilty that she is unable to provide for her family and mentioned that she has had some fleeting suicidal ideation. She endorsed some significant symptoms of anxiety that appeared to be a result of trying to deal with financial pressures and worries over being out of work. She recently received a prescription for alprazolam (Xanax) from her primary care doctor, which she has been taking on a daily basis to help her deal with anxiety symptoms. She endorsed some signs of problematic alcohol use, including drinking four to five mixed drinks per night.

Regarding objective measures, Ms. M.'s MMPI–2 was valid, and she exhibited clinically significant elevations on the Hysteria, Hypochondriasis, and Depression subscales. Her Beck Depression Inventory—II reflected severe depression and her State–Trait Anxiety Inventory reflected moderately severe state and trait anxiety.

Results of the presurgical evaluation suggested significant risk of poor surgical CTS surgical outcomes for multiple reasons: workers' compensation case; litigation; presence of depression, anxiety, and somatization; propensity for hypochondriasis; problematic alcohol abuse; low work social support; and low job control. A course of brief cognitive–behavioral therapy designed to help Ms. M. cope with her depression and anxiety in more adaptive ways was recommended. A brief controlled-drinking intervention was provided, as was information about what to expect in terms of realistic symptom relief after the surgery. She was also referred to a psychiatrist for a medication evaluation and was placed on an SSRI, with a good result. She discontinued using Xanax. Ms. M. was able to complete a 3-month course of presurgical psychological intervention, and her depression and anxiety decreased significantly. She developed more adaptive coping skills. She became educated about her CTS symptoms and learned what to expect after her surgery. She reduced her alcohol use significantly. She was urged to communicate with her employer about returning to a lighter duty position after surgery. She ultimately had a successful surgery and was able to return to lighter duty work at the manufacturing plant. Six months later, she returned to her former production job. She continued to have some minor CTS symptoms but was able to cope with these through prompt visits to her physical therapist.

CONCLUSION

The use of PPS with CTS surgery patients is not currently a routine practice. Yet, given the increasing prevalence of, high cost of, and significant risk for poor outcomes after this procedure, it is important to understand which patients might be at higher risk for poor outcomes before the operation. PPS is one possible method that allows for such identification of higher risk patients. Once a CTS patient is identified as having high risk for a poor outcome, then the clinician, surgical team, and patient can work together to come up with an appropriate plan to proceed with surgery, temporarily delay surgery in favor of psychosocial intervention, or decide against surgery. In this chapter, we have identified possible prognostic indicators for poor outcomes among CTS surgery patients on the basis of a review of the current literature. The available studies have suggested that psychosocial variables are relevant in predicting surgical outcomes. Further studies examining the prognostic value of such studies are clearly needed, as are eventual studies demonstrating the value for PPS among CTS surgery patients.

REFERENCES

Agee, J. M., McCarroll, H. R., Jr., Tortosa, R. D., Berry, D. A., Szabo, R. M., & Peimer, C. A. (1992). Endoscopic release of the carpal tunnel: A randomized prospective multicenter study. *Journal of Hand Surgery, 17,* 987–995. doi:10.1016/S0363-5023(09)91044-9

American Academy of Neurology, American Association of Electrodiagnostic Medicine, & American Academy of Physical Medicine and Rehabilitation. (1993). Practice Parameter for electrodiagnostic studies in carpal tunnel syndrome (summary statement). *Neurology, 43*, 2404–2405.

Amick, B. C., III, Habeck, R. V., Ossmann, J., Fossell, A. H., Keller, R., & Katz, J. N. (2004). Predictors of successful work role functioning after carpal tunnel release. *Journal of Occupational and Environmental Medicine, 46*, 490–500. doi:10.1097/01.jom.0000126029.07223.a0

Atroshi, I., Johnsson, R., & Ornstein, E. (1998). Patient satisfaction and return to work after endoscopic carpal tunnel surgery. *Journal of Hand Surgery, 23*, 58–65. doi:10.1016/S0363-5023(98)80090-7

Beck, A. T., & Steer, R. A. (1993). *BDI–II: Beck Depression Inventory: Manual*. San Antonio, TX: Harcourt Brace.

Beck, A. T., Ward, C. H., Mendelson, M., Mock, J., & Erbaugh, J. (1961). An inventory for measuring depression. *Archives of General Psychiatry, 4*, 561–571. doi:10.1001/archpsyc.1961.01710120031004

Bell, P. M., & Crumpton, L. (1997). A fuzzy linguistic model of the prediction of carpal tunnel syndrome risks in an occupational environment. *Ergonomics, 40*, 790–799. doi:10.1080/001401397187784

Ben-Porath, Y., & Tellegen, A. (2008). *Minnesota Multiphasic Personality Inventory—2 Restructured Form: Technical manual*. Minneapolis: University of Minnesota Press.

Block, A. R., Gatchel, R. J., Deardorff, W. W., & Guyer, R. D. (2003). *The psychology of spine surgery*. Washington, DC: American Psychological Association.

Braun, R. M., Doehr, S., Mosqueda, T., & Garcia, A. (1999). The effect of legal representation on functional recovery of the hand in injured workers following carpal tunnel release. *Journal of Hand Surgery, 24*, 53–58. doi:10.1053/jhsu.1999.jhsu24a0053

Brooks, J. J., Schiller, J. R., Allen, S. D., & Akelman, E. (2003). Biomechanical and anatomical consequences of carpal tunnel release. *Clinical Biomechanics, 18*, 685–693. doi:10.1016/S0268-0033(03)00052-4

Butterfield, G., Spencer, P. S., Redmond, N., Rosenbaum, R., & Zirkle, D. F. (1997). Clinical and employment outcomes of carpal tunnel syndrome in Oregon workers' compensation recipients. *Journal of Occupational Rehabilitation, 7*, 61–73. doi:10.1007/BF02765877

Cantatore, F. P., Dell'Accio, F., & Lapadula, G. (1997). Carpal tunnel syndrome: A review. *Clinical Rheumatology, 16*, 596–603. doi:10.1007/BF02247800

DeBerard, M. S., LaCaille, R. A., Spielmans, G. A., & Parlin, M. (2009). Outcomes and pre surgery correlates of lumbar discectomy in Utah workers' compensation patients. *The Spine Journal, 9*, 193–203. doi:10.1016/j.spinee.2008.02.001

DeBerard, M. S., Masters, K. S., Colledge, A., Schleusener, R., & Schlegel, J. (2001). Outcomes of posterolateral lumbar fusion in Utah patients receiving workers compensation: A retrospective cohort study. *Spine, 26,* 738–746. doi:10.1097/00007632-200104010-00007

Derogatis, L. R. (2000). *The Brief Symptom Inventory—18 (BSI–18): Administration, scoring and procedures manual.* Minneapolis, MN: National Computer Systems.

Descatha, A., Dale, A. M., Franzblau, A., Coomes, J., & Evanoff, B. (2011). Comparison of research case definitions for carpal tunnel syndrome. *Scandinavian Journal of Work, Environment, and Health, 37,* 298–306.

Franklin, G. M., Haug, J., Heyer, N., Checkoway, H., & Peck, N. (1991). Occupational carpal tunnel syndrome in Washington state, 1984–1988. *American Journal of Public Health, 81,* 741–746. doi:10.2105/AJPH.81.6.741

Gimeno, D., Amick, B. C., III, Habeck, R. V., Ossman, J., & Katz, J. N. (2005). The role of job strain on return to work after carpal tunnel surgery. *Occupational and Environmental Medicine, 62,* 778–785. doi:10.1136/oem.2004.016931

Goodson, J. T. (2005). *Occupational and biopsychosocial risk factors for carpal tunnel syndrome: A case-control study.* Doctoral dissertation, Utah State University. Retrieved August 18, 2011, from http://library.usu.edu/etd/index.php

Hamlin, C., Hitchcock, M., Hofmeister, J., & Owens, R. (1996). Predicting surgical outcome for pain relief and return to work. *Best Practices and Benchmarking in Healthcare, 1,* 311–314.

Hansen, T. B., Dalsgaard, J., Meldgaard, A., & Larsen, K. (2009). A prospective study of prognostic factors for duration of sick leave after endoscopic carpal tunnel release. *BMC Musculoskeletal Disorders, 10,* 144. doi:10.1186/1471-2474-10-144

Harris, I., Mulford, J., Soloman, M., van Gelder, J. M., & Young, J. (2005). Association between compensation status and outcome after surgery: A meta-analysis. *JAMA, 293,* 1644–1652. doi:10.1001/jama.293.13.1644

Higgs, P. E., Edwards, D. F., Martin, D. S., & Weeks, P. M. (1997). Relation of preoperative nerve-conduction values to outcome in workers with surgically treated carpal tunnel syndrome. *Journal of Hand Surgery, 22,* 216–221. doi:10.1016/S0363-5023(97)80154-2

Hobby, J. L., Venkatesh, R., & Motkur, P. (2005). The effect of psychological disturbance on symptoms, self-reported disability and surgical outcome in carpal tunnel syndrome. *The Journal of Bone and Joint Surgery, 87,* 196–200. doi:10.1302/0301-620X.87B2.15055

Jarvik, J. G., & Yuen, E. (2001). Diagnosis of carpal tunnel syndrome: Electrodiagnostic and magnetic resonance imaging evaluation. *Neurosurgery Clinics of North America, 12,* 241–253.

Jeng, O.-J., Radwin, R. G., & Rodriquez, A. A. (1994). Functional psychomotor deficits associated with carpal tunnel syndrome. *Ergonomics, 37,* 1055–1069. doi:10.1080/00140139408963718

Jensen, M. P., Turner, J. A., Romano, J. M., & Strom, S. E. (1995). The Chronic Pain Coping Inventory: Development and preliminary validation. *Pain, 60(2),* 203–216.

Katz, J. N., Amick, B. C., III, Keller, R., Fossel, A. H., Ossman, J., Soucie, V., & Losina, E. (2005). Determinants of work absence following surgery for carpal tunnel syndrome. *American Journal of Industrial Medicine, 47,* 120–130. doi:10.1002/ajim.20127

Katz, J. N., Keller, R. B., Fossel, A. H., Punnett, L., Bessette, L., & Simmons, B. P. (1997). Predictors of return to work following carpal tunnel release. *American Journal of Industrial Medicine, 31,* 85–91. doi:10.1002/(SICI)1097-0274(199701)31:1<85::AID-AJIM13>3.0.CO;2-3

Katz, J. N., Keller, R. B., Simmons, B. P., Rogers, W. D., Bessette, L., & Fossel, A. H. (1998). Maine Carpal Tunnel Study: Outcomes of operative and non-operative therapy for carpal tunnel syndrome in a community based cohort. *The Journal of Hand Surgery, 23,* 697–710. doi:10.1016/S0363-5023(98)80058-0

Katz, J. N., Losina, E., Amick, B. C., III, Fossel, A. H., Bessette, L., & Keller, R. B. (2001). Predictors of carpal tunnel release. *Arthritis and Rheumatism, 44,* 1184–1193. doi:10.1002/1529-0131(200105)44:5<1184::AID-ANR202>3.0.CO;2-A

Leigh, J. P., & Miller, T. R. (1998). Occupational illness within two national data sets. *International Journal of Occupational and Environmental Health, 4,* 99–113.

Lozano Calderón, S., Piava, A., & Ring, D. (2008). Patient satisfaction after open carpal tunnel release correlates with depression. *The Journal of Hand Surgery, 33,* 303–307. doi:10.1016/j.jhsa.2007.11.025

Mayfield, D., McLeod, G., & Hall, P. (1974). The CAGE questionnaire: validation of a new alcoholism screening instrument. *American Journal of Psychiatry, 131,* 1121–1123.

Miller, F. G., & Lazowski, L. E. (1999). *The Adult SASSI—3 manual.* Springville, IN: SASSI Institute.

Padua, L., Padua, R., LoMonaco, M., Rommanini, E., & Tonali, P. (1998). Italian multicentre study of carpal tunnel syndrome: Study design. *Italian Journal of Neurological Sciences, 19,* 285–289. doi:10.1007/BF00713854

Palazzo, J. J. (1994). Clinical electrophysiology in CTD: Nerve conduction tests protocols for prevention and early diagnosis. *Journal of Rehabilitation Management, 12,* 53–55.

Palmer, D. H., Paulson, J. C., Lane-Larsen, C. L., Peulen, V. K., & Olson, J. D. (1993). Endoscopic carpal tunnel release: A comparison of two techniques with open release. *Arthroscopy, 9,* 498–508. doi:10.1016/S0749-8063(05)80396-2

Porter, P., Venkateswaran, B., Stephenson, H., & Wray, C. C. (2002). The influence of age on outcome after operation for the carpal tunnel syndrome: A prospective study. *The Journal of Bone and Joint Surgery British Volume, 84,* 688–691. doi:10.1302/0301-620X.84B5.12266

Pryse-Phillips, W. E. (1984). Validation of a diagnostic sign in CTS. *Journal of Neurology, Neurosurgery, and Psychiatry, 47,* 870–872. doi:10.1136/jnnp.47.8.870

Rosenbaum, R. B., & Ochoa, J. L. (2002). *Carpal tunnel syndrome and other disorders of the median nerve* (2nd ed.). Woburn, MA: Butterworth & Heinemann.

Rosenstiel, A. K., & Keefe, F. J. (1983). The use of coping strategies in chronic low back pain patients: Relationship to patient characteristics and current adjustment. *Pain, 17*, 33–44

Silverstein, B. A., Fan, Z. J., Bonauto, D. K., Bao, S., Smith, C. K., Howard, N., & Viikari-Juntara, E. (2010). The natural course of carpal tunnel syndrome in a working population. *Scandinavian Journal of Work, Environment, and Health, 356*, 384–393. doi:10.5271/sjweh.2912

Smith, W. L., & Duerksen, D. L. (1979). Personality and the relief of chronic pain: Predicting surgical outcome. *Clinical Neuropsychology, 1*, 35–38.

Spielberger, C. D., Gorsuch, R. L., Lushene, R., Vagg, P. R., & Jacobs, G. A. (1983). Manual for the State–Trait Anxiety Inventory. Palo Alto, CA: Consulting Psychologists Press.

Sullivan, M. J. L., Bishop, S., & Privik, J. (1995). The Pain Catastrophizing Scale: Development and validation. *Psychological Assessment, 7*, 524–532. doi:10.1037/1040-3590.7.4.524

Szabo, R. M. (1998). Carpal tunnel syndrome as a repetitive motion disorder. *Clinical Orthopaedics and Related Research, 351*, 78–89. doi:10.1097/00003086-199806000-00011

Tanaka, S., Wild, D. K., Seligman, P., Behrens, V., Cameron, L., & Putz-Anderson, V. (1994). The US prevalence of self-reported carpal tunnel syndrome: 1988 national health interview survey data. *American Journal of Public Health, 84*, 1846–1848. doi:10.2105/AJPH.84.11.1846

Turk, D. C., & Robinson, J. P. (2011). Assessment of patients with chronic pain: A comprehensive approach. In D. C. Turk & R. Melzack (Eds.), *Handbook of pain assessment* (pp. 188–210). New York: NY: Guilford Press

Turner, A., Kimble, F., Gulyás, K., & Ball, J. (2010). Can the outcome of open carpal tunnel release be predicted? A review of the literature. *ANZ Journal of Surgery, 80*, 50–54. doi:10.1111/j.1445-2197.2009.05175.x

Turner, J. A., Herron, L., & Weiner, P. (1986). Utility of the MMPI Pain Assessment Index in predicting outcome after lumbar surgery. *Journal of Clinical Psychology, 42*, 764–769. doi:10.1002/1097-4679(198609)42:5<764::AID-JCLP2270420515>3.0.CO;2-H

Viikari-Juntura, E., & Silverstein, B. (1999). Role of physical load in carpal tunnel syndrome. *Scandinavian Journal of Work, Environment, and Health, 25*(3), 163–185. doi:10.5271/sjweh.423

Ware, J. E., & Sherbourne, C. D. (1992). The MOS 36-Item Short-Form Health Survey (SF-36): I. Conceptual framework and item selection. *Medical Care, 30*, 473–483. doi:10.1097/00005650-199206000-00002

Who gets carpal tunnel syndrome? (2009). Retrieved from http://www.umm.edu/patiented/articles/who_gets_carpal_tunnel_syndrome_000034_4.htm

Wolf, J. M., Mountcastle, S. B., & Owens, B. D. (2009). The epidemiology of carpal tunnel syndrome in a military population. *Hand, 4*, 289–293. doi:10.1007/s11552-009-9166-y

12

COSMETIC SURGERY

DAVID B. SARWER

The past 2 decades have witnessed a dramatic increase in the number of people who undergo cosmetic surgery as well as minimally invasive cosmetic treatments designed to improve their appearance. Even before this increase, plastic surgeons had long been interested in the psychological factors that motivate individuals to undergo these procedures as well as the psychological changes that frequently occur postoperatively. Early reports in the literature from decades ago, published by research teams of plastic surgeons and psychiatrists, characterized most people interested in changing their appearance through surgery as typically having mood or anxiety disorders, schizophrenia, and personality disorders. These early reports, however, have not been confirmed by more recent studies, nor by plastic surgeon's clinical impressions. More recent investigations of patients have focused on psychopathology but also on other motivations for surgery, of which body image dissatisfaction is commonly believed to be one of the strongest. For some patients, however, this dissatisfaction may be severe and suggestive of the presence of body

DOI: 10.1037/14035-013
Presurgical Psychological Screening: Understanding Patients, Improving Outcomes, Andrew R. Block and David B. Sarwer (Editors)

dysmorphic disorder (BDD) or other forms of psychopathology. These conditions are likely of greatest relevance to plastic surgeons because of their likely association with poor postoperative outcomes, including dissatisfaction with the aesthetic result or untoward changes in psychosocial status. They are also the conditions for which plastic surgeons will most frequently ask patients to undergo a consultation with a mental health professional before surgery.

I begin this chapter with an overview of the literature on psychological aspects of cosmetic procedures. Most of this research has been conducted with patients who have undergone traditional surgical procedures, such as rhinoplasty, breast augmentation, and liposuction, and is the focus of the chapter. The review includes a discussion of the sociocultural factors that have contributed to the popularity of cosmetic surgery as well as the psychological factors that motivate the individual patient. The psychiatric conditions most commonly seen among cosmetic surgery patients are detailed, and I then use the research in these areas to provide recommendations to the mental health professional who is asked to conduct a psychological evaluation of patients interested in these procedures.

POPULARITY OF COSMETIC TREATMENTS

In 2011, 13.8 million cosmetic surgery and minimally invasive treatments were performed in the United States, a 87% increase in such treatments since 2000 (American Society of Plastic Surgeons, 2012). The vast majority (12.2 million) of these treatments were minimally invasive procedures such as Botox injections and chemical peels. Approximately 1.6 million surgical procedures were performed, the most popular of which was cosmetic breast augmentation (American Society of Plastic Surgeons, 2012).

Many potential explanations exist for the dramatic increase in the popularity of cosmetic surgery (Crerand, Infield, & Sarwer, 2007; Sarwer, Crerand, & Gibbons, 2007; Sarwer & Magee, 2006). Technological advances have made many of these surgical treatments safer, and more general advances in medicine have decreased the length of most postoperative recovery periods. Furthermore, cosmetic surgery, unlike other forms of medicine, readily lends itself to direct-to-consumer advertisements. The mass media and entertainment industries have likely contributed to the growth of cosmetic surgery as well. Cosmetic surgery has long been a very popular topic for women's (and men's) beauty magazines, which often tout the latest advances in the field. The past decade also witnessed unprecedented coverage of cosmetic surgery on television, from informative health programs on channels such as Discovery Health to reality-based patient contests (e.g., Extreme Makeover) and surgeon-focused shows (e.g., Dr. 90210) to a fictional television drama

(Nip/Tuck). At the same time, a growing number of celebrities have publicly shared their experiences with cosmetic surgery. These more overt influences play against a backdrop of relentless images of physical perfection depicted in magazines, television programs, movies, and the Internet. The end result is that consumers cannot help but be exposed to depictions of physical perfection as well as the message that cosmetic surgery is the path to that perfection.

At the same time, other potential explanations for the growth of cosmetic surgery can be found. Evolutionary theories of physical attractiveness, which suggest that those individuals with the most physically attractive characteristics have the most reproductive potential, can be applied to cosmetic surgery (Sarwer & Magee, 2006). Many surgical and minimally invasive treatments performed on the face are undertaken to help an individual look more youthful or to enhance facial symmetry. Both of these traits are well-established markers of facial attractiveness and are thought to convey messages of physical health to potential partners. At the same time, procedures such as liposuction and abdominoplasty can decrease an individual's waist-to-hip ratio, another marker of reproductive potential (Geary, 2010). Although these physical characteristics are thought to signal health, and thus the health of the resulting offspring, little relationship exists between the appearance of these characteristics and health status.

Social psychological research on the importance of physical appearance in daily life can also be used to understand the growth of cosmetic surgery. Over the past 4 decades, this body of research has suggested that individuals who are more physically attractive are perceived by others as having more positive personality traits and receiving preferential treatment in a range of social situations across the life span (Sarwer & Magee, 2006). Thus, whether people like to acknowledge it or not, physical appearance does seem to matter. Although decades ago an individual's interest in improving his or her appearance may have been seen by mental health professionals as being symptomatic of excessive vanity, narcissism, or other deep-seated psychopathology, today, and with these theories in mind, it can also be seen as a more adaptive and potentially psychologically healthy strategy. For some individuals, it may be akin to other self-improvement strategies such as eating a healthy diet and exercising regularly (Sarwer, Wadden, Pertschuk, & Whitaker, 1998a).

PREOPERATIVE PSYCHOSOCIAL CHARACTERISTICS OF COSMETIC SURGERY PATIENTS

A now sizable body of research has investigated the psychosocial characteristics of people who present for cosmetic surgery. This literature is discussed in detail in other reviews (Crerand et al., 2007; Sarwer, 2007; Sarwer

& Crerand, 2002). The discussion in this section provides an overview of patients' motivations and expectations for surgery as well as the most common forms of psychopathology likely to be seen by the mental health professional asked to consult on candidates for cosmetic procedures.

Motivations for Surgery

Patients present for cosmetic surgery with a variety of motivations for treatment and expectations regarding the impact of the surgery on their lives. Motivations for surgery have been described as internal (e.g., desire to improve one's self-confidence) or external (e.g., undergoing surgery to obtain a romantic partner or a promotion at work; Edgerton & Knorr, 1971; Pruzinsky, 1996). Although both patients (and surgeons) may struggle to articulate or identify specific motivations for surgery, Honigman, Phillips, and Castle (2004), in their review of the literature, concluded that patients with internal motivations are thought to be more likely to have their postoperative expectations met.

Body image dissatisfaction is considered to be a primary motivation for cosmetic surgery (Sarwer, 2007; Sarwer & Crerand, 2004; Sarwer, Crerand, & Gibbons, 2005; Sarwer, Pertschuk, Wadden, & Whitaker, 1998; Sarwer, Wadden, et al., 1998b) and has been the focus of much of the study of cosmetic surgery patients over the past 2 decades (Crerand et al., 2007; Sarwer, 2007; Sarwer, Crerand, & Magee, 2011). Studies of cosmetic surgery patients have found that patients report heightened preoperative body image dissatisfaction (Frederick, Lever, & Peplau, 2007; Pertschuk, Sarwer, Wadden, & Whitaker, 1998; Sarwer, Bartlett, et al., 1998; Sarwer, Wadden, Pertschuk, & Whitaker, 1998b; Sarwer, Whitaker, Wadden, & Pertschuk, 1997; Simis, Verhulst, & Koot, 2001). For example, candidates for breast augmentation report greater dissatisfaction with their breasts than other small-breasted women who do not seek breast augmentation (Didie & Sarwer, 2003; Sarwer et al., 2003). Thus, some degree of body image dissatisfaction is believed to be a prerequisite for cosmetic surgery. However, this dissatisfaction may also be representative of several forms of formal psychopathology that should be evaluated by both the cosmetic surgeon and the consulting mental health professional, as discussed later.

Preoperative Psychopathology

The first studies of preoperative psychopathology among cosmetic surgery patients, conducted decades ago, relied heavily on clinical interviews of cosmetic surgery candidates and described them as having high rates of psychopathology, including mood and anxiety disorders as well as personality disorders (e.g., Baker, Kolin, & Bartlett, 1974; Beale, Lisper, & Palm,

1980; Edgerton & McClary, 1958). All of these conditions were believed to be associated with poor postoperative psychological outcomes.

More contemporary studies included the use of standardized psychometric measures rather than or in addition to clinical interviews. These studies have typically found less psychopathology (e.g., Didie & Sarwer, 2003; Kjøller et al., 2003; Sarwer et al., 2003; Young, Nemecek, & Nemecek, 1994). Unfortunately, both sets of studies have methodological problems that have made interpretation of these conflicting findings difficult (Sarwer, Didie & Gibbons, 2006; Sarwer, Pertschuk, et al., 1998; Sarwer, Wadden, et al., 1998b). As a result, the rate of psychopathology among cosmetic surgery patients remains poorly understood. Perhaps more important, the relationship between preoperative psychopathology and postoperative outcomes, with few exceptions, is unknown.

Given the number and diversity of individuals who now seek cosmetic surgery and its related treatments, all of the psychiatric diagnoses can likely be found within the patient population. Three disorders in particular—BDD, eating disorders, and depression—warrant the greatest attention from plastic surgeons as well as mental health professionals asked to consult on a patient's psychological appropriateness for surgery.

Body Dysmorphic Disorder

Body dysmorphic disorder is defined as a preoccupation with a slight or imagined defect in appearance that leads to substantial distress or impairment in social, occupational, or other areas of functioning (American Psychiatric Association, 2000). Although the incidence rate in the general population is believed to be between 1% and 2%, several studies conducted throughout the world have found that 5% to 15% of cosmetic surgery patients appear to have some form of the disorder (for a detailed review, see Crerand, Franklin, & Sarwer, 2006, and Sarwer & Crerand, 2008). Although people with BDD typically report concerns with their skin, hair, and nose, any body part can become a source of preoccupation (Veale, De Haro, & Lambrou, 2003).

People with BDD frequently seek cosmetic treatment as a means of improving their perceived defects (Crerand, Phillips, Menard, & Fay, 2005). In contrast to most cosmetic surgery patients, individuals with BDD are typically dissatisfied with the outcome of such treatments (Veale et al., 1996). Two retrospective studies have found that more than 90% of people with BDD report either no change or a worsening in their BDD symptoms after cosmetic treatment (Crerand, Menard, & Phillips, 2010; Crerand et al., 2005). Of even greater concern, studies have documented high rates of suicidal ideation, suicide attempts, and self-harm behaviors (e.g., "do-it-yourself" surgery) among patients with BDD (Phillips & Menard, 2006; Veale, 2000). There have also been reports of patients with BDD who have threatened to sue or physically harm their treatment providers (Sarwer, 2002). In light of these issues, consensus is growing that cosmetic treatments should be contraindicated for people with BDD (Crerand et al., 2006; Phillips, 2004; Sarwer & Crerand, 2004; Sarwer, Wadden, et al., 1998a).

Eating Disorders

Given the disproportionate amount of concern that patients with eating disorders have with their appearance, these disorders may be common among those who seek cosmetic surgery. Individuals with eating disorders may erroneously believe that surgery will improve their immense dissatisfaction with their bodies. Eating disorders may be a particular concern with women (and men) who seek body contouring procedures, including liposuction, abdominoplasty, and breast augmentation. Such patients may mistakenly believe that these procedures can reshape their bodies in a way that restrictive eating or maladaptive compensatory behaviors cannot. Women who present for cosmetic breast augmentation are frequently of below-average weight (Beale et al., 1980; Didie & Sarwer, 2003; Sarwer et al., 2003; Simis et al., 2001) and report more exercise than physically similar women not seeking breast augmentation (Sarwer, Wadden, et al., 1998a), both of which may also be suggestive of eating psychopathology. Unfortunately, the study of the relationship between eating disorders and other cosmetic procedures has been restricted to case reports.

Depression

The presence of major depression or other mood disorders also warrants particular attention. At least one study has suggested that approximately 20% of people presenting for cosmetic surgery are engaged in mental health treatment, most typically the use of an antidepressant or other psychiatric medication (Sarwer, Zanville, et al., 2004). Women considering breast augmentation or who have breast implants have been found to report a higher rate of outpatient psychotherapy (Sarwer et al., 2003), psychopharmacologic treatments (Sarwer, Zanville, et al., 2004), and psychiatric hospitalizations (Jacobsen et al., 2004) than other cosmetic surgery patients or women from the general population. Although these studies have suggested that the rate of psychopathology may be higher among patients with breast implants, the investigations provided no information on the specific psychiatric diagnoses of these women.

Of even greater concern is the association between cosmetic surgery and suicide. Seven epidemiological studies that investigated the relationship between silicone gel–filled breast implants and all-cause mortality have found an association between cosmetic breast implants and suicide (see Sarwer,

Brown, & Evans, 2007, for a detailed review of this literature). These studies have suggested that the rate of suicide among women with breast implants is two to three times higher than estimated rates in the general population.

Explanations of the relationship between breast implants and suicide have primarily focused on the women's preoperative psychosocial status and functioning (McLaughlin, Wise, & Lipworth, 2004; Sarwer, 2003, 2007; Sarwer, Gibbons, et al., 2005). As detailed in these reviews, women who undergo breast augmentation have been shown to have several distinguishing demographic characteristics. They are more likely to report more lifetime sexual partners and more use of oral contraceptives, be younger at the time of their first pregnancy, and have a history of terminated pregnancies. They have been found to be more frequent users of alcohol and tobacco. As noted earlier, many have below-average body weight. Many of these characteristics are, in and of themselves, risk factors for suicide.

At present, the most intuitively consistent explanation of the relationship between cosmetic breast implants and suicide appears to be the presence of preexisting psychopathology before implantation. However, only one of the epidemiological studies (Jacobsen et al., 2004) provided any information on the psychiatric history of the women studied and documented a higher rate of previous psychiatric hospitalizations among women with breast implants than among both women who received other cosmetic procedures and women who underwent breast reduction. A history of psychiatric hospitalizations is one of the strongest predictors of suicide among women in the general population (Appleby et al., 1999; Goldacre, Seagroatt, & Hawton, 1993; Qin, Agerbo, & Mortensen, 2003). Unfortunately, Jacobsen et al. (2004) did not report information on diagnosis, history of illness, or other psychiatric treatments for the women in their sample.

PSYCHOSOCIAL STATUS AFTER COSMETIC SURGERY

Despite the concerns regarding the psychosocial status of some patients described earlier, the vast majority of cosmetic surgery patients report satisfaction with their postoperative result in the first few years after surgery (Park, Chetty, & Watson, 1996; Sarwer, Gibbons, et al., 2005; Schlebusch & Marht, 1993; Young et al., 1994). Studies have also suggested that within the first 2 years after cosmetic surgery, most women report improvements in body image (Banbury et al., 2004; Cash, Duel, & Perkins, 2002; Sarwer, Gibbons, et al., 2005; Sihm, Jagd, & Pers, 1978; Young et al., 1994). However, the impact of cosmetic surgery on other areas of functioning, such as self-esteem, depressive symptoms, and quality of life, is less well understood. Although some studies have shown postoperative improvements in these domains, other studies have found no significant improvements in these areas after surgery. With the exception of studies of patients with BDD, little evidence has demonstrated a clear relationship between preoperative status and postoperative outcomes.

An issue that has received surprisingly little attention is the relationship between postoperative complications, such as excessive scarring or infection, and psychosocial outcomes after surgery. Intuitively, one would assume that postoperative satisfaction and the psychological benefits associated with cosmetic surgery might be negatively affected by the occurrence of a postoperative complication (Honigman et al., 2004). At least one study has found that breast augmentation patients who experienced postoperative complications reported less favorable changes in body image in the first 2 years after surgery (Cash et al., 2002). Unfortunately, little else is known about these relationships.

PREOPERATIVE PSYCHOLOGICAL ASSESSMENT OF COSMETIC SURGERY PATIENTS

Despite the mental health issues detailed earlier, it is unlikely that any cosmetic surgeon currently requires that all patients undergo a mental health evaluation before undergoing cosmetic surgery. In the competitive market-place of cosmetic medicine, such a practice would likely drive patients to other practices. More important, given the lack of current evidence suggest-ing a relationship between preoperative psychosocial status and postoperative outcomes, recommendations for such routine evaluations are not warranted. Rather, cosmetic surgeons should, as should all medical professionals, assess and screen for the presence of psychopathology as part of taking a medical history and completion of physical examination. Unfortunately, most plastic surgeons (or their delegates) likely skip this part of the assessment and, as a result, fail to identify patients who may exhibit symptoms of psychopathology. That the vast majority of patients interested in cosmetic surgery are thought to be psychologically appropriate for such treatments is encouraging (Sarwer, 2006; Sarwer & Magee, 2006). These patients typically have specific appear-ance concerns, internal motivations, and realistic postoperative expectations. Thus, most patients do not need a psychological evaluation before undergoing a cosmetic treatment. The patients most likely to be referred for presurgical psychological screening are those who display symptoms of psychopathology during their initial consultation with the physician offering cosmetic surgery, as well as those with a history of psychopathology.

Because no evidence has suggested that unconscious conflicts or poor parental relationships are related to the decision to seek cosmetic surgery, a detailed assessment of patients' parental relationships and decades-old historical experiences is unlikely to provide useful information to either the mental health professional or the referring surgeon in determining appropriateness for surgery. Rather, a more straightforward evaluation of patients' current functioning, as found in the more general cognitive–behavioral assessment (Sarwer & Sayers, 1998), is recommended.

A trusted mental health professional can be a valuable consultant to a plastic surgery practice. This mental health professional should have a good understanding of the psychological aspects of cosmetic surgery, as well as knowledge of disorders with a body image component, such as BDD and eating disorders. In most cases, the mental health professional will be called on to assess a patient's psychological appropriateness for a procedure at a given point in time. Patients may react to a referral to a mental health professional with anger and defensiveness, believing that they will only feel better if they look better. Some may refuse to go to the consultation. To increase the likelihood that patients will accept the referral, it should be treated just as would a referral to any other health professional. Patients should be informed of the specific areas of concern and the reason for the referral. This information should also be shared with the mental health professional.

Patients interested in cosmetic surgery may represent a unique, interesting, and challenging experience for the mental health professional. Before agreeing to conduct these consultations, professionals should examine their own beliefs about cosmetic surgery and its ability to have a positive impact on patients' lives. Professionals who do not believe that changing one's outward appearance can improve one's internal perceptions of oneself should probably not conduct these assessments. Thus, consulting professionals should either believe in or be open to the idea that cosmetic treatments can produce psychological benefits. Additionally, these professionals should also understand that such treatments are not beneficial to everyone.

Before the onset of the consultation, mental health professionals should remind patients that, as consultants, they will be sharing the results of their evaluation and their recommendations of the appropriateness of treatment with the referring physician. The cognitive–behavioral assessment of cosmetic medicine patients will focus on the patients' thoughts, behaviors, and experiences that have contributed to their dissatisfaction with their appearance as well as the decision to seek treatment, which involves the assessment of the "ABCs" of patients' interest in surgery (Sarwer, 2006): the antecedents (A) to the decision to seek a cosmetic treatment, the behavioral responses (B) to patients' concerns about their appearance, and the consequences (C) of their decision to seek surgery. In addition, the evaluation should determine whether the patients' thoughts and behaviors are maladaptive (e.g., patients who believe that others are taking special notice of their appearance) to the point that they reflect some form of psychopathology that would contraindicate cosmetic treatment.

In addition to using the basic principles of cognitive–behavioral assessment, the mental health professional's assessment should focus on patients' psychiatric status and history, their appearance and body image concerns, and their motivations for and expectations of the procedure. Although these areas of assessment overlap with those recommended for the treating physician, the mental health professional's expertise will allow for a more detailed assessment of these areas than is typically undertaken in the initial consultation with the physician.

Psychiatric History and Status

The assessment of patients' psychiatric history and current status, as would be done in any mental health consultation, is a central part of the evaluation. With the exception of BDD, no conclusive data currently exist on the prevalence of psychiatric diagnoses among people who seek or undergo cosmetic surgery. As noted earlier, all of the major psychiatric diagnoses are likely to be found in this patient population. Particular attention should be paid to disorders with a body image component, such as eating disorders and somatoform disorders, as well as mood and anxiety disorders. The presence of these disorders, however, may not be an absolute contraindication for cosmetic surgery. In the absence of sound data on the relationship between psychopathology and surgical outcome, appropriateness for surgery should be made on a case-by-case basis.

As discussed earlier, approximately 20% of patients who seek cosmetic treatment report using a psychiatric medication at the time of treatment (Sarwer, Zanville, et al., 2004). As mental health professionals frequently observe, patients who receive these medications from a primary care physician often do not experience complete relief from their symptoms. Thus, a psychopharmacologic evaluation should be considered if symptoms do not appear to be well controlled. If a patient is in treatment with another mental health professional, the consultant should contact this professional and, as appropriate, discuss the patient's appropriateness for cosmetic treatment.

Physical Appearance and Body Image

Pruzinsky (1996) has suggested the use of Lazarus's (1973) BASIC ID—Behavior, Affect, Sensation, Imagery, Cognition, Interpersonal, and Drugs—as a template to assess the body image concerns of patients interested in cosmetic surgery. In addition, Cash's (2002) model of the historical and proximal influences on body image can provide an additional framework for this part of the assessment. The mental health professional may also want to consider the use of more specific body image measures to assist with providing a more comprehensive assessment. Valid and reliable measures such as the Multidimensional Body Self Relations Questionnaire (Brown, Cash, & Mikula, 1990) or the Deriford Appearance Scale (Carr, Harris, & James, 2000) can provide the mental health professional with detailed information on the symptoms of body image dissatisfaction or BDD.

Prospective patients should be able to articulate specific concerns about their appearance. Patients who are markedly distressed about slight defects that are not readily visible to the mental health professional may have BDD. At the same time, the nature of the appearance defect may be difficult for mental health professionals to assess. Ethical care would prohibit mental health professionals from asking patients to remove article of clothing to observe the defect. Furthermore, the judgment of an appearance defect as slight or imagined is highly subjective. What a mental health professional judges to be a slight defect well within the range of normal may be a defect that a physician offering cosmetic treatments judges to be observable and easily correctable. As a result, the degree of emotional distress and impairment, rather than the specific nature of the defect, may be a more accurate indicator of BDD among these patients (Sarwer, 2006; Sarwer & Crerand, 2004; Sarwer, Crerand, & Gibbons, 2005; Sarwer et al., 2003; Sarwer, Magee, & Crerand, 2004; Sarwer & Pertschuk, 2002).

The degree and psychosocial consequences of the dissatisfaction should also be assessed. Asking about the amount of time spent thinking about a feature or the activities missed or avoided may indicate the degree of distress and impairment a person is experiencing and may help determine the presence of BDD. Self-report measures of BDD symptoms, such as the Body Dysmorphic Disorder Questionnaire (Cash, Phillips, Santos, & Hrabosky, 2004), may also be helpful in this regard.

Motivations and Expectations

The mental health professional should also inquire about patients' motivations and expectations for cosmetic treatment. In assessing patients' motivations for surgery, the mental health professional may want to begin by asking, "When did you first think about changing your appearance?" Similarly, asking "What other things have you done to improve your appearance?" may be instructive. In addition to providing important clinical information, these questions may also reveal the presence of some obsessive or delusional thinking, as well as bizarre or compulsive behaviors, related to physical appearance. Cosmetic surgery patients not uncommonly report that they have tried several "do-it-yourself" treatments, such as treatments not approved by the Food and Drug Administration, in an attempt to improve their appearance (Veale, 2000), many of which may be not helpful and may potentially be dangerous.

Patients should be asked how romantic partners, family members, and close friends feel about the decision to change a physical feature. Although these individuals likely influence patients' decision-making process, their role may not be as great as has been thought. Breast augmentation patients have reported that their decision to seek surgery was influenced more by their own feelings about their appearance than by those of their romantic partner (Cash et al., 2002; Didie & Sarwer, 2003). Nevertheless, patients who seek treatment specifically to please a current partner, or attract a new one, are thought to be less likely to be satisfied with their postoperative outcomes. Thus, the mental health professional should inquire about patients' general expectations about how the change in appearance, which may be rather subtle and potentially unnoticed by others, will influence their lives.

No current evidence has suggested that cosmetic procedures directly affect interpersonal relationships. Therefore, patients should be reminded that predicting how others will respond to their changed appearance is impossible. Some patients may find that few people notice the change in their appearance, and others may find that everyone seems to notice. Although some patients may find this attention pleasurable, others may find it uncomfortable. To assess this issue, patients should be asked how they anticipate their lives will be different after surgery. The experience of unmet postoperative expectations is another possible explanation of the relationship between cosmetic breast augmentation and suicide (Sarwer, 2007; Sarwer, Brown, & Evans, 2007). Some women may present for breast augmentation surgery with unrealistic expectations of the effect that the procedure will have on their romantic relationship or daily functioning. When these expectations are not met, they may become despondent, depressed, and potentially suicidal.

Concluding the Evaluation

At the conclusion of the evaluation, mental health professionals should share their clinical impressions with the patient, as well as their ultimate recommendation to the referring physician about the appropriateness of cosmetic surgery. The results of the evaluation can be communicated to the referring physician in a letter summarizing the assessment and including the mental health professional's recommendations. Obviously, referring physicians will make the ultimate decision about whether to go forward with a given treatment. Nevertheless, it is good practice to share the results of the consultation with patients.

Postoperative Consultations

Mental health professionals may also be asked to consult with patients postoperatively. This request typically occurs in two scenarios: The patient is dissatisfied with a technically successful procedure or the patient is experiencing an exacerbation of psychopathology that was not detected preoperatively. Each of these scenarios typically warrants psychotherapeutic care. Cognitive–behavioral models of body image therapy (Cash, 2002) are often useful with these individuals, although more diagnosis-specific treatments may also be required (e.g., for depression or social or generalized anxiety disorders).

CASE EXAMPLE

C. A. was a 55-year-old, European American woman who presented to a plastic surgeon with concerns about wrinkling around her mouth and eyes.[1] She was married, worked as a high school teacher, and had two high-school-age children. She came to her initial appointment well dressed and well groomed. She indicated that the wrinkling around her mouth made a scar from a childhood accident more visible than it had been earlier in her life. The surgeon had little difficulty observing some modest wrinkling but believed that the scar had healed well and was more or less invisible from conversational distance.

The day after the consultation, C. A. phoned the surgeon's office and spent 30 minutes on the phone with his nurse asking her opinion of the consultation. As customary to his practice, the surgeon subsequently sent C. A. a letter detailing his impression and his recommended course of treatment. On receiving the letter, C. A. called the surgeon and, in a long phone conversation, went over the letter with the surgeon line by line. In response to her apparent preoccupation with a slight defect in her appearance, as well as her obsessive behavior regarding his impressions, the surgeon referred C. A. for a psychological evaluation before treatment.

C. A. accepted the surgeon's referral to the mental health professional with some reluctance, believing that she was not "crazy" and telling the surgeon that she was considering a consultation with another surgeon. She arrived at her psychological consultation well dressed and well groomed but clearly anxious. She indicated that she had been self-conscious about the scar on her lip since the time of the accident. She believed the scar left her looking deformed, although it was not visible from a conversational distance. C. A. indicated that her concern with the scar had affected both her professional and her personal life. She indicated that, in the past, she was frequently late to teach her first class of the day because she would often get stuck at home applying and reapplying her makeup to hide her scar. She also indicated that she would only approach her students from her left side, the side away from

---

[1]Details of this case have been altered to protect the patient's identity.

the scar. C. A. also reported that she essentially did not leave her house on the weekends because of concerns about her appearance. She recalled one recent instance when, while buying some popcorn at the movies, she was convinced that the employee behind the counter was staring at her scar.

The mental health professional concluded that C. A. was experiencing symptoms of BDD of mild to moderate severity. In response to this impression, C. A. agreed to delay surgery and engage in psychotherapy to address her preoccupation with her appearance and disruption in daily functioning.

CONCLUSION

Given the increasing popularity of cosmetic surgery, most mental health professionals will likely encounter patients interested in changing their bodies through these procedures. In addition to using the basic principles of cognitive–behavioral assessment, clinicians should focus on several additional areas in preoperative assessments. The mental health professional should complete a detailed assessment of the patient's psychiatric status and history, body image concerns, and motivations and expectations for surgery. Successful collaboration between medical and mental health professionals can increase the likelihood that the greatest number of patients receive appropriate treatment for their appearance and body image concerns.

REFERENCES

American Psychiatric Association. (2000). *Diagnostic and statistical manual of mental disorders* (4th ed., text rev.). Washington, DC: Author.

American Society of Plastic Surgeons. (2012). *National plastic surgery procedural statistics, 2011.* Arlington Heights, IL: Author.

Appleby, L., Shaw, J., Amos, T., McDonnell, R., Harris, C., McCann, K., . . . Parsons, R. (1999). Suicide within 12 months of contact with mental health services: National clinical survey. *British Medical Journal, 318,* 1235–1239. doi:10.1136/bmj.318.7193.1235

Baker, J. L., Kolin, I. S., & Bartlett, E. S. (1974). Psychosexual dynamics of patients undergoing mammary augmentation. *Plastic and Reconstructive Surgery, 53,* 652–659. doi:10.1097/00006534-197406000-00007

Banbury, J., Yetman, R., Lucas, A., Papay, F., Graves, K., & Zins, J. E. (2004). Prospective analysis of the outcome of subpectoral breast augmentation: Sensory changes, muscle function, and body image. *Plastic and Reconstructive Surgery, 113,* 701–707. doi:10.1097/01.PRS.0000101503.94322.C6

Beale, S., Lisper, H., & Palm, B. (1980). A psychological study of patients seeking augmentation mammoplasty. *The British Journal of Psychiatry, 136*, 133–138. doi:10.1192/bjp.136.2.133

Brown, T. A., Cash, T. F., & Mikula, P. J. (1990). Attitudinal body-image assessment: Factor analysis of the Body-Self Relations Questionnaire. *Journal of Personality Assessment, 55*, 135–144.

Carr, T., Harris, D., & James, C. (2000). The Derriford Appearance Scale (DAS-59): A new scale to measure individual responses to living with problems of appearance. *British Journal of Health Psychology, 5*, 201–215. doi:10.1348/135910700168865

Cash, T. F. (2002). Cognitive-behavioral perspectives on body image. In T. F. Cash & T. Pruzinsky (Eds.), *Body image: A handbook of theory, research, and clinical practice* (pp. 38–46). New York, NY: Guilford Press.

Cash, T. F., Duel, L. A., & Perkins, L. L. (2002). Women's psychosocial outcomes of breast augmentation with silicone gel-filled implants: A 2-year prospective study. *Plastic and Reconstructive Surgery, 109*, 2112–2121. doi:10.1097/00006534-200205000-00049

Cash, T. F., Phillips, K. A., Santos, M. T., & Hrabosky, J. I. Measuring "negative body image": Validation of the Body Image Disturbance Questionnaire in a nonclinical population. (2004). *Body Image, 1*, 363–3723. doi:10.1016/j.bodyim.2004.10.001

Crerand, C. E., Franklin, M. E., & Sarwer, D. B. (2006). Body dysmorphic disorder and cosmetic surgery. *Plastic and Reconstructive Surgery, 118*, 167e–180e. doi:10.1097/01.prs.0000242500.28431.24

Crerand, C. E., Infield, A. L., & Sarwer, D. B. (2007). Psychological considerations in cosmetic breast augmentation. *Plastic Surgical Nursing, 27*, 146–154.

Crerand, C. E., Menard, W., & Phillips, K. A. (2010). Surgical and minimally invasive cosmetic procedures among persons with body dysmorphic disorder. *Annals of Plastic Surgery, 65*, 11–16. doi:10.1097/SAP.0b013e3181bba08f

Crerand, C. E., Phillips, K. A., Menard, W., & Fay, C. (2005). Nonpsychiatric medical treatment of body dysmorphic disorder. *Psychosomatics, 46*, 549–555. doi:10.1176/appi.psy.46.6.549

Didie, E. R., & Sarwer, D. B. (2003). Factors which influence the decision to undergo cosmetic breast augmentation surgery. *Journal of Women's Health, 12*, 241–253. doi:10.1089/154099903321667582

Edgerton, M. T., & Knorr, N. J. (1971). Motivational patterns of patients seeking cosmetic (esthetic) surgery. *Plastic and Reconstructive Surgery, 48*, 551–557. doi:10.1097/00006534-197112000-00005

Edgerton, M. T., & McClary, A. R. (1958). Augmentation mammoplasty: Psychiatric implications and surgical indications. *Plastic and Reconstructive Surgery, 21*, 279–305. doi:10.1097/00006534-195804000-00005

Edgerton, M. T., Meyer, E., & Jacobson, W. E. (1961). Augmentation mammoplasty II: Further surgical and psychiatric evaluation. *Plastic and Reconstructive Surgery, 27*, 279–302. doi:10.1097/00006534-196103000-00005

Frederick, D. A., Lever, J., & Peplau, L. A. (2007). Interest in cosmetic surgery and body image: Views of men and women across the lifespan. *Plastic and Reconstructive Surgery, 120*, 1407–1415. doi:10.1097/01.prs.0000279375.26157.64

Geary, D. C. (2010). *Male, female: The evolution of human sex differences* (2nd ed.). Washington, DC: American Psychological Association. doi:10.1037/12072-000

Goldacre, M., Seagroatt, V., & Hawton, K. (1993). Suicide after discharge from psychiatric inpatient care. *The Lancet, 342*, 283–286. doi:10.1016/0140-6736(93)91822-4

Honigman, R. J., Phillips, K. A., & Castle, D. J. (2004). A review of psychosocial outcomes for patients seeking cosmetic surgery. *Plastic and Reconstructive Surgery, 113*, 1229–1237. doi:10.1097/01.PRS.0000110214.88868.CA

Jacobsen, P. H., Holmich, L. R., McLaughlin, J. K., Johansen, C., Olsen, J. H., Kjøller, K., & Friis, S. (2004). Mortality and suicide among Danish women with cosmetic breast implants. *Archives of Internal Medicine, 164*, 2450–2455. doi:10.1001/archinte.164.22.2450

Kjøller, K., Holmich, L. R., Fryzek, J. P., Jacobsen, P. H., Friis, S., McLaughlin, J. K., . . . Olsen, J. H. (2003). Characteristics of women with cosmetic breast implants compared with women with other types of cosmetic surgery and population-based controls in Denmark. *Annals of Plastic Surgery, 50*, 6–12. doi:10.1097/00000637-200301000-00002

Lazarus, A. A. (1973). Multimodal behavior therapy: Treating the "BASIC ID." *Journal of Nervous and Mental Disease, 156*, 404–411. doi:10.1097/00005053-197306000-00005

McLaughlin, J. K., Wise, T. N., & Lipworth, L. (2004). Increased risk of suicide among patients with breast implants: Do the epidemiologic data support psychiatric consultation? *Psychosomatics, 45*, 277–280. doi:10.1176/appi.psy.45.4.277

Park, A. J., Chetty, U., & Watson, A. C. H. (1996). Patient satisfaction following insertion of silicone breast implants. *British Journal of Plastic Surgery, 49*, 515–518. doi:10.1016/S0007-1226(96)90127-7

Pertschuk, M. J., Sarwer, D. B., Wadden, T. A., & Whitaker, L. A. (1998). Body image dissatisfaction in male cosmetic surgery patients. *Aesthetic Plastic Surgery, 22*, 20–24. doi:10.1007/s002669900160

Phillips, K. A. (2004). Treating body dysmorphic disorder using medication. *Psychiatric Annals, 34*, 945–953.

Phillips, K. A., & Menard, W. (2006). Suicidality in body dysmorphic disorder: A prospective study. *The American Journal of Psychiatry, 163*, 1280–1282. doi:10.1176/appi.ajp.163.7.1280

Pruzinsky, T. (1996). Cosmetic plastic surgery and body image: Critical factors in patient assessment. In J. K. Thompson (Ed.), *Body image, eating disorders, and obesity: An integrative guide for assessment and treatment* (pp. 109–127). Washington, DC: American Psychological Association. doi:10.1037/10502-005

Qin, P., Agerbo, E., & Mortensen, P. B. (2003). Suicide risk in relation to socioeconomic, demographic, psychiatric, and familial factors: A national register-based study of all suicides in Denmark, 1981-1997. *The American Journal of Psychiatry, 160,* 765–772. doi:10.1176/appi.ajp.160.4.765

Sarwer, D. B. (2001). Psychological considerations in cosmetic surgery. In R. M. Goldwyn & M. N. Cohen (Eds.), *The unfavorable result in plastic surgery* (pp. 14–23). Philadelphia, PA: Lippincott Williams & Wilkins.

Sarwer, D. B. (2002). Awareness and identification of body dysmorphic disorder by aesthetic surgeons: Results of a survey of American Society for Aesthetic Plastic Surgery members. *Aesthetic Surgery Journal, 22,* 531–535. doi:10.1067/maj.2002.129451

Sarwer, D. B. (2003). Discussion of causes of death among Finnish women with cosmetic breast implants, 1971-2001. *Annals of Plastic Surgery, 51,* 343–344. doi:10.1097/01.sap.0000093120.25257.29

Sarwer, D. B. (2006). Psychological assessment of cosmetic surgery. In D. B. Sarwer, T. Pruzinsky, T. F. Cash, R. M. Goldwyn, J. A. Persing, & L. A. Whitaker (Eds.), *Psychological aspects of reconstructive and cosmetic plastic surgery: Clinical, empirical and ethical perspectives* (pp. 267–283). Philadelphia, PA: Lippincott Williams & Wilkins.

Sarwer, D. B. (2007). The psychological aspects of cosmetic breast augmentation. *Plastic and Reconstructive Surgery, 120,* 110S–117S. doi:10.1097/01.prs.0000286591.05612.72

Sarwer, D. B., Bartlett, S. P., Bucky, L. P., LaRossa, D., Low, D. W., Pertschuk, M. J., . . . Whitaker, L. A. (1998). Bigger is not always better: Body image dissatisfaction in breast reduction and breast augmentation patients. *Plastic and Reconstructive Surgery, 101,* 1956–1961. doi:10.1097/00006534-199806000-00028

Sarwer, D. B., Brown, G. K., & Evans, D. L. (2007). Cosmetic breast augmentation and suicide: A review of the literature. *The American Journal of Psychiatry, 164,* 1006–1013. doi:10.1176/appi.ajp.164.7.1006

Sarwer, D. B., & Crerand, C. E. (2002). Psychological issues in patient outcomes. *Facial Plastic Surgery, 18,* 125–134. doi:10.1055/s-2002-32203

Sarwer, D. B., & Crerand, C. E. (2004). Body image and cosmetic medical treatments. *Body Image, 1,* 99–111. doi:10.1016/S1740-1445(03)00003-2

Sarwer, D. B., & Crerand, C. E. (2008). Body dysmorphic disorder and appearance enhancing medical treatments. *Body Image, 5,* 50–58. doi:10.1016/j.bodyim.2007.08.003

Sarwer, D. B., Crerand, C. E., & Gibbons, L. M. (2005). Body dysmorphic disorder. In F. Nahai (Ed.), *The art of aesthetic surgery* (pp. 33–57). St. Louis, MO: Quality Medical.

Sarwer, D. B., Crerand, C. E., & Gibbons, L. M. (2007). Cosmetic Procedures to Enhance Body Shape and Muscularity. In J. K. Thompson & G. Cafri (Eds.), *The muscular ideal: Psychological, social, and medical perspectives* (pp. 183–198). Washington, DC: American Psychological Association. doi:10.1037/11581-009

Sarwer, D. B., Crerand, C. E., & Magee, L. (2011). Cosmetic surgery and changes in body image. In T. F. Cash & L. Smolak (Eds.), *Body image: A handbook of science, practice, and prevention* (2nd ed., pp. 394–403). New York, NY: Guilford Press.

Sarwer, D. B., Didie, E. R., & Gibbons, L. M. (2006). Cosmetic surgery of the body. In D. B. Sarwer, T. Pruzinsky, T. F. Cash, R. M. Goldwyn, J. A. Persing, & L. A. Whitaker (Eds.), *Psychological aspects of reconstructive and cosmetic plastic surgery: Clinical, empirical, and ethical perspectives* (pp. 251–266). Philadelphia, PA: Lippincott Williams & Wilkins.

Sarwer, D. B., Gibbons, L. M., Magee, L., Baker, J. L., Casas, L. A., Glat, P. M., . . . Young, V. L. (2005). A prospective, multi-site investigation of patient satisfaction and psychosocial status following cosmetic surgery. *Aesthetic Surgery Journal, 25,* 263–269. doi:10.1016/j.asj.2005.03.009

Sarwer, D. B., LaRossa, D., Bartlett, S. P., Low, D. W., Bucky, L. P., & Whitaker, L. A. (2003). Body image concerns of breast augmentation patients. *Plastic and Reconstructive Surgery, 112,* 83–90. doi:10.1097/01.PRS.0000066005.07796.51

Sarwer, D. B., & Magee, L. (2006). Physical appearance and society. In D. B. Sarwer, T. Pruzinsky, T. F. Cash, R. M. Goldwyn, J. A. Persing, & J. A. Whitaker (Eds.), *Psychological aspects of reconstructive and cosmetic plastic surgery: Clinical, empirical, and ethical perspectives* (pp. 23–36). Philadelphia, PA: Lippincott Williams & Wilkins.

Sarwer, D. B., Magee, L., & Crerand, C. E. (2004). Cosmetic surgery and cosmetic medical treatments. In J. K. Thompson (Ed.), *Handbook of eating disorders and obesity* (pp. 718–737). Hoboken, NJ: Wiley.

Sarwer, D. B., & Pertschuk, M. J. (2002). Cosmetic surgery. In S. G. Kornstein & A. H. Clayton (Eds.), *Textbook of women's mental health* (pp. 481–496). New York, NY: Guilford Press.

Sarwer, D. B., Pertschuk, M. J., Wadden, T. A., & Whitaker, L. A. (1998). Psychological investigations in cosmetic surgery: A look back and a look ahead. *Plastic and Reconstructive Surgery, 101,* 1136–1142. doi:10.1097/00006534-199804040-00040

Sarwer, D. B., & Sayers, S. L. (1998). Behavioral interviewing. In A. S. Bellack & M. Hersen (Eds.), *Behavioral assessment: A practical handbook* (4th ed., pp. 63–78). New York, NY: Pergamon Press.

Sarwer, D. B., Wadden, T. A., Pertschuk, M. J., & Whitaker, L. A. (1998a). Body image dissatisfaction and body dysmorphic disorder in 100 cosmetic surgery patients. *Plastic and Reconstructive Surgery, 101,* 1644–1649. doi:10.1097/00006534-199805000-00035

Sarwer, D. B., Wadden, T. A., Pertschuk, M. J., & Whitaker, L. A. (1998b). The psychology of cosmetic surgery: A review and reconceptualization. *Clinical Psychology Review, 18,* 1–22. doi:10.1016/S0272-7358(97)00047-0

Sarwer, D. B., Whitaker, L. A., Wadden, T. A., & Pertschuk, M. J. (1997). Body image dissatisfaction in women seeking rhytidectomy or blepharoplasty. *Aesthetic Surgery Journal, 17,* 230–234. doi:10.1016/S1090-820X(97)80004-0

Sarwer, D. B., Zanville, H. A., LaRossa, D., Bartlett, S. P., Chang, B., Low, D. W., & Whitaker, L. A. (2004). Mental health histories and psychiatric medication usage among persons who sought cosmetic surgery. *Plastic and Reconstructive Surgery, 114,* 1927–1933. doi:10.1097/01.PRS.0000142999.86432.1F

Schlebusch, L., & Marht, I. (1993). Long-term psychological sequelae of augmentation mammoplasty. *South African Medical Journal, 83,* 267–271.

Sihm, F., Jagd, M., & Pers, M. (1978). Psychological assessment before and after augmentation mammoplasty. *Scandinavian Journal of Plastic and Reconstructive Surgery, 12,* 295–298. doi:10.3109/02844317809013009

Simis, K. J., Verhulst, F. C., & Koot, H. M. (2001). Body image, psychosocial functioning, and personality: How different are adolescents and young adults applying for plastic surgery? *Journal of Child Psychology and Psychiatry, 42,* 669–678. doi:10.1111/1469-7610.00762

Veale, D. (2000). Outcome of cosmetic surgery and "DIY" surgery in patients with body dysmorphic disorder. *Psychiatric Bulletin, 24,* 218. doi:10.1192/pb.24.6.218

Veale, D., Boocock, A., Gournay, K., Dryden, W., Shah, F., Willson, R., & Walburn, J. (1996). Body dysmorphic disorder. A survey of fifty cases. *British Journal of Psychiatry, 169,* 196–201. doi:10.1192/bjp.169.2.196

Veale, D., De Haro, L., & Lambrou, C. (2003). Cosmetic rhinoplasty in body dysmorphic disorder. *British Journal of Plastic Surgery, 56,* 546–551.

Young, V. L., Nemecek, J. R., & Nemecek, D. A. (1994). The efficacy of breast augmentation: Breast size increase, patient satisfaction, and psychological effects. *Plastic and Reconstructive Surgery, 94,* 958–969. doi:10.1097/00006534-199412000-00009

AFTERWORD

DAVID B. SARWER AND ANDREW R. BLOCK

This book has described the development of presurgical psychological screening (PPS) and its application across a broad range of medical conditions. In editing this book, we have reached the conclusion that the text would have been much shorter, and had fewer chapters, even 5 years ago. We also believe that subsequent texts in this area will be larger and more comprehensive as advances in surgical specialties lead to even greater use of PPS in the future. For example, the past decade has witnessed a greater recognition of the psychological challenges faced by individuals who consider themselves to be transgendered and may consider or present for sexual reassignment surgery (e.g., Bockting & Fung, 2006). Although these surgical procedures remain somewhat rare and are performed at only a handful of specialty centers throughout the country, PPS is already considered to be a critically important part of treatment. Mental health evaluations are

DOI: 10.1037/14035-014
Presurgical Psychological Screening: Understanding Patients, Improving Outcomes, Andrew R. Block and David B. Sarwer (Editors)

required of all patients, and those interested in the genital procedures must undergo two mental health evaluations and 12 months of psychotherapy before surgery.

Modern warfare, and advances in military health care, may also affect the field of PPS in both the near and distant future. For many reasons, a growing number of military personnel are returning from combat with devastating injuries—significant burns, amputation of limbs, and so forth—that they would not previously have survived. These individuals often face an exhaustive number of medical and surgical procedures as well as significant residual disfigurement, as described in Chapter 8 by Crerand and Magee. Both the original injuries and resulting treatments have the potential to severely compromise psychosocial functioning and long-term adaptation to civilian life. Obviously, PPS cannot be performed before the initial trauma or surgical procedure. However, mental health professionals are often involved in the evaluation of patients as they go through subsequent surgical procedures and rehabilitation. They also have an already-established role on treatment teams that are working in the rapidly developing areas of composite tissue allographs for hand and face transplantation. At the same time, mental health professionals will continue to play an important role in helping individuals who have traumatic injuries that affect their appearance adapt to this significant psychosocial stressor.

Although mental health professionals are participating in the evaluation and care of a growing number of surgical patients, PPS, as a specialty, needs to strive for the use of evidence-based practice. Most, if not all, of the specialties detailed in this book rely on a cognitive–behavioral foundation for the conduct of the preoperative evaluations. All have a body of research that examines the relationship between preoperative psychosocial issues and postoperative outcomes. Obviously, some of these programs of research are more fully developed than others. Professionals working in these areas are encouraged to conduct clinical research to further investigate the relationship between the relevant psychosocial and surgical issues in the respective specialties.

One of the keys to such research will be the use of psychometric testing. Such testing can provide objective, quantified measurements of personality, emotion, and health-related behaviors. As described in the Introduction to this volume, testing allows for definition of psychosocial concerns through convergent validity. At present, however, consensus is lacking regarding the use of psychometric testing before surgical interventions. Some specialties (and professionals) augment their clinical interviews with personality inventories such as the Minnesota Multiphasic Personality Inventory—2 (Butcher, Dahlstrom, Graham, Tellegen, & Kaemmer, 1989) or its newer version, the Minnesota Multiphasic Personality Inventory—2 Revised Form

(Ben-Porath, 2012). Many professionals use paper-and-pencil symptom inventories or tests of health-related behaviors to further assess specific symptom areas. Others perform or refer a patient for formal neuropsychological testing when relevant to the patient's particular case, such as when there is concern about brain damage or limited intellectual functioning. Regardless of the specific rationale, because of their quantitative results, the relationship of preoperative psychometric tests to surgical outcomes can be directly assessed. Such assessment will help determine both which (combinations of) tests are most effective in identifying psychosocial risk factors for adverse surgical results and how these tests can augment information obtained in clinical interviews. As such research continues to develop, the clinician conducting PPS must draw conclusions on the basis of the most current, empirically determined, and face-valid measures available.

One intuitive question that often arises is whether PPS can be used to predict postoperative outcomes. This question, which has probably been asked of most mental health professionals conducting PPS, is often the biggest issue for most surgeons. However, the reality is that the question of prediction sets an unrealistically high bar for the mental health professional compared with other medical health professionals who are asked to conduct preoperative screening. When the treating surgeon refers a patient for preoperative cardiac clearance, the surgeon is not asking the cardiologist to predict a postoperative outcome. Rather, the referral is made to assess the risk of the patient vis-à-vis the surgical procedure. In its simplest terms, is the patient's heart healthy enough to survive the operation? The surgeon subsequently takes the information from the referral and makes a decision about whether he or she is comfortable assuming that risk if the decision is to go forward with surgery. PPS should be seen in the same manner—that the evaluation is designed to assess risk and not to predict outcome, as though the mental health professional has access to a crystal ball.

A related issue revolves around the multiple goals of many surgical procedures. Although all surgeries aim to correct or mitigate an aberrant medical condition, often many other results are desired. For example, although deep brain stimulation in Parkinson's disease aims to directly reduce muscular tremors, the surgeon also hopes that this procedure will lead to improvements in quality of life, emotional stability, and social interaction. Particular psychosocial factors may be differentially associated with specific types of outcome. Chronic depression, for example, may bode poorly for improvements in emotional stability after a procedure but may not reduce the direct physical effects of the surgery. Continued investigations linking specific psychosocial measures to the full range of desired surgical outcomes will both improve the effectiveness of PPS and demonstrate its limitations and qualifications.

Evidence has suggested that even patients with significant psychopathology can benefit from the procedures detailed in this book. In the area of bariatric surgery, one of us (David B. Sarwer) has seen patients with schizophrenia and dissociative identity disorder obtain good postoperative results. In these cases, the patients had long-standing relationships with mental health professionals in the community and were stable at the time of surgery. Thus, although the primary goal of the evaluation is to assess for the presence of psychopathology, some evidence from some of the specialties discussed in this book has shown that severe psychopathology may not always be associated with suboptimal postoperative outcomes. At the same time, in other specialties the concern is that patients with significant psychopathology may be the ones most likely to have poor postoperative outcomes. Not only are some of these patients more likely to experience complications, but some appear to be more likely to bring legal action against their surgeons. Thus, there is a strong need for research demonstrating conditions under which patients with severe mental disorders, such as psychosis, bipolar disorder, or major personality disorders, may achieve appropriate surgical results.

The need for continued investigation leads inevitably to a discussion of standards of care in PPS. Presently, well-established standards of mental health care are available related to the assessment of children born with craniofacial conditions and of adults disfigured by burns (see Chapter 8). Even newer specialties under the PPS umbrella, such as bariatric care, are coming closer to standards of care, which have also been introduced for the anesthesia and nutritional care of patients in the past few years. We anticipate that as PPS continues to evolve, we will see standards of care develop in a greater number of specialties. What is unclear at present is the potential methods for credentialing of mental health professionals who work in these areas. Specialty credentials or certification is a relatively popular phenomenon in many areas of medicine and nursing. It is less common in psychology, although the growth of specialty certification by the American Board of Professional Psychology points to its increasing value. The combination of well-established standards of care and advanced credentialing in specialty areas is appealing, particularly when the advancement of high-quality research and clinical care is considered. At the same time, such credentialing may be difficult in some of the higher volume specialties in PPS, such as bariatric surgery, in which the availability of a small number of credentialed professionals may actually limit access to quality care. However, our hope is that this text may contribute to the development of a general set of certifications for mental health professionals and the conduct of PPS.

One additional major issue for the field of PPS concerns reimbursement. Although PPS is coming into increasing use, it does not fit well into any existing coding scheme for billing. Traditionally, clinicians bill for evaluation services, under mental health codes, for a diagnostic interview (Code 90801) and psychometric testing (Code 96101). These codes present two problems for PPS. First, they require the evaluator to give the patient a mental health diagnosis. Because many patients sent for PPS do not fit the criteria for any mental health diagnosis and, moreover, because the goals of PPS are to determine psychosocial risk for surgery and adjust medical treatment plans accordingly, billing using Codes 90801 and 96101 is often inappropriate.

Also, some major health insurers will not reimburse for these codes when the patient is sent for PPS. Rather, these carriers require providers to bill under the Health and Behavior Codes, Initial Assessment Code 96150. This code is billed in 15-minute segments. Thus, a 90-minute evaluation would bill for six units of Code 96150. The advantage of this code is that it does not require the evaluator to give the patient a psychological diagnosis, because it is specifically designed to reimburse for mental health services connected with a medical condition. The major disadvantage is that there is no Health and Behavior code for psychometric testing. As this text has repeatedly demonstrated, testing is a major component of PPS because it provides objective data to provide convergent validity for the patient's psychosocial concerns and risk factors. Testing entails significant time and expense to the provider and should be reimbursed. Given that PPS has the potential to provide significant cost savings to insurers through avoidance of likely unsuccessful surgery and more efficient and effective treatment, it is incumbent on insurers to either develop a new reimbursement code for PPS or allow clinicians to bill for psychometric testing as a component of the evaluation.

These issues can represent significant challenges for mental health professionals who work in private practice settings or who perform PPS as a small part of their clinical work. Reimbursement can be less of an issue for professionals working in larger hospitals, academic medical centers, or other situations in which the mental health professional may be housed within the Department of Surgery or other specialty groups. In these situations, the provider may be a salaried employee, and the revenues for services may be generated and salary supported as part of a bundled payment for the surgical procedure. This model is often seen in areas such as solid organ transplant and bariatric surgery.

Another important aspect of PPS that is often overlooked is the role of risk management for the treating surgeon and institution. For the past decade, one of us (Sarwer) has taught an instructional course focused on the identification and management of psychological issues seen in cosmetic surgery patients at the annual meeting of the American Society of Plastic Surgeons. As detailed in Chapter 12, PPS is not required before cosmetic procedures but is often requested when the cosmetic surgeon has identified potential psychological issues in an individual interested in surgery. Nevertheless, the American Society of Plastic Surgeons believes strongly in the appropriate management of mental health issues among plastic surgery patients and offers the seminar as one of its risk management courses. From the society's perspective, proper identification and management of psychosocial issues is an important part of quality care and may also help surgeons identify patients who may have postoperative psychological problems that may contribute to a medical malpractice lawsuit. As noted in many chapters throughout this text, psychological and behavioral issues may interfere with a patient's ability to follow postoperative recommendations from the treatment team, which may contribute to the development (or maintenance) of postoperative complications and poor outcomes, both of which are often the linchpins of medical malpractice cases.

The use of PPS is growing at a time when several government agencies have begun to recognize and appreciate the important role of psychosocial factors in illness and treatment. At the National Institutes of Health, federal funding for grants with a psychosocial component, if not focus, now occurs at institutes other than the National Institute of Mental Health. Similarly, the Food and Drug Administration (FDA) has issued guidance documents on the appropriate use of Patient Reported Outcomes, encompassing psychometric measures to assess changes in psychological symptoms after a treatment being considered for FDA approval. In this regard, a treatment cannot claim to have an impact on psychosocial functioning, such as quality of life, if the investigators have not used a specific, valid, and reliable measure of the construct of interest. These changes at the federal level, although not specifically related to PPS, further suggest that recognition of the importance of psychosocial outcomes after medical treatment can only further bolster the acceptance of PPS.

As the use of PPS continues to grow, we anticipate that we will also see growth in research and clinical application of psychological interventions during postoperative treatment. Although the surgical treatments described in this book can have a tremendous impact on the physical and psychological pain and suffering experienced by patients, many individuals continue to struggle with residual issues that are not resolved by surgery. PPS may well provide a road map not only for the timing of surgery and the exploration of alternatives to surgical intervention but also for the potential psychological challenges that patients may face during recovery—a road map that can be used by other mental health professionals who are involved in the postoperative care of patients.

REFERENCES

Ben-Porath, Y. S. (2012). *Interpreting the MMPI-2-RF*. Minneapolis: University of Minnesota Press.

Bockting, W. O., & Fung, L. C. T. (2006). Genital reconstruction and gender identity disorders. In D. B. Sarwer, T. Pruzinsky, R. F. Cash, R. M. Goldwyn, J. A. Persing, & L. A. Whitaker (Eds.), *Psychological aspects of reconstructive and cosmetic plastic surgery: Clinical, empirical, and ethical perspectives* (pp. 207–232). Philadelphia, PA: Lippincott Williams & Wilkins.

Butcher, J. N., Dahlstrom, W. G., Graham, J. R., Tellegen, A, & Kaemmer, B. (1989). *The Minnesota Multiphasic Personality Inventory-2 (MMPI-2): Manual for administration and scoring*. Minneapolis: University of Minnesota Press

INDEX

Psychological factors
    with carpal tunnel surgery, 238–240
    with cosmetic surgery, 277–278
    with disfigurement, 175–176
    with face or hand transplants,
        180–181
    with hand surgeries, 179
    for pre- and post-operative HSCT
        patients, 107–109
    with reconstructive procedures,
        174–177, 186–187
    with stimulator and intrathecal
        pump therapy, 89–90
Psychological history
    of carpal tunnel surgery candidate,
        243–244
    with hematopoietic stem cell
        transplant, 111
    of reconstructive surgery candidates,
        186–187
Psychological interventions
    for anxiety, 138–139
    for apathy, 139–140
    for depression, 134–135
    for high-risk CTS patients, 245–246
    for noncompliance, 12
    for organ transplant candidates, 32
    for pre- or post-operative
        gynecologic patients, 222–225
Psychological–psychosocial disease axis
    (AXIS II of RDC–TMD), 157
Psychological risk factors, 52
Psychometric testing
    consensus on, 274–275
    in presurgical psychological
        screening, 10
    of reconstructive surgery candidates,
        188
Psychopathology. See Preoperative
    psychopathology
Psychopharmacotherapy, 135–136, 139
Psychosocial factors
    with bariatric surgery, 64–67
    with chronic pain, 85
    with cosmetic surgery, 255–259
    with deep brain stimulation,
        142–144
    with gynecologic surgery, 224–227
    with hematopoietic stem cell
        transplant, 104–111

instruments for measurement of,
    33–34, 114–115
interpersonal relationships as, 14
for organ recipients, 27–35
in pain perception, 158–159
with Parkinson's disease, 142–144
of patients unsuitable for organ
    transplant, 37
with pediatric reconstructive
    procedures, 181–184
with physical appearance, 174–175
with reconstructive surgery, 177–181
with spine surgery, 44–49, 53
in surgical outcome, 13–17
PTSD. See Posttraumatic stress disorder
Public health policy, 20–21

Quality of life (QOL)
    with bariatric surgery, 66
    measures for risk factors with, 158,
        160
    with Parkinson's disease, 127, 142
Quality of Life instrument, 200
Questionnaires, 65, 244. See also specific
    headings

Radical hysterectomy, 216, 219
Radical vulvectomy, 221
Randomized control trial (RCT),
    129–130
RDC–TMD (research diagnostic
    criteria for temporomandibular
    disorders), 157–160
Reconstructive procedures, 173–190
    in adult populations, 177–181
    pediatric, 181–184
    psychological assessment for,
        184–188
    psychological factors with, 174–177
    self-report questionnaires for, 189
"Red flags," 243
Referrals
    framing of, 18
    for mental health treatment, 166
    ongoing relationships for, 163–165
    sources of, 91
Reimbursement, 276–277
Reinforcement, 48
Reproductive organs, 215–217. See also
    Gynecologic surgery

Research diagnostic criteria for
    temporomandibular disorders
    (RDC–TMD), 157–160
Respect for People's Rights and Dignity
    (APA Ethics Code), 18
Response expectancies, 205–206
Rest difficulties, 200
Results
    of cosmetic surgery evaluation, 264
    disclosure of, 166–167, 245, 261
    of organ transplant recipient PPS,
        34–35
Richardson, A., 203
Richlin, D. M., 48–49
Risk assessment, 5
Risk factor(s)
    with carpal tunnel syndrome, 245–246
    combined, with spine surgery, 51–53
    and cultural differences, 226
    employment as, 241
    for gynecologic surgery candidates,
        225
    with hematopoietic stem cell
        transplant, 110–112
    with implantable devices, 88
    in information gathering stage, 8
    legal representation as, 241
    minimal standards for, 11
    in PPS algorithm, 53
    psychological and medical, 52
    suicidality as, 166
    with temporomandibular disorder
        surgery, 157, 168
Robinson, J. P., 243
Robinson-Whelen, S., 154
Rohl, J., 217
Roles, social, 109–110, 143–144
Romantic partners, 264
Rosenbaum, R. B., 238
Roux-en-Y gastric bypass (RYGB), 63–64
Rub, U., 128

Salpingo-oophorectomy, 216
Scar revision, 178–179
Scarring, 183
Schofferman, J., 47
SCID-I (Structured Clinical Interview
    for the *Diagnostic and Statistical
    Manual of Mental Disorders
    III–R*), 67, 156

SCS (spinal cord stimulation), 86–90,
    93–94
Self-determination, 18–19
Self-esteem, 66
Self-report measures
    for breast cancer surgery candidates,
        204–207
    for pain, 91, 158–159
    for Parkinson's disease patients, 135
    for reconstructive procedures, 189
Semistructured interviews, 185
Sensitivity
    to pain, 45–46, 155
    somatic, 16
Sensory experience, 90
Sentinel node biopsy, 197
Setting, 202
Sexual abuse, 47, 71–72
Sexual relationships
    and bariatric surgery, 66–67
    of gynecologic surgery candidates,
        218–219, 224
Short Form–12, 242
Short Form–36, 158, 160, 239
Short-Form Health Survey, 92
Shulman, L. M., 135
Sitzia, J., 203
Sleep difficulties, 200, 206
Smith, G., 47
Smoking, 51
Social Comfort Questionnaire, 189
Social context
    chronic pain in, 91
    disfigurement in, 176–177
    of medical conditions, 14
    pain in, 48
Social roles, 109–110, 143–144
Social Security Disability, 17
Social support
    for organ transplant candidate,
        30–31
    of Parkinson's disease patients,
        143–144
    for reconstructive surgery candidates,
        187–188
Sogg, S., 71
Somatic sensitivity, 16
Somatization, 239
Sparkes, E., 90
Spengler, D. M., 46

Spielberger State–Trait Anxiety
     Inventory, 138
Spinal cord stimulation (SCS), 86–90,
     93–94
Spinal infusion, 87
Spine surgery, 43–56. *See also* Stimulator
     and intrathecal pump therapy
     in case study, 54
     medical risk factors with, 49–53
     overview of, 43–44
     psychosocial risk factors with, 44–49,
          53
State–Trait Anxiety Inventory, 178,
     199, 244
Steege, J., 217
Stem cell transplant. *See* Hematopoietic
     stem cell transplant
Stepped approach, 113
Stern, M. B., 134
Stigmatization
     and bariatric surgery, 67
     with depression, 117
     with disfigurement, 187–188
Stimulator and intrathecal pump
     therapy, 85–97
     in case study, 94–96
     future research directions for, 96–97
     outcomes with, 88–90
     overview of, 86–88
     psychological evaluations with, 90–91
     psychological measures with, 91–94
STN (subthalamic nucleus), 129, 141
Stressors, 216–217. *See also* Distress
Structured Clinical Interview for the
     *Diagnostic and Statistical Manual of
     Mental Disorders III–R* (SCID-I),
     67, 156
Substance use/abuse
     assessment of, 116
     by bariatric surgery candidates,
          70–71
     measures for risk factors of, 158, 160
     by organ transplant candidate, 32–33
     by spine injury patients, 47
Subthalamic nucleus (STN), 129, 141
Suicidality
     in bariatric surgery patients, 64, 69
     of breast implant patients, 258–259
     liabilities with, 165
     as risk factor, 166

Support. *See* Social support
Surgical breast biopsy, 197
Surgical interventions
     for carpal tunnel syndrome, 237–238
     decision making about, 10–12
     goals for, 275
     ineffective, 4
     informed consent for, 21–22
     recommendation to avoid, 12–13
     scarring after, 179
     with spine surgery, 49–50
     for temporomandibular disorder,
          152–153
     timing of, 73
Surgical outcomes
     benefits of PPS for, 6–7
     and individualized treatment, 12
     and informed consent, 22
     mental health clinicians in, 4–5
     possibilities for, 11
     and presurgical psychological
          screening, 3–6
     psychosocial factors in, 13–17
Surgical team, 4–7
Survey of Pain Attitudes, 93
Survival rates, 26, 106–107
Symptom Checklist—90, 161
Symptom Checklist—90—Revised, 92
Symptom Checklist—90 Somatization
     scale, 159
Syrjala, K. L., 109
Szabo, R. M., 236

Tan, G., 154
Temporomandibular disorder (TMD),
     151–168
     biopsychosocial conceptualizations
          with, 154–156
     in case study, 161–167
     overview of, 151–154
     presurgical screening for, 156–161,
          168
Temporomandibular joint (TMJ), 151
Tension–Anxiety subscale, 199, 204
Thornby, J. J., 154
Thought disorders, 71
Timing, 73, 201–202
Tissue flap procedure, 197
TMD. *See* Temporomandibular disorder
TMJ (temporomandibular joint), 151

ABOUT THE EDITORS

Andrew R. Block, PhD, received his bachelor's degree from Haverford College and his doctorate from Dartmouth College. He is a board-certified clinical health psychologist and fellow of Division 38 (Health Psychology) of the American Psychological Association. He has worked for more than 20 years with the Texas Back Institute in Plano, Texas, and, before that, with the Spine Institute in Carmel, Indiana. He specializes in presurgical psychological screening and perioperative treatment of candidates for spine surgery and pain control procedures (implantable stimulators and pumps), as well as candidates for bariatric surgery. He serves on the Conservative Care Committee and the Clinical Outcomes Committee of the North American Spine Society.

Dr. Block has many peer-reviewed research publications in the areas of chronic pain and presurgical psychological screening, beginning in the 1970s. He has written two books, most recently *The Psychology of Spine Surgery*, of which he was lead author. He was also the editor-in-chief of the *Handbook of Pain Syndromes: Biopsychosocial Perspectives*. This is his fourth book.

David B. Sarwer, PhD, is professor of psychology, Departments of Psychiatry and Surgery, Perelman School of Medicine, University of Pennsylvania, and director of clinical services, Center for Weight and Eating Disorders. He received his bachelor's degree in 1990 from Tulane University, his master's degree in 1992 from Loyola University Chicago, and his doctorate in clinical psychology in 1995 from Loyola University Chicago.

Dr. Sarwer's research interests focus on the assessment and treatment of obesity. He is principal or coprincipal investigator on several grants from the National Institutes of Health, investigating the psychological and behavioral aspects of obesity and, more specifically, bariatric surgery. Dr. Sarwer is also a consultant to the Edwin and Fannie Gray Hall Center for Human Appearance, University of Pennsylvania Medical Center, where he conducts research on the psychological aspects of cosmetic and reconstructive surgery.

Clinically, Dr. Sarwer is the director of the Albert J. Stunkard Weight Management Program and is actively involved in the Bariatric Surgery Program, Perelman School of Medicine, University of Pennsylvania. He conducts behavioral and psychological evaluations of patients before surgery and treats individuals with eating or other psychological concerns after bariatric surgery. Dr. Sarwer also provides psychotherapeutic treatment to people who have body dysmorphic disorder or other appearance concerns.